Science, the Self, and Survival after Death

Science, the Self, and Survival after Death

Selected Writings of Ian Stevenson

Edited by Emily Williams Kelly

ROWMAN & LITTLEFIELD PUBLISHERS, INC.
Lanham • Boulder • New York • Toronto • Plymouth, UK

Published by Rowman & Littlefield Publishers, Inc.
A wholly owned subsidiary of The Rowman & Littlefield Publishing Group, Inc.
4501 Forbes Boulevard, Suite 200, Lanham, Maryland 20706
www.rowman.com

10 Thornbury Road, Plymouth PL6 7PP, United Kingdom

British Library Cataloguing in Publication Information Available

Library of Congress Cataloging-in-Publication Data Available

ISBN 978-1-4422-2114-7 (cloth : alk. paper)

The paper used in this publication meets the minimum requirements of American National Standard for Information Sciences Permanence of Paper for Printed Library Materials, ANSI/NISO Z39.48-1992.

Printed in the United States of America

Contents

General Introduction

EWK

> I do not believe science has heard the last of the mind or the soul.
>
> —Ian Stevenson, 1954

The purpose of this volume is to provide an introduction to Ian Stevenson, M.D. (1918–2007), and his work. There are many people who have never heard of him but could benefit greatly from knowing him and how he approached certain questions about life and death that most thinking persons ask themselves at one time or another in their lives. Many others have heard of him, but may have only a limited perspective on what he accomplished in his long, multifaceted, and distinguished career. For many of these latter people, the name "Ian Stevenson" is inevitably linked with the word "reincarnation"—and rightly so, since he was the first person to identify the widespread occurrence of what he called "cases of the reincarnation type." In so doing, he singlehandedly launched the empirical study of what previously had been a religious belief alone. Nevertheless, Ian's research on reincarnation was only part—albeit a major part—of a career that focused more generally on large questions about the nature of human personality. In providing a collection of his writings, taken from different periods in his career, that illustrate the questions and issues that guided him and his research throughout his life, I hope that even those people who knew him and his work well will gain a larger perspective on who he was.

Ian Stevenson was a philosopher—but not in the sense in which we in the modern era have come to understand that word. In the past few centuries humankind's pursuit of knowledge has bifurcated, broadly speaking, into the flora and fauna of science and the humanities, each subdivided into almost innumerable species and subspecies. Professional scientists and academics specialize in increasingly focused areas, so that a philosopher, for example, has become someone who studies, say, specific topics in logic or ethics or epistemology. Moreover, as the species of knowledge occupy increasingly specialized niches, they, like biological species, have become more isolated from each other and less able to mingle and interbreed.

Ian Stevenson was the antithesis of the specialist. He was instead a philosopher in the original, ancient sense of the word—one who seeks the wisdom that comes from knowledge of the cosmos and understanding our place in it. For Ian, as for other such philosophers, there are no more important questions to ask than who we as individuals are and what our lives mean. Where did we come from? How did each of us become the completely unique individuals that we are? What is our destiny? And for philosophers such as Ian, questions such as these are not exclusively the province of religion or metaphysics or the humanities. They are—or should be—central to all efforts to understand the world we live in—including the efforts of scientists. Too often in the modern era, scientists have neglected basic questions about the nature of consciousness and its place in the physical universe, whether because they have assumed such questions to be beyond the reach of science or because they have assumed that the fundamental relationship of consciousness and brain is already known.

What distinguished Ian, however, was not just the large questions that guided him but his understanding of *how* one pursues answers to such questions. Knowledge is not merely an accumulation of information; it is a growth in understanding. It does not grow simply by the addition of more and more facts, but it grows by a continuing expansion of the framework into which we fit those facts. It is, in short, not so much a quantitative process as a qualitative one. For Ian, therefore, the indispensable—and inseparable—tools of knowledge are science and history, the former because it increases the depth and accuracy of our observations of ourselves and the world around us, the latter because it provides the wider view that encourages the development of a framework that can make sense of those observations.

Ian was born in Montreal, Canada, on October 31, 1918. His father had been born in Scotland and his mother in England, but they moved to Canada when his father was offered a position as a political journalist for the *Toronto Star*. Several years later he became the chief correspondent of the London *Times*—the most prestigious journalism job in Canada—as well as Canadian correspondent for *The Economist, Boston Transcript, Baltimore Sun, Detroit Free Press, New York Times, The Scotsman,* and several Australian and South African papers. Ian's older brother, Kerr, was born in 1917, their younger siblings, Ronald and Edith, in 1926.

Ian had been born during the Great Flu Epidemic of 1918 and, perhaps as a consequence, he had in infancy developed bronchiectasis, a chronic lung condition that caused frequent bouts of bronchitis. His illness had the paradoxical effect of both shrinking and expanding the horizons of his early childhood experiences. On the one hand, he was housebound for long periods of time, a confinement that fostered his lifelong habit of insatiable reading.[1] On the other hand, when Ian was five, he, his mother, and his brother Kerr traveled by train across the continent from

Ottawa to Los Angeles, in part to find a climate that might improve Ian's health. They remained in Los Angeles for two years, during which time Ian was exposed not only to a part of the world and a kind of life quite different from that of Ottawa but also to some of the unorthodox ideas and people to which his mother was drawn.

Ian's love of history and his unmatched skill in writing almost certainly owe much to his father. History—both the past and its unfolding in the present—and writing were the lifeblood of his father's profession, journalism. To Ian's mother, however, may be attributed his interest in the larger philosophical and spiritual questions that ultimately became the lifeblood of *his* career—and, indeed, his life. She had a longstanding interest in Eastern religions and philosophy, including Theosophy and reincarnation, and she had a large library that included books on comparative religion, occultism, and medicine, including alternative practices such as homeopathy, osteopathy, and herbalism.[2]

After his early schooling in Canada, Ian left in 1931 to attend Bryanston, an innovative boarding school in England, and in 1937 he enrolled at St. Andrew's University in Scotland, where he began majoring in history. In 1939, however, with the threat of World War II, he returned to Canada and enrolled that fall at McGill University, where in one year he completed a bachelor of science degree with studies in physics, chemistry, and biology, as well as history. In 1940, perhaps influenced by his father's sister Mary, who was a physician in Scotland, Ian enrolled in McGill's School of Medicine, where his brother Kerr was already pursuing a medical degree. Working under an accelerated wartime program, he completed in three years both an M.D. and C.M. (master of surgery), graduating not only first in his class but with the further distinction of being considered one of the most gifted students at the medical school in anyone's memory.

After internships and residencies in Montreal and in Phoenix, Arizona, Ian went to New Orleans as a fellow in internal medicine at the Alton Ochsner Medical Foundation and as a fellow in biochemistry at Tulane University. He then spent two years at Cornell University Medical College and the New York Hospital, training and doing research in psychosomatic medicine. He returned to New Orleans, where from 1949 to 1957 he was assistant and then associate professor of psychiatry and medicine at Louisiana State University School of Medicine. During these years he also completed training in psychoanalysis. In 1957, not quite 39 years old, Ian was appointed professor and chairman of the Department of Psychiatry at the University of Virginia, a position he held until 1967, when he became Carlson Professor of Psychiatry. Then, in 1969, he founded the Division of Parapsychology (now the Division of Perceptual Studies in the Department of Psychiatry and Neurobehavioral Sciences).

The various stages of Ian's career reflect his dissatisfaction with the limitations he felt at each step and his attempts to go beyond those limits by challenging the assumptions that set them. His career was built on his observation that "advances must start with dissent" (Stevenson, 1963, p. 523). The mechanistic, reductionist assumption that he encountered from his earliest years in medicine—that health and disease can be understood as malfunctioning of parts of a machine, the body[3] —led him to turn to areas of medicine that ostensibly took mental factors more seriously as part of the etiology of disease, that is, psychosomatic medicine, psychoanalysis, and psychiatry. Even in these areas, however, he encountered other restrictive assumptions. When he turned to psychosomatic medicine, for example, he found that the then-prevailing theory was that physical symptoms are symbolic conversions of underlying psychological problems; and some of the attempts to apply this theory could become rather amusing. Chronic diarrhea, he noted wryly, might be the result of the patient's "wish to be rid of some unpleasant problem or person" (Stevenson & Matthews, 1953, p. 294). Ian began instead to seek a broader understanding of why different people develop different illnesses or symptoms in response to stress or other factors weakening the body. Similarly dissatisfied with the assumption in psychoanalysis that personality is fixed by early childhood experiences (Stevenson, 1957), he sought a broader approach to psychiatry and psychotherapy based on his belief that change, growth, and improvement of oneself are possible at any time in one's life (Stevenson, 1955 [reprinted in part 5]).

Finally, Ian began pursuing topics that challenge the biggest assumption of all: the assumption of most modern scientists and philosophers that human personality is the product solely of genes, the brain, and environmental influences that have shaped that brain. Beginning in the mid-1950s, he began to read widely in the area of psychical research. Founded in the late 19th century, this field has long been misperceived as dealing with "occult" or "anomalous" phenomena in an effort to undermine "rational" science and replace it with a "mystical" view. Ian instead recognized the aim of psychical research as being precisely his own: to apply the methods of science to the still unanswered question of the relationship of mind and brain, a problem about which "we know no more . . . than Aristotle did" (Stevenson, 1954, p. 34).[4]

During the 1950s Ian published several papers in which he began to describe what he saw as the importance of psychical research (see, e.g., Stevenson, 1959). A major turning point in his life, however, came in 1960 when he published a two-part paper titled "The Evidence for Survival from Claimed Memories of Former Incarnations" (Stevenson, 1960). In his wide reading, both in his mother's library and elsewhere, he had over the years come across isolated reports of persons, usually children, who seemed to remember the life of someone who had lived and died before the child's birth. In this paper he described recurrent features of the cases and provided brief reports of some of them, and he then evaluated various possible explanations for the cases and proposed some directions for further research. The paper was read by several people who provided Ian with information about additional, more contemporary cases; but most importantly it was read by Chester Carlson, the inventor of the Xerox process. Just as Ian's mother had done for Ian, Carlson's wife, Dorris, had exposed Carlson to topics such as Eastern religions and psychical research and had aroused his interest in them. When he read Ian's paper, he clearly recognized someone who was capable of applying the scientific methods with which he was intimately familiar to the spiritual topics in which he had become interested. As a result, he began providing financial support for Ian to continue this line of research, and when he died in 1968 he left Ian sufficient funds to pursue full time the avenues of research on the topics that he and Carlson had both considered so important—in particular, questions about the origins of individual differences, the relationship of mind and brain, and the question of survival after death.

The next nearly 40 years of Ian's life can be traced by examining his list of publications.[5] His life basically alternated between (1) periods of extensive travel—to Southeast Asia, Africa, Europe, the Middle East, and South and North America—to interview witnesses and collect documents related to the cases he learned about, cases not only of what he called "the reincarnation type" but also of apparitions, mediums, telepathic impressions, poltergeists, xenoglossy, near-death experiences, and death-bed visions; and (2) periods spent at home in Charlottesville or at Darwin College in Cambridge, England, when he would write up reports of individual cases and analyses of groups of cases. During the last 40 years of his life, Ian logged hundreds of thousands of miles of travel, some to extremely dangerous parts of the world, and published nearly 200 papers and 15 books. At age 78 he published a massive 2,268-page monograph reporting over two hundred cases of the reincarnation type in which the children had unusual birthmarks or birth defects closely resembling fatal wounds or other marks on the body of the person whose life the child seemed to remember (Stevenson, 1997a). In the fall of 1997, when Ian was nearly 79, a *Washington Post* editor, Tom Shroder, accompanied him on research trips in Lebanon, India, and the United States, later noting (in a fascinating book about Ian and his research [Shroder, 1999]) how difficult it was for him to keep up with this man twice his age. Ian worked well into his 80s, making his last research trip to India in October 2002 when he was nearly 84. Despite his lifelong bronchial illness, Ian overcame the limitations of his body with sheer will and drive, just as he sought to overcome the limitations of 20th-century science. His mind never gave out, but his body finally did, on February 8, 2007.

I must not end this introduction, however, by leaving the impression that Ian was a lone maverick, his life and work primarily matters of a solitary pursuit of knowledge. As with all great individuals, he was single-minded in this endeavor, and he believed, as he wrote in a tribute to

Chester Carlson, that "all great achievements come only from the efforts of *individual* persons, never from those of groups" (Stevenson, 1969, p. 120). Nevertheless, he fully recognized that the achievements of those individuals are not constructed ex nihilo, and an important theme that he referred to repeatedly in his writings is the collective nature of the scientific enterprise. He frequently emphasized that all advances in knowledge depend on, and are influenced by, what has come before; that all work is improved by the critiques of knowledgeable persons and, conversely, is prone to error if carried out in isolation without the correcting influence of the wider purview of others; and, finally, that new ideas can contribute to the expansion of knowledge only when they become accepted by the larger scientific community. This collective nature of knowledge, whether in science or any other area, clearly has its dark side—another frequent theme in Ian's writings—when the "thought-collective" becomes too rigidly fixed around certain systems and the assumptions behind them.[6] Nonetheless, he understood that overcoming the inherent—and necessary—conservatism built into science requires a continuing dialogue and collaboration with colleagues, to improve the quality of the work supporting new observations and ideas and thereby eventually to convince others to accept them. During his years as a psychical researcher, he came to lament the isolation of parapsychologists[7] who, he felt, were increasingly speaking only to each other, at specialist conventions or in specialist parapsychology journals (Stevenson, 1984a, 1988). Conversely, he spoke approvingly of his colleague J. G. Pratt, who, like his predecessor at Duke University, the psychologist William McDougall, believed that parapsychology and psychical research belong in universities, where researchers can interact with qualified persons in other disciplines, rather than in private institutes where isolation is more likely (Stevenson, 1980, p. 279).

Ian practiced what he preached. Throughout his career, he sought the advice of colleagues in other disciplines and encouraged them to read the literature of, and even participate in, psychical research. He submitted many of his papers to mainstream scientific journals. He encouraged and supported younger colleagues who showed serious interest in psychical research. And in the early 1980s he was instrumental in founding the Society for Scientific Exploration (SSE), an organization whose purpose was (and is) to encourage scientists with new, frequently unorthodox ideas to share them with scientists from other disciplines. These efforts, not surprisingly, met with mixed success. Although his papers in psychiatry were routinely accepted by mainstream journals, some of his papers in psychical research were accepted by them, others not.[8] Some younger colleagues have taken up careers in psychical research, others have dropped out. Even the SSE, he later worried, may have done more to foster isolation than to break it down (Stevenson, 1999 [reprinted in part 1], p. 268).

It is also evident that Ian was not successful in convincing the mainstream scientific community of the validity of his ideas about either psychical research in particular or the nature of human personality in general; in fact, he was not successful in getting many mainstream scientists even to *look* at his research. We still live in a society dominated by the assumptions of a materialistic, reductionistic view of life, and too often those who hold those assumptions see no need to examine the work of someone who challenges them. Ian, however, would be the first to say that the enterprise to which he tried to contribute—the expansion of scientific knowledge of ourselves and the world around us—is a slow, cumulative, collective, and never-ending process. My purpose in this volume, therefore, is not just to give readers a sampling of the research that Ian conducted during his more than 60-year career. It is, more importantly, to lay out the large issues and themes inciting and guiding that work—ideas and approaches that are essential to the expansion of knowledge, whatever the validity of Ian's specific endeavors turns out to be.

No one can hope to express Ian's ideas and research better than he himself did, and so, rather than write a biography summarizing his work, I have chosen to let him tell the tale. The remainder of this volume therefore consists primarily of selections from his own published work, either full papers or excerpts from papers and books, that I think convey most effectively what he was trying to do and why. I particularly want to emphasize here, however, the overall approach behind most of Ian's work, one that might be called the "tertium quid" approach. Since about the middle of the 19th century there has been increasing polarization of religion and science, of faith and reason, of free will and determinism, of a view of the world as primarily one of personal forces versus one of impersonal mechanisms. In the 21st century we are seeing a proliferation of fundamentalisms, among religious and scientistic zealots alike, and the voices of those like Ian who are trying to move beyond the polarization are too often drowned out by the strident clashing. Ian's career, in fact, exemplifies a rejection of an "either-or" approach to science and religion. For him, like his predecessors in psychical research such as Frederic Myers and William James, religion is not primarily the sectarian, often dogmatic cultural systems of faith that we see outwardly but more broadly the human sense of, and striving toward, something transcending individual finite existence. Similarly, science was for him not a metaphysical belief in the primacy of the physical world but a method of observation leading to publicly shared knowledge. For those who subscribe to a "tertium quid" approach to science and religion, the methods of science can be applied to certain questions traditionally considered metaphysical or spiritual, particularly those related to the relationship between physical processes of the brain and the subjective experiences that we call mental.

The remainder of this general introduction consists of an autobiographical talk that Ian gave in 1989, in which he himself introduces most of the central themes and "leitmotifs" of his career. In part 1, the selections focus on Ian's ideas about the nature of the scientific enterprise in general. In particular, the most fundamental and consistent themes in Ian's career grew out of his awareness of the dangers to science of closure around fixed theoretical systems and the resistance to new ideas, observations, and methods that almost inevitably results.

In part 2, I turn more specifically to his ideas about the nature of human personality and their implications for psychology and medicine. Ian rejected what William James (1898/1900) called the "production" model of mind, namely, that physical processes have, through the evolutionary process, produced consciousness, which is thus wholly dependent on the state of the biological organism. In medicine as well as psychical research, Ian found, in contrast, much evidence for the influence of mental processes on the physical body, evidence that suggested to him the need for a different model of mind-brain relations than the "production" model.

In part 3, I have chosen writings illustrating Ian's ideas about psychical research, including not only what that is, in itself, but more importantly how it embodies methodological and theoretical issues of general importance to science. The themes raised in parts 1 and 2—namely, the need to maintain the view of science as a neutral method and not a system of fixed assumptions, and the need to keep open the question of the relationship of mind and body—come together most fully in psychical research, where the phenomena observed, not only in the laboratory but even more strongly *outside* the laboratory, challenge assumptions currently prevailing among scientists about the mind-brain relationship.

Part 4, the largest section, provides an overview of Ian's work on the question of survival after death, including papers in which he reviewed large areas of research as well as papers reporting specific cases that he investigated. The survival question was of central importance in Ian's work because it most directly confronts the question of the relationship of consciousness to the physical organism. If consciousness is the product of the brain, it cannot survive death; but if there are phenomena suggesting that consciousness *does* survive death, then our understanding of mind and brain needs revision. Moreover, the notion of survival, suggesting as it does that consciousness may not be confined to one relatively brief life span, opens up new possibilities for understanding the etiology of individual human differences, both physical and psychological. In particular, Ian's research on cases of the reincarnation type led him to suggest that, in addition to the important contributing factors of genes and the environment, a third factor—the experiences of a previous existence—might also be operating in the formation of human personality.

In the final section I present some of Ian's comments about certain implications of his work. This section is relatively brief. Ian himself dwelled very little on those implications, other than to remind his readers continually that there are major gaps in our present state of knowledge about human personality, gaps that are too often ignored in contemporary science and that his work was intended to help fill. His emphasis was on pushing the boundaries of scientific knowledge, not on suggesting firm conclusions to be drawn, because one of his most strongly held convictions was that the answers we may think we have found are *always* provisional.

NOTES

1. After his death I discovered a notebook in which he had kept a record from 1935 until 2003 of every book that he read. It contained 3,535 entries.

2. For a delightful account of Ian's childhood written by his older brother, see White, 2008.

3. See, for example, Stevenson, 1948, 1984b, and 1985 (excerpts from the latter are reprinted in part 2 of this volume).

4. Many will argue that in the more than fifty years since Ian wrote this statement, things have changed, and that now we *do* understand the general nature of the relationship of mind and brain, even if not the actual details and specifics. For example: "During the last three decades, the pace of discovery in neuroscience has been breathtaking," and as a result "the mind-body problem has ceased to be the reliably tangled conundrum it once was." "Now we understand" that thoughts, feelings, intentions, and the subjective sense of self are "events happening in the physical brain" (Churchland, 2002, pp. 2, 1).

Others, however, are more humble in the face of the enormity of the so-called hard problem of consciousness, that is, "how physical processes in the brain give rise to subjective experience" (Chalmers, 1995, p. 81): "In the process of reducing mentality to physical/biological properties, we may well lose the intrinsic, subjective character of our mentality—arguably, the very thing that makes the mental mental" (Kim, 1998, p. 237).

5. A list of his publications, organized by topic, may be found in the appendix.

6. Ian wrote two papers (1958 [reprinted in part 1], 1965) about scientists' resistance—sometimes alarming, sometimes amusing—to new ideas.

7. I am making a deliberate distinction here between the terms "psychical research" and "parapsychology," although the two are often treated as synonyms. The former is the older designation for the field that, in my view, denotes the broader scope that its founders intended, namely, as the study of all phenomena suggesting the causal efficacy of mind, using the scientific method broadly conceived as observational, whether in experiments, individual case studies, or field research. The latter term, in contrast, refers specifically to that narrower aspect of it that is limited to experimental studies of "psi" ("paranormal" phenomena such as extrasensory perception and psychokinesis).

8. For a discussion of the reception of Ian's work, see the conclusion of this volume.

REFERENCES

Chalmers, D. J. (1995). The puzzle of conscious experience. *Scientific American, 273*, 80–86.

Churchland, P. S. (2002). *Brain-Wise: Studies in Neurophilosophy*. Cambridge, MA: Bradford.

James, W. (1900). *Human Immortality: Two Supposed Objections to the Doctrine* (2nd ed.). Boston & New York: Houghton, Mifflin. (Original work published 1898)

Kim, J. (1998). *Philosophy of Mind*. Boulder, CO: Westview.

Shroder, T. (1999). *Old Souls: The Scientific Evidence for Past Lives*. New York: Simon & Schuster.

Stevenson, I. (1948). The constitutional approach to medicine. *New York State Journal of Medicine, 48*, 2156–2159.

Stevenson, I. (1954). Psychosomatic medicine. Part I. What we know about illness and the emotions. *Harper's Magazine, 209*, 34–37.

Stevenson, I. (1955). Assumptions of religion and psychiatry. *Bulletin of the Menninger Clinic, 19*, 199–209.

Stevenson, I. (1957). Is the human personality more plastic in infancy and childhood? *American Journal of Psychiatry, 114*, 152–161.

Stevenson, I. (1958). Scientists with half-closed minds. *Harper's Magazine, 217*, 64–71.

Stevenson, I. (1959). The uncomfortable facts about extrasensory perception. *Harper's Magazine, 219*, 19–25.

Stevenson, I. (1960). The evidence for survival from claimed memories of former incarnations. Part I. Review of the data; Part II. Analysis of the data and suggestions for further investigations. *Journal of the American Society for Psychical Research, 54*, 51–71, 95–117.

Stevenson, I. (1963). The preservation of a vanishing species: The part-time chairman. *Journal of Nervous and Mental Disease, 137*, 521–524.

Stevenson, I. (1965). On the irrational among the rational: Incredulity in scientists. *Virginia Quarterly Review, 41*, 40–57.

Stevenson, I. (1969). Some implications of parapsychological research on survival after death. *Proceedings of the American Society for Psychical Research, 28*, 18–35.

Stevenson, I. (1980). Gaither Pratt: An appreciation. *Journal of the American Society for Psychical Research, 74*, 277–295.

Stevenson, I. (1984a). Guest editorial: Are parapsychology journals good for parapsychology? *Journal of the American Society for Psychical Research, 78*, 97–104.

Stevenson, I. (1984b). On preserving the healing power of hope. *Pharos, 47*, 20–22.

Stevenson, I. (1985). The end of patient abuse in medical care. *Virginia Quarterly Review, 61*, 565–583.

Stevenson, I. (1988). Guest editorial: Was the attempt to identify parapsychology as a separate field of science misguided? *Journal of the American Society for Psychical Research, 82*, 309–317.

Stevenson, I. (1997a). *Reincarnation and Biology: A Contribution to the Etiology of Birthmarks and Birth Defects* (2 Vols.). Westport, CT: Praeger.

Stevenson, I. (1997b). *Where Reincarnation and Biology Intersect*. Westport, CT: Praeger.

Stevenson, I. (1999). What are the irreducible components of the scientific enterprise? *Journal of Scientific Exploration, 13*, 257–270.

Stevenson, I., & Matthews, R. I. (1953). Fact and theory in psychosomatic medicine. *Journal of Nervous and Mental Disease, 118*, 289–306.

White, K. L. (2008). Ian Stevenson: Recollections. *Journal of Scientific Exploration, 22*, 11–17.

ONE

Some of My Journeys in Medicine

1989[1]

I noticed with some misgivings the announcement that this is the Levy Lecture *in the Humanities*. It may seem tactless therefore for me to state at the beginning of the lecture that after intending to study history and indeed doing so for several years, I abandoned history for medicine. History became for me Robert Frost's "the road not taken." Frost's metaphor does not fully suit my case, because I have continued to have a strong interest in history and other humanities. If I shall later seem to have accomplished something original in science, I may owe this to my study of history. Let me explain. I do not believe that what history teaches is that history teaches nothing. What it has taught me is the transience, not of our aspirations, but of our material accomplishments and, even more, of our ideas about the nature of man. In particular, the history of medicine shows a humbling succession of ideas about disease, each appearing infrangible for a short period only to prove degradable by the next idea that—at first also hailed as ultimate—is overthrown in its turn. Knowledge in science, as Whitehead said, keeps like fish. An awareness from my reading of history of the ephemeral nature of most concepts about the nature of things freed me to challenge received opinions in medicine. For me everything now believed by scientists is open to question, and I am always dismayed to find that many scientists accept current knowledge as forever fixed. They confuse the product with the process.

Before I give an account of some of my journeys in medicine I wish to extend my tribute to the humanities by emphasizing that with their heritage and their present dialectics we have our only resources for improving our conduct. A few scientists have presumed to declare how we should live on the basis of alleged scientific knowledge, but most scientists believe that scientific knowledge is itself neutral about values. A tiny handful—in which I include myself—dare to hope that scientific knowledge may one day contribute to decisions about values. However, no one now living can foretell when that day may come. In the meantime we must continue searching the humanities for the wisdom that, as T. S. Eliot told us, we have lost in knowledge.

Early in my medical career I undertook (while at Tulane University) some research in biochemistry. To this I brought some ideas, but the success of our experiments on aspects of the oxidation of rat kidney tissue must largely have been due to the technical expertise of my collaborator, who later went on to become a distinguished biochemist (Stevenson & Smith, 1948). An unexpected result of our experiments was the destruction by our data of a dogma concerning oxidation that the great German chemist Otto Warburg had pronounced. I thought little of that and was astonished one day when a German biochemist who learned of our results told me that it would have been impossible to publish them in Germany. He meant that the awe in which Warburg was held would have led to editorial rejection of our report. From this episode I may date my strong interest in all the obstacles that confront the conduct of original research and the communication of its results.

Sir Peter Medawar described reductionism as "the most successful research stratagem ever devised: it has been the making of science and technology." Quite so, but science can study more than parts considered separately. While killing harmless rats (in order to use their kidneys in the experiments on oxidation mentioned earlier) I experienced a revulsion for this kind of scientific activity and decided that I wanted to devote myself to something more than the study of parts and to something closer to whole human beings.

My mother had believed strongly in the influence of thoughts on physical well-being, and I may owe to her my initial interest in psychosomatic medicine. Even as a medical student I was keenly interested in the physical accompaniments of emotion. One of the first patients assigned to me had angina pectoris, the dreadful pain of which comes when the heart, through blockage or spasm of the coronary arteries, receives insufficient oxygen. One day I was on this patient's ward when he became angry at a nurse and instantly gripped his chest in the agony of this disease. By this time I may have read what John Hunter, the great eighteenth-century surgeon, had said about his own angina pectoris: "My life is at the mercy of any rogue who cares to provoke me." (One later did, and he died as a consequence.) However, I only *read* about Hunter; I *saw* my patient and can still recall vividly the suffering in his face.

The impression from this and similar observations led me, when I abandoned reductionism, to take up research on the physical accompaniments of stress and the emotions it induced. The group with which I was associated in this at the New York Hospital in the late 1940s showed for almost every organ of the body that strong emotions induced by life stresses, and even by talking about such stresses, included markedly altered physical functions, often to the point of experienced symptoms (1949a, 1949b).

In these researches we thought of ourselves as pioneers, but we could not long sustain this view unless we stopped reading and also forgot what we had already read. Solomon had said in Proverbs: "A merry heart doeth good like a medicine: but a broken spirit drieth the bones." References to what we call psychosomatic medicine occur frequently in Shakespeare and in many other writers outside the medical profession. One can find reports of psychosomatic symptoms in Defoe's *A Journal of the Plague Year*, Burton's *The Anatomy of Melancholy*, and Wesley's *Journal*. This is to mention three authors only. However, what needs emphasis is not the frequency of references to the effect of the mind on the body, but the acceptance without question through centuries of this relationship. Doubts and neglect of this knowledge came later, at least within the medical profession, with the discovery of the role of microorganisms in disease. Louis Pasteur said as he was dying, "[Claude] Bernard was right. The *terrain* is everything." He was wiser than many who built on his discoveries, and it was the middle of this century before physicians discovered again the power of the mind on the body.

If our group at the New York Hospital has a rightful claim to originality, it may lie in our having asked (and provisionally tried to answer) the question: "Why during stress does one person develop asthma, another high blood pressure, and a third a peptic ulcer?" W. B. Cannon had already shown that many of the physiological accompaniments of fear and rage correspond to those that occur during strenuous physical exertion; the body reacts as if the person is going to respond to the provocation by fighting or running away. This rarely happens in civilized society, but the atavistic physical changes occur anyway. Some of my colleagues extended Cannon's hypothesis with conjectures about the symbolic meaning of various localized psychosomatic symptoms. For example, a woman who reacted to her stresses with a running nose was said to be trying to wash away her troubles; the man whose bronchi closed in the spasms of asthma was trying to shut out the truth of some unpleasant aspect of his situation. This kind of thinking led on to even wilder surmises from the more ridiculous examples of which I shall spare you. More seriously, some of my colleagues sought to delineate certain attitudes toward stressful situations that would predictably induce particular symptoms, other attitudes leading to other symptoms. However, these concepts seemed to me teleological also.

None of these interpretations seemed satisfying to me. The organ whose psychosomatic relationships I investigated was the heart, and I published numerous papers about our observations.[2] However, I could never believe that arrhythmias have any purposeful function for those afflicted by them. My discontent with teleological interpretations of psychosomatic phenomena became greater when I became aware that not infrequently the same physical symptoms occurred in a person not only when he was angry or frightened, but also when he was unusually happy or joyful. I began to collect instances of physical symptoms that had occurred during pleasurable emotional states. Here my habit of reading outside medicine brought me some useful examples. I learned that both Beethoven and Goya could be fairly described as having died of joy. They had been ill, to be sure, but their final relapses occurred just after they had received news that made them excitedly happy. In Beethoven's case a letter from London brought him 100 pounds that eased his financial embarrassment and in effect commissioned his tenth symphony; in Goya's case the happy news came in a letter from his son, who announced his imminent visit to his father, then exiled in France. Other examples occurred among the appallingly emaciated prisoners held in German concentration camps at the end of World War II. Some of them literally died of joy when they saw the Red Cross buses approach the camps to bring them food and liberty.

In trying to publish these and similar reports I encountered another instance of the resistance to deviant ideas on the part of otherwise first-rate scientists.[3] I owe more to H. G. Wolff than I can take time here adequately to acknowledge. He has had few equals in the standards of rigorous investigation and clarity in the presentation of results that he demonstrated himself and demanded of his associates. However, he was much attached to the teleological interpretation of psychosomatic symptoms. He believed they must have some meaning, some protective purpose in the economy of persons manifesting them. Not surprisingly he reacted with noticeable coolness to my data on the occurrence of physical symptoms during pleasurable emotional states. A crisis was avoided, because it was time for me to move to another position, and I published my results in two papers after I left the New York Hospital (1950, 1970).

Although our studies at the New York Hospital failed to answer the question of why a person develops one particular disease or another, I have never lost interest in this problem. If my professional work has a *leit-motif* this is it, and I shall have more to say about the subject later.

In the 1950s there seemed some prospect that a medical specialty or subspecialty of psychosomatic medicine would develop. This did not happen, and eventually all physicians who had been active in this field had to move decisively toward either internal medicine or psychiatry. Psychiatry then seemed to offer a better opportunity than internal medicine for the further study of the effects of mental states on bodily ones. So I chose psychiatry and accepted an appointment in a Department of Psychiatry. However, I had had comparatively little training in psychiatry; and it was partly to remedy this deficiency that I enrolled in a psychoanalytic institute and in due course graduated from it. Some of this training was beneficial, but the atmosphere of a psychoanalytic institute was foreign to my eclecticism. The Arabs have a proverb: "Beware of the man with a single book." This may sound strange coming from a group of people who seem more than most groups to restrict themselves to a single book. However, there is a truth to it, and I enlarge the proverb to say "Beware of those who read only the works of a single man." In the psychoanalytic institutes the works of Freud and a few of his disciples were treated as having oracular authority. The works of other authors were not read, let alone discussed. "Where all men think alike, few men think at all."

Having left the reductionism of the biochemistry laboratory, I found that of psychoanalysis equally uncongenial. Given the concepts of Freud it might follow that art and religion could be reduced to expressions of infantile cravings and frustrations. But what was the factual basis for his concepts? A reading of Malinowski's *Sex and Repression in Savage Society* in which Malinowski reported his failure to find the allegedly universal Oedipus complex among the matrilineal Trobrianders stimulated me to look more closely at psychoanalytic evidence. Ernest Jones's inability to accept Malinowski's evidence, if only as an exception to a generalization, made me realize that psychoanalysis had lost its right to reduce religion because it had itself taken on the negative attributes of a religion: the uncritical acceptance of what its founder says.

Freud had begun his studies of the psychological factors in illness in company with other investigators of the same subject. He studied with Charcot, translated Bernheim's work, and wrote his own first work in psychiatry with Breuer. Thereafter, however, he seems to have isolated himself for many years from persons who could help him correct his ideas. He ignored Eugen Bleuler's advice to keep meetings of psychoanalysts open and chose instead to develop first a coterie and then a movement of choric followers.

Ideas about unconscious mental processes were widely discussed in the second half of the nineteenth century. We can easily learn about these in the reviews by Whyte and Ellenberger. Freud was aware of this current, but separated himself from it. He wrote in his autobiography, almost with smugness, that he avoided reading Nietzsche because he was concerned "with keeping my mind unembarrassed." This attitude suits a philosopher, and I have much sympathy with Thomas Hobbes's remark "that if I had read as much as other men, I should have known no more than other men." However, the way of philosophers is not that of scientists. Whitehead was correct in characterizing the scientific revolution initiated around the turn of the seventeenth century as anti-rationalist. It sought to replace abstract reasoning with observations.

There are other means of attaining knowledge besides the scientific method. Art, music, poetry, and other types of literature give us knowledge. I can also believe that in mystical experiences we may have direct access to important truths or, more specifically, to the most important truth of all, which is that we ourselves are part of a Great All. I do not know whether you would call William James's *The Varieties of Religious Experience* a work of the humanities or one of science. It partakes of the best of both, and for me is one of the greatest books ever written; I know no better defense of the value of mystical experiences. However, inspirational and mystical experiences are, *qua* experiences, incommunicable, whereas scientific observations are and must be; there is no science without public demonstrability. This means independent verification of a patient's (or informant's) statements. Independent verification has been almost entirely lacking in psychoanalysis. Thus for me, Freud's greatest mistake was in not attempting to inquire into the truth of his patients' claims about sexual seduction in childhood. To say that there is no difference between being sexually abused and imagining that you have been sexually abused is to take oneself out of science.

As if all the foregoing were not enough to turn me away from psychoanalysis, I found unconvincing its assertion that a person's later character depends almost exclusively on the events of infancy. This seems to me like smuggling in predestination; for what infant can avail against the follies of his parents? But then these wicked parents must have been mistreated during their infancies by their parents, and so on back to Adam. One of my earliest papers in psychiatry questioned whether human personality is more plastic in infancy and childhood than it is in the later years of life (1957). This provoked much annoyance among psychoanalysts; and because they were then the dominant force in American psychiatry, Sir Aubrey Lewis, who was professor of psychiatry at the Institute of Psychiatry in London, asked me (soon after the paper's publication) whether I could go about on the streets unarmed.

In sum, Freud now appears to me to have been an emperor without clothes, and I am less surprised that he developed the concepts he espoused than that he succeeded in persuading so many persons to accept them. We must leave to the historians of science the task of explaining why of the several contemporaneous concepts of unconscious mental processes, including those of Pierre Janet, Morton Prince, William James, C. G. Jung, and F. W. H. Myers, Freud's moved ahead in popular acceptance and almost crushed the others into oblivion. The concepts of the unconscious mind developed by the other thinkers I have named, especially James, Jung, and Myers, allowed for unconscious mental processes to be the sources or the conduits of man's higher creative achievements (as well as some of his pathological aberrations); they allowed also for the experiences we call paranormal and even for a soul. How the facts on which they based their larger concepts of the unconscious mind became overlooked during the Freudian period remains a mystery. Perhaps the very extravagance of Freud's claims—to be able to explain psychopathology, art, war, and religion—made his ideas attractive to uncritical thinkers craving for certitude. Be that as it may, the widespread acceptance of psychoanalytic ideas among psychiatrists and anthropologists (and many humanists, too) shows that the social sciences cannot yet claim to be obtaining cumulative knowledge, as physics, chemistry, and biology are doing. I do not mean to be querimonious about Freud, but it is necessary to learn from mistakes in scientific method if we are to progress.

Psychoanalysis did not decline only because the weaknesses I have mentioned (and others) became exposed to damaging criticism. It received challenges from new observations about the nature and treatment of mental disease in psychology, genetics, and neurobiology. I do not regard these replacements as unmixed blessings. Psychoanalysis, despite its taint of determinism from infantile experiences, had preserved an awareness of the importance of *mental* processes in human disease. This element is minimized or openly denied by most investigators in psychology, genetics, and neurobiology. For them mind is an epiphenomenon of cerebral processes and free will an illusion.

While I was still involved with psychoanalysis, I began experimenting with hallucinogenic (perhaps better called psychedelic) drugs. I have taken or had administered to me a number of drugs and anesthetics as part of a search for drugs that would assist psychiatrists in interviewing or in psychotherapy. However, here I shall speak only of the effects on me of mescaline and LSD.

The sensory apparatus of my body is defective: I have had poor eyesight since youth, my hearing is imperfect, and my sense of smell extremely dull. My first wife was a gifted amateur artist and also a lover of natural beauty, especially that of forests and jungles. Her senses were extraordinarily acute, and I was often aware that she could perceive aspects of the world that I did not. Mescaline could not improve my vision, but it vastly bettered my appreciation of what I saw. The beauty of the colors that I inwardly saw under the influence of mescaline made me ever afterward far more sensitive to color both in nature and in art than I had been before. From my experience with mescaline I also became more aware than I had been of the subjective element in our sense of the passage of time.

With LSD I had less experience of beautiful colors and much more of memories of my early life. With one of my experiences with LSD I also had a mystical experience by which I mean a sense of unity with all beings, all things. After the second of my LSD experiences I passed three days in perfect serenity. I believe that many persons could benefit as much as I did through taking psychedelic drugs under proper medical supervision, which is the only sensible way to take them.

I have mentioned these experiences here to say that they increased my conviction of the dual natures of mind and body. This may seem paradoxical, because if a small amount of a drug acting on the brain can markedly alter our mental experiences does this not prove that our thoughts are only our subjective awareness of our brain's activity? For me it does not. I admit certainly that the chemical changes in my brain that the drugs induced released the extraordinary images and feelings that entered my consciousness. However, this does not account for the images themselves, which (apart from those that I could identify as memories) had no correspondence to anything that I had earlier experienced. Here I need to add that my experiences included nothing that I could prove to have originated outside my mind and, if you like, my brain. I had no verifiable extrasensory experience when under the influence of drugs. My interest in extrasensory perception did not derive from my experiences with drugs, although they enhanced it.

For many years I had had a keen interest in extrasensory experiences and kindred phenomena. My dissatisfaction with prevailing theories of human personality led me to extend this interest, and in the 1950s I began to read systematically in the literatures of theosophy and psychical research. These had both arisen in the last quarter of the nineteenth century, but their methods were altogether different. Theosophists presented a potted version of Buddhism to the Western world, but they alloyed this with the teachings of alleged Masters channeled through the imperfect minds of frail humans. Like psychoanalysts, theosophists eschewed verifications of their claims, and however valuable the moral teachings of theosophy are, it forms no part of science.

Psychical research, on the other hand, does. The Society for Psychical Research was founded in 1882 in London, and within a few years a sister society, the American Society for Psychical Research, was established in New York. They exist "to examine without prejudice or prepossession and in a scientific spirit those faculties of man, real or supposed, which appear to be inexplicable on any generally recognized hypothesis." In simpler words, the Societies study evidence of communication without the known sensory organs and of movements occurring without the usual motor forces. Implicit in their programs is the possibility of obtaining evidence—to replace or supplement faith—that human personality survives bodily death. However, the societies hold no corporate views, and a belief in mind/body dualism or even a belief in extrasensory perception are not requirements of membership in them. A member need only believe that the question of paranormal phenomena is worthy of inquiry and amenable to scientific investigation.

Investigators of these phenomena have two different methods of studying them. One group of researchers has sought to produce or observe the phenomena in laboratories, which provide conditions for excluding normal means of communication and which also, at times, permit varying the conditions in order to learn more about the requirements for the occurrence of the phenomena and their processes. There have been important successes with the experimental method, and I could list for anyone interested a dozen experiments for which I am satisfied that normal explanations fail to explain the observations. However, it must be admitted that experimental results in psychical research are unpredictable. Although experiments have been successfully repeated, they are not voluntarily repeatable as are most experiments in the more developed branches of science. A further weakness of laboratory experiments is that (with rare exceptions) the positive effects are meager and only detectable by statistical methods. A large number of trials are required in order to show an effect, but then one cannot say which successes are due to chance and which to paranormal processes. This necessarily limits what one can learn about processes from experiments. Hopes once held that laboratory experiments in extrasensory perception would convince the majority of scientists to take the phenomena seriously have not been fulfilled.

Nevertheless, an appreciable number of scientists (thirty percent in one recent survey) do believe that something like extrasensory perception is either an undoubted fact or a likely possibility. However, it seems that most of them have reached this judgment through personal experiences instead of from reading reports of laboratory experiments. The study of such experiences—those that occur spontaneously in everyday life—forms the second division of psychical research, and it is the one to which I have given nearly all my attention for the past twenty years.

The study of spontaneous cases of extrasensory perception sometimes needs defending against the disapproval of those who have come to equate science with the controlled conditions that laboratories can offer and naturalistic situations cannot. Here the first point to make is that some important phenomena, such as the weather, volcanoes, fossils, earthquakes, and meteorites, do not occur in laboratories under controlled conditions, and yet we study them with scientific methods. We do this because science is not a physical location where we obtain evidence, but instead a process for appraising evidence wherever we find it.

In the study of spontaneous paranormal phenomena we must usually interview and cross-question informants about events that have happened before we arrive on the scene. In principle, the methods are those that lawyers use in reconstructing a crime and historians use in understanding the past. Having the best account possible of the events in question one considers one by one the alternative explanations and tries to eliminate them until only the single most probable one remains. One then tries with further observations to confirm or reject the initially preferred explanation. In addition, series of apparently similar phenomena are searched for recurrent features that may provide clues to causative conditions and processes of occurrence.

The investigators of paranormal phenomena have tried to find a middle way between the gullible and the skeptical, the former saying (usually from the perspective of a religion) that everything relevant is already known, the latter that there are no genuine phenomena to be investigated. Nevertheless, although psychical researchers have never been more than a handful in number and never possessed of adequate resources, they have managed somehow to survive. They have now passed on a tradition of systematic inquiry through four generations. With quiet persistence they adhere to Bacon's assertion that "rarities and reports that seem incredible are not to be suppressed or denied to the memory of men." In my library the publications of the British and American Societies for Psychical Research almost fill one large bookcase. What distinguishes the work of these societies is an almost ruthless insistence on corroboration of an experient's statements and equal insistence on independent verification of the correspondence between these statements and the apparently related event of which the percipient claimed paranormal knowledge. "Were I asked," William James wrote, "to point to a scientific journal where hard-headedness and never-sleeping suspicion of sources of error might be seen in their full bloom, I think I should have to fall back on the *Proceedings* of the Society for Psychical Research. The common run of papers, say on physiological subjects, is apt to show a far lower level of critical consciousness."

I have had some interest in nearly all the phenomena subsumed under the term "psychical research." However, I have concentrated most of my effort in examining the evidence for the survival of human personality after death. I have studied and written reports on apparitions, the visions of dying persons and of persons recovered from near death, and certain types of mediumistic communications. The evidence that I have found most promising has been that provided by children who claim to remember previous lives. I have studied their cases more than those of any other group in this field.

From my childhood reading I had become familiar with the idea of reincarnation. The concept made sense to me, but I never thought until many years later that there could ever be any evidence to support a belief in it. Certainly the theosophists had offered none. Here again, my habit of wide reading proved useful. In the course of this reading I came across accounts of persons who actually claimed to remember the details of previous lives. These accounts mostly appeared as individual case histories or in small groups of case reports. Moreover, I found most of them in newspapers and magazines or in books for general readers. Still, there seemed to be more than a few of them, and I decided to tabulate and analyze them for recurrent features. They had some. For example, the great majority of the persons who claimed to remember previous lives were very young children when they first spoke about these lives; and in most instances the children stopped speaking about the previous lives when they were still young children of between five and eight years. I could tell also that although some of the reports I had collected were of low quality and little more than journalistic anecdotes, this was not true of all. In several cases cautious adults had inquired searchingly into the claims of the children, and in three instances someone had made a written record of what the child had been saying before its statements had been verified.

In 1960 I published in the *Journal* of the American Society for Psychical Research an essay reporting these observations (1960a, 1960b). My report discussed the various interpretations of the cases and recommended accepting reincarnation only after excluding all others. My main conclusion was that if more cases of the same general type could be found and investigated carefully, we might obtain better evidence of survival after death. I added that "in mediumistic communications [and this is true of apparitions also] we have the problem of proving that someone clearly dead still lives. In evaluating apparent memories of former incarnations, the problem consists in judging whether someone clearly living once died. This may prove the easier task."

I do not think that it occurred to me then that I would be the person to undertake the task.[4] Although the American Society for Psychical Research awarded a prize to me for the essay, its journal was (and still is) one of the most obscure journals in the whole of science. Nevertheless, the Essay attracted some attention, and within a few months I received a telephone call from Eileen Garrett, who had (about ten years before) established the Parapsychology Foundation. She had learned of a case in India that seemed to resemble the ones whose reports I had reviewed, and she asked me whether I would be interested in going to India to investigate it. I was indeed interested, and the following summer (August 1961) I made my first visit to India, where I spent about five weeks before going on to Ceylon (as Sri Lanka was then called) for another week. Before leaving for India I had learned of some other cases of fairly recent origin, and I also had the addresses of some subjects figuring in cases I had reviewed in my essay. I thought they might still be alive, and I wanted to meet them if I could.

On reaching India I underwent considerable culture shock; yet this was less than the shock of learning how little I knew about India and Sri Lanka. I have subsequently thought that if I had known how ignorant I was of Asia I should never have had the nerve to begin these investigations. However, shielded by this ignorance I pushed on with them. I soon found that the cases were much more numerous than I had been led to expect from the scattered reports I had summarized for my essay. (Altogether, during this first trip, I learned about and studied—not all with the same thoroughness—about twenty cases in India and five in Sri Lanka.)

Also unexpected by me were the informants' often lively reports of the unusual behavior that most of the subjects showed—behavior that harmonized with the child's statements about the previous life it claimed to remember. I had expected that the cases would consist exclusively of statements the subjects would express neutrally about the previous lives. Instead, I found that the children often talked with strong emotions about the previous lives, and they sometimes behaved as if still living in the past life. For them it seemed still present, not past. For example, a child of low-caste parents who said that he remembered the life of a Brahmin would show snobbish behavior toward his own family and might even refuse to eat their food; from his perspective it was polluted. A child remembering a previous life as a person of the opposite sex might dress for that sex and play its games. One who remembered being shot would show a fear of guns and loud noises. As I mentioned, many of the reports I had used for my essay had appeared in newspapers or other popular publications, and one expects that journalistic accounts will exaggerate the basic facts of an event; however, this example shows that such accounts may also miss important details.

Back in Virginia after this first trip to Asia I tried to assimilate a mass of information about the cases that far exceeded my initial expectations. I wrote and had accepted for publication in 1964 a monograph about some of the cases that I had investigated. At this point doubts were publicly expressed about the honesty of the man who had been my interpreter for several of the stronger cases in India. Learning of these suspicions, the publisher halted the publication of my monograph. Although the man in question undoubtedly had been dishonest in some matters—something I did not know during my first journey to Asia—I did not think he had deceived me as an interpreter. However, rather than lose the extensive work involved in the cases in which this man had helped me, I decided to return to India and study again these cases (and some others) with new interpreters. The happy side of this misfortune was that the cases I investigated again proved to be even stronger than they had earlier seemed to be. Moreover, I learned the value of repeated interviews. From this experience I date my habit of trying to return to cases for second and third interviews whenever possible. Too often after leaving the site of a case I think of questions that I should have asked when I was there; I can ask them on a second or later visit.

After my second visit to India I revised my monograph, and it was published, in 1966, without further difficulty (1966/1974). If I were inclined to equate market success with scientific worth, I should be more than satisfied with this book. It has been translated into seven foreign languages, has sold about 50,000 copies since 1966, and is still in print. However, I am well aware that these sales figures reflect public interest in the subject of reincarnation and little else. In 1977 I achieved what was for me a more gratifying success. In that year I published in a scientific journal an article entitled "The Explanatory Value of the Idea of Reincarnation" (1977). For this I had more than 1,000 requests for reprints from scientists all over the world. This was far more than I had ever had for any of my numerous articles derived from what I call orthodox research. In this paper I drew attention to reincarnation as a hypothesis of explanatory value for a wide variety of unsolved problems in psychology and medicine. The interest it evoked among other scientists assured me that I was not alone in my discontent with psychoanalytic and other current theories of human personality.

At about the time of my first visit to India, Chester Carlson, the inventor of xerography, (encouraged by his wife, Dorris) began to offer me funds with which to expand my investigations. I remember being at first conscientiously unable to accept as much money as Chester Carlson offered, because I was then heavily involved in administrative and teaching duties as Chairman of the University of Virginia's Department of Psychiatry. However, I was able gradually to change my situation, and Chester Carlson then offered matching funds for an endowed chair that would enable me to devote myself full-time to psychical research. The risks of giving up the secure position I then had were obvious; but the unique opportunity offered warranted the risks, and I have never regretted my decision to engage full-time in this research.

I am sometimes asked what my colleagues at the University of Virginia think about my research. It has had a mixed reception among them. A few have openly disapproved of having such research at the University, but the majority (at least of those whose opinions have reached me) adhere to the maxim of the University's founder, Thomas Jefferson: "Here we are not afraid to follow truth wherever it may lead, nor to tolerate any error so long as reason is left free to combat it."

Since 1967 I have widened and deepened the research as much as available time and financial resources have permitted. I have published some sixty-five[5] detailed case reports, mostly in books. And I have published each year three or four articles about various aspects of these cases and about other types of cases that I have studied. In late 1987 I published a book written for general readers in which I described my methods of investigation and summarized the results and my present conclusions about children who say they remember previous lives (1987/2001). Before telling you about these conclusions I should briefly describe for you the scope of the research.

Between my first visit to India and the publication, finally, of my monograph reporting, as its title says, twenty cases suggestive of reincarnation, I had extended my investigations to the tribal peoples of northwest North America, and to Lebanon, Brazil, Turkey, and Thailand. In the 1970s I began investigating cases in Burma and West Africa. I have also investigated whatever cases came to my attention in Europe and in North and South America (1983).[6] The number of cases now available for our analysis has gradually increased to about 2,500; but I wish to stress that the cases are of varying quality and we have not investigated all of them with the same thoroughness.

Adults sometimes claim to remember previous lives, but with rare exceptions their cases have much less value than those of young children and most, in my view, are worthless. This is because in the case of a young child of only two or three years of age one can reach reasonably satisfactory conclusions concerning the information to which it might have been normally exposed. In contrast, the mind of an adult and even that of an older child has been filled with a large amount of information that becomes available for the ingredients of an imagined previous life. Accordingly, I have concentrated my efforts increasingly on the cases of young children.

I mentioned earlier that in the cases I first reported in 1960 I had discerned some recurrent features. We have since found other recurrent features. One of these is a high incidence of violent death in the persons whose lives the children remember. This feature occurs in the cases of all the ten cultures for which we have examined groups of cases; although the incidence of violent death in the cases varies from one culture to another, it is far higher among the cases than in the general populations from which they are drawn. Other recurrent features also vary from culture to culture. These include the occurrence of dreams in which a deceased person seems to announce to the dreamer the intention of being reborn (usually in the family of the dreamer), the incidence of claims to have been a person of the opposite sex in the previous life, and the interval between the concerned deceased person's death and the subject's birth.

These and other variations in the cases tell us that culture—by which I mean here the beliefs of a group of people—powerfully influences the features of the cases. This being so, it may fairly be asked whether beliefs are not the sufficient causes of the cases. We do not know the actual prevalence of cases (except from one survey in India), but we do know that the cases can be found much more readily in cultures having a belief in reincarnation than in ones not having this belief.[7] Critics of the cases have therefore suggested that a child's fantasies, perhaps of an imaginary playmate, may become shaped by its parents and peers, through their questions and suggestions, until the child assumes an identification with a deceased person. In this way the child becomes the subject of a factitious case suggestive of reincarnation. This argument has considerable force, and its cogency can hardly be denied when we consider the numerous cases in which the subject of a case and the deceased person with whom he or she identifies belong to the same family or same village. However, it will not suffice to explain the smaller, but not negligible number of cases in which the two families live widely separated and, from all the evidence, have had no acquaintance with each other before the case developed. Moreover, in the stronger of such cases the child has furnished specific details (sometimes written down before verification) about the deceased person; there can be no question in such cases of imaginings, confused memories, and pseudoidentification. In examining the cases of this group we are almost forced to believe that the child has somehow acquired knowledge about a deceased person by other than normal means. If this be granted, one has still a choice among several explanations all of which suppose some paranormal process; and reincarnation is only one of these.

Journalists have sometimes incorrectly (and unjustly) described me as trying to *prove* that reincarnation occurs. This allegation is wrong as a description both of my motive and of science. Outside of mathematics there is no proof in science; scientists make judgments about probabilities, and they rarely express themselves in statements of certainty. It is true that I search for stronger evidence than we now have for paranormal processes in the cases I study, and if that evidence points toward reincarnation I am not displeased. I have never hidden my interest in the results of my research. William James pointed out that "if you want an absolute duffer in an investigation, you must, after all, take the man who has no interest in its results . . . the most useful investigator . . . is always he whose eager interest in one side of a question is balanced by an equally keen nervousness lest he become deceived." The search for stronger evidence is therefore not with an aim at developing some coercive proof. Instead, it recognizes that different persons require different amounts and qualities of evidence before they alter their opinions. Although most educated Westerners have some acquaintance with the idea of reincarnation from at least a slight knowledge of Hinduism and Buddhism, few are familiar with concrete instances of children's claims to remember a previous life. It is not surprising that the truth of the claims seems to them antecedently improbable. As Charles Richet, a great French physiologist (and psychical researcher) observed: "Pour croire complètement à un phénomène it faut y être habitué." Perhaps my main contribution will be that of making Western persons familiar, not with the idea of reincarnation—it must be one of the oldest ideas in the world—but with evidence tending to support a belief in reincarnation.

I am frequently asked whether I myself believe in reincarnation. I decline to answer this question, because my beliefs should make no difference to anyone asking such a question. As Leonardo da Vinci said, "Whoever in discussion adduces authority uses not intellect but rather memory." Everyone should examine the evidence and judge it for himself. As I have just said, the evidence that my colleagues and I have obtained gives some support to a belief in reincarnation. Before the modern investigations a belief in reincarnation had to rest on the basis of faith, usually inculcated by the scriptures or oral teachings of a traditional religion. Now, one may, if one wishes, believe in reincarnation on the basis of evidence. However, the evidence is not flawless and it certainly does not compel such a belief. Even the best of it is open to alternative interpretations, and one can only censure those who say there is no evidence whatever.

Has then an impasse been reached without a way forward? I do not think so, because I believe we will advance further with the publication of reports of cases the subjects of which have birthmarks or birth defects that seem to derive from previous lives. These marks and defects correspond closely in size and location to wounds (occasionally other marks) on the deceased person whose life the child later claims to remember. Apart from their relevance to medicine the cases with birthmarks and birth defects raise the standard of evidence for the cases in which most of them occur: the birthmarks (or defects) can be photographed, and for many of the corresponding wounds we have obtained medical records, such as autopsy reports. These are important steps toward greater objectivity in the research. You can readily understand how these cases have brought me back to my principal interest in medicine: psychosomatic relationships. However, now we are talking about a mind's influence on a body across the gap of death.

Most of the marks and defects of these cases are on the skin or extremities. However, in a small number of cases the subject has had some internal disease similar or identical to one which the person whose life the child remembers had had. For such a case to be significant the disease must be one from which the subject alone of all members of his family has suffered. We have a few such cases, and they have returned me to another topic in which I have never lost interest: Why does a person acquire one particular disease instead of another?

I think that for most scientists today this last question is absurd. They believe that there is no person apart from a body. For them, any disease a person acquires derives from the combination of the genes he draws in the lottery of parenthood modified by the environment into which he is born and in which he later lives. No one is more aware than I of how subversive it is to talk in the West today[8] of a soul that may survive the death of one physical body and later become associated with another, which second body it may influence, at least to some extent, in form and function. Nevertheless, the accumulated evidence, which I shall be publishing in detail next year,[9] warrants conjectures of this kind.

Here I need to add and to emphasize that the evidence suggestive of reincarnation imperils no present knowledge. I do not question the findings of genetics or even that environments have some effect on us (although I do deny any primacy for the events of infancy among all environmental influences). I am suggesting that instead of a single line of evolution—the one of our physical bodies—we also participate in a second line of evolution—that of our minds or, if you prefer, our souls.

The claim to have evidence of a second line of evolution is, I need hardly say, a large one, and if it does not challenge any substantial knowledge it certainly does throw into question many common assumptions about the nature of man, especially those concerning the relationship between mind and brain. To this I add the heterodox idea that certain birth defects and even some internal diseases may have mental causes anteceding the conception of a person's body. In presuming to doubt the ideas about the nature of man that most Western scientists hold, I can take comfort in an aphorism of the great French neurologist Charcot: "La théorie, c'est bon, mais ça n'empêche pas d'exister." Those who would judge my conclusions should first examine the evidence that has led me to them.

It is tempting to conclude this lecture by invoking the names of the many great philosophers and poets who have believed in reincarnation and thereby obliquely exhort you to believe in it yourself. I have already said that such a path is closed to me; authority has no place in science. Yet science acknowledges leaders, and it particularly pleases me to remember that some of the greatest encouragement for the scientific methods of psychical research has come from humanists like William James and Henri Bergson. Each of these great men accepted the Presidency of the Society for Psychical Research, and James was for many years at least a part-time investigator of psychical phenomena. I venerate them less for the particular views they held than for their endorsement of the scientific method applied to paranormal experiences as a means of attaining important new knowledge of man's nature.

Such are some of my journeys in medicine with occasional wanderings in the humanities. I do not agree with a great writer who said that "to travel hopefully is a better thing than to arrive." Certainly those who do not travel hopefully may never arrive, but hope alone cannot long sustain a journey in science. Accordingly, I have tried to describe for you some of the choices that I made of roads to take during my journeys.

NOTES

1. The Flora Levy Lecture in the Humanities 1989, Lafayette, LA: The University of Southwestern Louisiana.—Ed.
2. References to these papers may be found in the appendix, where I have listed by topic all Ian's publications (excluding most book reviews and published correspondence).—Ed.
3. This is a subject in which I have never lost interest, and I later published two papers about it (1958 [reprinted in part 1], 1965).
4. In 1923 an Indian (R. B. Sunderlal), who had studied four of the cases that I later included in my 1960 Essay, offered reports of them for publication by the American Society for Psychical Research. The Research Officer (W. F. Prince) sent a polite note of rejection in which he said "it is difficult to see how, unless such cases could be multiplied, and attested by various evidences, such a claim . . . could be proved true." Another member of the Society's staff commented in a memorandum that the cases were "worthy of following up by some Western scientific methods and investigators." Sunderlal published his report in India and also, in 1924, in the French journal of psychical research *Revue métaphysique*.
5. Particularly with the publication of *Reincarnation and Biology* (1997a) and *European Cases of the Reincarnation Type* (2003), this number has since grown to over 300.—Ed.
6. I have published detailed reports or analyses of cases from all these regions except Western Europe. [In 2003, Ian published *European Cases of the Reincarnation Type*.—Ed.]

7. I am not halting here to discuss why the cases are found more readily in some parts of the world than in others. The question is certainly an extremely important one, and I have made a beginning attempt to consider the factors involved in my book for general readers (1987/2001).

8. If heretics were burned alive today, the successors in science of the theologians who, in the sixteenth century, burned anyone who denied the existence of souls would today burn those who affirm their existence.

9. The scope of the project of publishing cases of the reincarnation type with birthmarks and birth defects kept expanding. Instead of "next year," the monograph was not actually published for another 8 years (Stevenson, 1997a, 1997b).—Ed.

REFERENCES

(1948). The influence of oxygen tension upon the respiration of rat kidney slices. *Archives of Biochemistry, 17*, 61–73. (with L. Smith)

(1949a). Circulatory dynamics before and after exercise in subjects with and without structural heart disease during anxiety and relaxation. *Journal of Clinical Investigation, 28*, 1534–1543. (with C. H. Duncan and H. G. Wolff)

(1949b). Life situations, emotions, and extrasystoles. *Psychosomatic Medicine, 11*, 257–272. (with C. H. Duncan, S. Wolf, H. S. Ripley, and H. G. Wolff)

(1950). Physical symptoms during pleasurable emotional states. *Psychosomatic Medicine, 12*, 98–102.

(1957). Is the human personality more plastic in infancy and childhood? *American Journal of Psychiatry, 114*, 152–161.

(1958). Scientists with half-closed minds. *Harper's Magazine, 217*, 64–71.

(1960a). The evidence for survival from claimed memories of former incarnations. Part I. Review of the data. *Journal of the American Society for Psychical Research, 54*, 51–71.

(1960b). The evidence for survival from claimed memories of former incarnations. Part II. Analysis of the data and suggestions for further investigations. *Journal of the American Society for Psychical Research, 54*, 95–117.

(1965). On the irrational among the rational: Incredulity in scientists. *Virginia Quarterly Review, 41*, 40–57.

(1970). Physical symptoms occurring with pleasurable emotional states. *American Journal of Psychiatry, 127*, 175–179.

(1974). *Twenty Cases Suggestive of Reincarnation* (2nd ed., rev.). Charlottesville: University Press of Virginia. (Originally published as *Proceedings of the American Society for Psychical Research, 26*, 1–362, 1966)

(1977). The explanatory value of the idea of reincarnation. *Journal of Nervous and Mental Disease, 164*, 305–326.

(1983). American children who claim to remember previous lives. *Journal of Nervous and Mental Disease, 171*, 742–748.

(1997a). *Reincarnation and Biology: A Contribution to the Etiology of Birthmarks and Birth Defects* (2 vols.). Westport, CT: Praeger.

(1997b). *Where Reincarnation and Biology Intersect*. Westport, CT: Praeger.

(2001). *Children Who Remember Previous Lives: A Question of Reincarnation* (rev. ed.). Jefferson, NC: McFarland. (Originally published in 1987, Charlottesville: University Press of Virginia)

(2003). *European Cases of the Reincarnation Type*. Jefferson, NC: McFarland.

1

New Ideas in Science

EWK

One of the most basic observations we can make about ourselves and the world around us is that there is constant tension between the desire for stability and security and the drive toward growth and change. In science in particular, the drive to understand our experience and control our environment leads us to systematize our observations into some kind of ordered form, and to the extent that we can successfully fit subsequent observations into that system we can feel secure in our understanding and control of events. On the other hand, there is an equally strong drive to improve and increase knowledge and understanding. As a result, science involves a delicate balancing act between the security of what we know and the lure of what we don't.

There is thus a constant tension in science between a necessary conservatism, which prevents collapse into the chaos and confusion that would result if every new idea were given an equal hearing, and the equally necessary novel thinking that prevents stagnation. Ian was not so much concerned with the former. There are, in principle if not always in practice, sufficient safeguards for maintaining high standards in science and keeping out the unhelpful or misleading ideas. For one thing, a would-be scientist must go through rigorous training and attain a certain level of proficiency before his or her ideas will be taken seriously. For another, to obtain research funds or publish one's ideas and research in professional journals, scientists must submit their ideas and work to the scrutiny of peers. What *did* concern Ian, from the beginning of his career until the end of his life, was that there are no similar mechanisms to allow new, especially unorthodox, ideas to get a *fair* hearing. The peer review process that prevents scarce funds and journal pages from going to worthless ideas also too often prevents them from going to potentially important new ideas that are unfamiliar or uncongenial to reviewers. Noting that there is a strong temptation for editorial boards and granting agencies to support work consistent with their own views, Ian several times proposed ideas for diversifying decisions about funding, such as setting aside a certain percentage of available funds for new and unorthodox approaches (e.g., Stevenson, 1963, 1966).

More fundamentally, however, Ian repeatedly warned about the dangers of forgetting what science really is. First, science is a method of observation, not a system of fixed assumptions and knowledge. As William James (1896) put it years earlier, "science means, first of all, a certain dispassionate method. To suppose that it means a certain set of results that one should pin one's faith upon and hug forever is sadly to mistake its genius, and degrades the scientific body to the status of a sect" (p. 6).

Second, science is a process for generating knowledge and understanding, not the data, facts, or technological devices that provide the building blocks for that process. Quoting T. S. Eliot, Ian asked: "Where is the knowledge we have lost in information?" (Stevenson, 1954, p. 87). Early in his career, Ian argued that medicine is not yet a science, because its emphasis has been on technology or a description of diagnostic categories, rather than on seeking an understanding of the basic laws and principles behind health and disease (Stevenson, 1949 [reprinted in part 2]; see also 1953). Moreover, because science is a process, it is ever-evolving and constantly changing. Established *facts* don't change, but, as new observations accumulate, our understanding or perception of those facts does. Ian argued, therefore, that the most fundamental characteristic of science is the transience of its ideas, assumptions, and theories. Even its laws are subject to revision—not because they are in any sense overthrown but because they reflect only the current state of our understanding and will become refined as knowledge increases (Stevenson, 1996, p. 299).

Like William James, therefore, Ian resisted strongly the temptation to accept any system or ideology as the final word on a given topic. With acceptance of a particular system often comes prejudice against anything that does not fit into that system. Early in his career—during the throes of desegregation in America—Ian published two papers on prejudice, which he characterized as the rigidity that can accompany the human tendency to categorize (Lief & Stevenson, 1958; Stevenson, 1956). Whether it was in psychiatry, psychosomatic medicine, psychical research, or science in general, he struggled against "forc[ing] one interpretation on [observations] that are somewhat similar but really diverse" (1983, p. 27). Ian explained that he subscribed to "Leavett's Law, which states: 'the authoritative pronouncement that something is definitely established will be immediately followed by evidence to the contrary'" (1985, pp. 98-99).

In the remainder of this section are two papers in which Ian drew on his wide-ranging knowledge of the history and philosophy of science to show the difficulties of bringing new ideas to the attention of scientists and perhaps into the scientific framework.

REFERENCES

James, W. (1896). Address by the President. *Proceedings of the Society for Psychical Research, 12,* 2–10. (Reprinted in 1986, F. H. Burkhardt [ed.], *The Works of William James: Essays in Psychical Research* [pp. 127–137]. Cambridge, MA: Harvard University Press.)

Lief, H. I., & Stevenson, I. (1958). Psychological aspects of prejudice with special reference to desegregation. *American Journal of Psychiatry, 114,* 816–823.

Stevenson, I. (1949). Why medicine is not a science. *Harper's Magazine, 198,* 36.

Stevenson, I. (1953). Sir James Mackenzie, 1853–1953. *American Heart Journal, 46,* 479–484.

Stevenson, I. (1954). As a man thinketh . . . psychosomatic medicine, Part II. *Harper's Magazine, 209,* 83–87.

Stevenson, I. (1956). Southern attitudes on desegregation. *The New Republic, 134,* 22.

Stevenson, I. (1963). The preservation of a vanishing species: The part-time chairman. *Journal of Nervous and Mental Disease, 137,* 521–524.

Stevenson, I. (1966). New channels for grants [letter to editor]. *Science, 153,* 816–817.

Stevenson, I. (1983). Cryptomnesia and parapsychology. *Journal of the Society for Psychical Research, 52,* 1–30.

Stevenson, I. (1985). The Kern City poltergeist: Comments on the critique by Hövelmann and Zorab. *Journal of the Society for Psychical Research, 53,* 96–99.

Stevenson, I. (1996). Guest column: On the necessity of medical documents in claims of paranormal phenomena in diseases. *Journal of Scientific Exploration, 10,* 299–306.

TWO

Scientists with Half-Closed Minds

1958[1]

A surprising number are scared to death of new ideas. They have attacked major discoveries without even glancing at the evidence. And their distrust of unconventional experiments may now be hampering scientific progress.[2]

A Dutchman living in the East Indies once tried to tell a native of Java that in his country the water sometimes becomes so hard you can walk on it. The Javan was immediately convulsed with laughter, and the Dutchman could make no progress with his explanation.

We find this an amusing story, but it would be even funnier if it did not really refer to us all. Ordinarily our reaction to new ideas does not harm us or others. But when we make the discovery of new facts and new concepts our business, then incredulity can prove costly. When humans become scientists they continue to experience some of the less rational qualities of being human. And with this part of them they can get in each other's way, and in the way of progress.

Pierre Gassendi, for example, made notable contributions to seventeenth-century physics. He devised the first atomic theory of matter since Democritus, and his works strongly influenced Newton. Yet when in 1627 someone reported the fall of a meteorite in Provence, Gassendi explained it as due to some unidentified volcanic eruption. This attitude toward meteorites was shared by nearly all astronomers and many other leading scientists for the next century and a half. Some insisted that the stones had been picked up somewhere and carried by the wind; others accused those who claimed to have seen the stones fall of lying. In the late eighteenth century the great Antoine Lavoisier, himself a radical innovator in chemistry, rejected accounts of meteorites as the products of malobservation. Stones could not fall out of the sky, he declared, because none were there. Finally, in April 1803, a shower of small meteorites on L'Aigle, France, persuaded the astronomers to change their attitudes.

In the same way the first reports of hypnotism—or mesmerism, as it was called in the eighteenth and early nineteenth century—evoked many denials that the reported phenomena had ever occurred. In London, Dr. John Elliotson was driven from the chair of medicine at University College for endorsing and promoting the study of hypnotism. The early accounts of surgical operations conducted under hypnosis encountered extraordinarily irrational opposition. Dr. James Esdaile reported from India in the 1840s the successful completion of over a thousand operations (one-third of them major operations) with the patients hypnotized and a death rate of only 6 per cent during or after the operations. Although this occurred before asepsis when almost 30 per cent of other surgeons' patients died, Esdaile had great difficulty in getting his work even published, much less accepted. His scientific critics alleged that he had bribed his patients to sham insensibility. According to one account "it was because they were hardened impostors that they let their legs be cut off and large tumors be cut out without showing any sign even of discomfort." In their opposition to hypnotism many of the most creative scientists of the period forgot the rules of their own calling. Lord Kelvin announced that "one-half of hypnotism is imposture and the rest bad observation."

Similar prejudices met Harvey's discovery of the circulation of the blood, Pasteur's work on microbes, and Semmelweis' discovery that physicians themselves spread the infection of puerperal or childbed fever from one mother to another. To the list of scientists who have suffered from the incredulity of their colleagues we can add Darwin, the several discoverers of anesthesia, and Freud.

Early in the nineteenth century a tragic example of resistance delayed the introduction of a life-saving medical treatment. An English physician, O'Shaughnessy, discovered evidence that patients with cholera died not of the infection directly, but of the depletion of salt and water carried off in the diarrhea. Another physician, Dr. Thomas Latta of Leith, boldly acted on these observations and snatched from the grave a number of patients desperately ill with cholera to whom he gave infusions of salt and water. He reported his almost miraculous success; a few other physicians tried and confirmed the value of his treatment; but still not enough interest could be aroused to promote the treatment further. Almost one hundred years later, twentieth-century physicians rediscovered it.

CONTEMPT PRIOR TO EXAMINATION

A common and astonishing feature of the opposition to scientific advance is the certainty with which it is offered. For the moment, and sometimes for years, the doubter forgets that he could be wrong. At the first demonstration of Edison's phonograph before the Paris Academy of Sciences, all the scientists present declared that it was impossible to reproduce the human voice by means of a metal disc. One man proposed to throttle the demonstrator. "Wretch!" said he. "Do you suppose that we are fools to be duped by a ventriloquist?"

Resistance to the new can reach into the highest places. We owe to Francis Bacon much of the foundation of scientific method. He said: "We have set it down as a law to ourselves that we have to examine things to the bottom; and not to receive upon credit or reject upon improbabilities, until these have passed a due examination." Yet Bacon could not believe that the Earth goes around the Sun. Galileo, who could not persuade fellow astronomers to look into his telescope, could not himself accept Kepler's evidence that the planets move in ellipses. Nor could he believe that witches suffered from mental illness, a view beginning to gain acceptance in his day.

Professor P. G. Tait, a contemporary and colleague of Lord Kelvin, made contributions to physics hardly less important than those of Kelvin. But when the news of the discovery of the telephone reached him, he said, "It is all humbug, for such a discovery is impossible." Another interesting conversation occurred between Sir William Hamilton and Sir George Airy, justly celebrated mathematicians of the nineteenth century. Hamilton had just published his discovery of quaternions and was explaining it to Airy. Airy said, "I cannot see it at all." Hamilton replied, "I have been investigating the matter for many months and I am certain of its truth." "Oh," rejoined Airy, "I have been thinking it over for the last two or three minutes and there is nothing to it."

Many great ideas have, to be sure, won rather easy acceptance. Einstein had his difficulties, but they did not include stupid hostility from fellow scientists. Still such hostility should not occur at all among scientists. For it was science that once fought religion for freedom of inquiry and belief. In its original victories—and some of its more recent ones too—science defeated attempts to censor ideas. The principle of expanding knowledge replaced that of closed revelation. What had seemed to be a body of established facts was challenged and succeeded by a new body of facts based on observation rather than on reason and authority. But in the process a confusion arose between science and that body of newly discovered facts.

As science has progressed, more and more facts have become established with reasonable certainty—with enough certainty unfortunately to stimulate the illusion that science is chiefly a body of knowledge. The current body of scientific knowledge differs markedly from that of the seventeenth century, and the comparison shows the transience of our concepts. Yet we frequently overlook this and identify science with current knowledge. Those who forget that science is fundamentally a method and not a collection of facts will righteously challenge new concepts which seem to question old facts.

Organized scientific activity as we know it goes back less than five hundred years. And during this time it has occupied the interest and attention of only a few people. I am not referring to the millions it has affected, but to the few thinkers who have affected the millions. These people had first to struggle with themselves to believe that things could be other than they appeared to be. When someone asked Einstein how he came to discover relativity, he replied: "By challenging an axiom."

To accomplish anything worthwhile in science (and in nearly everything else), one has first to persuade oneself that things may be different from what they seem. This is the most difficult step to take and we should not be surprised if those who have walked furthest have frequently slipped. A scientist is—perhaps fortunately—only capable of scientific thought for a small portion of his time. At other times he usually allows his wishes, fears, and habits to shape his convictions. The wish not to believe can influence as strongly as the wish to believe. Most of us most of the time practice Paley's recipe for obstruction: "There is a principle, proof against all argument, a bar against all progress . . . which if persisted in cannot but keep the mind in everlasting ignorance—and that is, contempt prior to examination."

Scientists may also become seduced by their own attainments and acquire the conviction that success in one matter makes them authorities in all. James Clerk Maxwell's genius achieved an advance in the theory of electromagnetism from which came radio, television, and radar. His imagination shattered previously impenetrable theoretical barriers. Yet today he would surely blush crimson to read what he said to the British Association in 1879: "Atoms are the foundation stones of the material universe, unbroken and unworn. They continue to this day as they were created, perfect in number and measure and weight."

Pasteur struggled as much as any important scientist against the uninformed opposition of orthodoxy. After he attained recognition and at the height of his fame, he addressed a distinguished group of scientists and gratuitously included in his speech an announcement that scientific methods would never be used successfully in the study of the emotions. Yet already living at the time of his speech were the two persons who later established the scientific study of the emotions—Ivan Pavlov and Walter B. Cannon.

Like lesser human beings, scientists have a proprietary affection for their own contributions. Having given the best of their lives, as many have, to new observations and concepts, they may defend these as devotedly as those who give their lives to material possessions. And this kind of psychological investment can carry the investor into the most ridiculous positions. About fifty years ago, for instance, a curious exchange took place between the great anthropologist Malinowski and Dr. Ernest Jones, one of Freud's most devout followers and his biographer.

Jones subscribed wholeheartedly to Freud's statement about the universality of little boys' attachment to their mothers, which he called the Oedipus complex. This occurred often enough in nineteenth-century Vienna, and Freud declared it an invariable feature of human development. When Malinowski studied the Trobriand Islanders in the South Pacific he found that their children were reared by their mothers and uncles and had little or no contact with their biological fathers. The domestic relations and psychological development of the Trobrianders differed considerably from those reported by Freud for Viennese families. Malinowski published his observations, but they did not convince Jones. From his office in London he insisted that Freud was right and urbanely reprimanded Malinowski for faulty observations. To this Malinowski patiently replied that he was compelled to accept the evidence of his own senses rather than statements made by those who had never visited the Trobriand Islands.

The tendency to erect "systems"—which are then marketed as a whole—affects particularly the less mature sciences of medicine and psychology. In these subjects we have had a succession of intellectual edifices originally made available only in their entirety. It is as if one cannot rent a room or even a suite in a new building, but must lease the whole or not enter. Starting with a substantial contribution to medicine the authors of such systems expand their theories to include ambitious explanations of matters far beyond the original validated observations. And after the first pioneer, later and usually lesser contributors to the system add further accretions of mingled fact and theory. Consequently systems of this kind—like homeopathy, phrenology, psychoanalysis, and conditioned reflexology (the last dominant for years in Russia)—eventually contain almost inextricable mixtures of sense and nonsense. They capture fervid adherents, and it may take a generation or several for those who preserve some objectivity to succeed in salvaging the best in them while discarding the dross.

Many such systems repeat the same story almost tediously. A few brilliant observations encounter fierce opposition from entrenched authorities. Despite this the new ideas slowly acquire adherents. Gradually opposition to much of the original propositions crumbles. But in the meantime the avant-garde of the enlightened have stiffened their doctrines into a sectarian orthodoxy. Instead of befriending further advances, they frequently attack and deride them. Certainly not all early adherents to a new discovery do this, but those who do not often find that loyalty to a group requires loyalty to a set of ideas which conflicts with dispassionate examination of later ideas and observations.

HARMFUL INCREDULITY

Rigid systems and their fanatical devotees have driven many scientists into the camp of the too incredulous. The querulous "schools" of psychiatry have by their own extravagance delayed the acceptance of the best in psychiatry by other physicians and laymen. However, physicians of all kinds are particularly guilty of failing to keep up with advances in their own specialty. This comes about because medicine is, to be frank, a trade as well as a science. Most medical students go into the practice of medicine, not research, and we all know worthy physicians who devotedly practice the medicine taught them twenty-five years ago, apparently uninfluenced by the events of intervening years. Yet these same men conscientiously trade in their old automobiles for new ones every two or three years.

Theoretically, physicians should have no more difficulty than, say, chemists or physicists in changing their habits to accommodate new advances. But to accomplish this, medical schools must change their principles in selecting students and try, first, to attract flexible minds into medicine, and, second, to avoid doing anything that will harden these minds against new ideas. Happily, medical educators have already recognized the need for this. When medical science moved slowly a man could write the same prescriptions for thirty or more years and still not fall far behind the times. The increasing pace of medical discovery has made such physicians not only foolish, but positively harmful. Whitehead's comment that "knowledge keeps like fish" applies to medicine as much as any subject.

However, research scientists, too, are bound by harmful incredulity, although it is harder to determine to exactly what extent. In some ways scientists today have more protection against uninformed authoritarian opposition than their predecessors. For one thing there are more scientists and they are constantly testing each other's work so that confirmation, revision, or rejection of new observations and concepts can come rather rapidly. Communications between scientists have improved, and many journals now spread new data and new theories quickly across the world. Thus many scientists and not merely a handful judge the work of a fellow scientist.

On the other hand, the vastness of our scientific activity tells us nothing about the number of genuinely open minds occupied with it. A few years ago, Dr. Lucien Warner surveyed a number of psychologists on extrasensory perception. He asked what they thought about the existence of extrasensory perception and how they had reached their conclusions. All who replied had convictions, but less than 20 per cent said they had studied the original reports of the work on this subject. Seventeen per cent had reached their opinions on the basis of hearsay. Twenty per cent had made up their minds entirely on a priori grounds.

One can only respect the candor of persons who have registered themselves as scientists and yet make public declaration of the fact that they can decide on a matter of extraordinary importance without examining the relevant published work. Perhaps parapsychology provides a special case and scientists do not feel so free to make up their minds on other matters. Certainly the implacable opposition parapsychology encounters among some scientists illustrates again the relationship between the heat of antagonism and the possible threat to established convictions from the new data or ideas. For the data of parapsychology portend, I believe, a conceptual revolution which will make the Copernican revolution seem trivial in comparison.

We may tell ourselves that this incredulity has no effect on creative achievement, but I personally do not believe it. I am convinced that deep conservatism strongly influences the approach of many scientists to new ideas. I have tested this frequently by throwing out into a group of them some new idea, especially one whose acceptance would fracture favorite concepts. Almost invariably they attack it like a school of piranhas. By the time it reaches the bottom of the discussion they have stripped off its flesh.

My friends are not ordinarily destructive people. They do not injure people, only ideas. And I think this behavior has to do with a mistaken concept of the role of scientist. Certainly the role includes skepticism and tough-mindedness, but these alone are not enough. The best part of science derives from the imagination and creativity which contribute to it no less than to the arts. A scientist should examine an idea as an artist might look at a delicately enameled vase—in many different lights and positions so as to bring out all its beauty and value.

Scientists frequently pride themselves on not being gullible. Sometimes they do not seem to realize that they cannot be incredulous about new ideas without at the same time being excessively credulous about old ones. Between the merits of accepting too much and not enough of what is new there is perhaps little to choose, but surely that little favors a receptivity to the new since we already know so little.

I believe our conservatism has infected the financial support of scientists. Although a lot of money flows toward scientific research we do not know how much runs in well-cut gorges and how much can irrigate new ground. But the system of project grants for research is a symptom. Nearly all the funds poured into research by foundations and the federal government reach scientists after they have submitted a project to a committee. Since a scientist must gain the approval of the committee for his project, he may not resist the temptation to design his project along the lines most likely to harmonize with the convictions of the committee. The committee in turn must account to a board of trustees or to Congress or the public for the success of the research it has supported. Who can blame the members if they behave like bankers and venture their money more readily on "good risks" than on "wild ideas"?

Once he has his money, the scientist feels committed to the project he has outlined. If he makes some interesting but unexpected discovery or observation, he cannot easily abandon his main object to pursue a new line. Nearly every year he must submit an account of progress to the committee. I have heard a number of scientists tell, half laughing, half crying, how they adjusted their applications or reports, or, worse still, adjusted their scientific projects, to the real or apparent expectations of a granting committee.

It matters little that often the scientist's fears are unjustified or exaggerated. Certainly most scientific members of committees evaluating projects consciously wish to give the working scientists the greatest possible freedom. Still possession of the power to make decisions can eventually persuade anyone that he also has the proper knowledge to do so. The fault, I think, lies in the system, but wherever the fault, I believe that our scientists and the tellers of their money can easily become mutually involved in timid projects which always succeed but never advance.

It is difficult to pin down instances of the withering effect of incredulity on budding ideas. Prejudice can rationalize itself as caution or be easily disguised by other appearances. A surveying committee may conceal from the applicant, and even from itself, the real reasons for turning down a request for funds. Yet there are grounds for believing that research in psychiatry in this country has become excessively influenced by the theories of psychoanalysis.[3] I know of two first-rate investigators who have had great difficulty in obtaining support for their projects because (so the available evidence strongly suggests) their ideas run counter to psychoanalytic concepts. One eminent psychiatrist, much experienced in such matters, told me in discussing one of these cases that it is now extremely difficult to obtain support for psychiatric research projects which are not psychoanalytical in orientation. (He was referring to psychological and psychotherapeutic projects, not biochemical or neurophysiological ones.)

Another leading American psychiatrist recently published a vigorous protest in one of our professional journals against the centralization of psychiatric research and its control by committees which permit a few persons to swing enormous funds toward a few favorite or fashionable themes of research. The one-sidedness of our approach evokes both horror and amusement in our European colleagues who have managed to preserve a better balance in planning psychiatric research. This state of affairs does not reflect adversely on the merits of psychoanalysis, only on those who insist that its assumptions must be the point of departure for all psychiatric research.

FREEDOM TO ACT FOOLISH

Defenders of grants for project research claim that they permit scientists to get funds long before they are sufficiently well known to receive support for themselves. This supposes that we can support scientists directly only when they have already become well known—certainly a most unsatisfactory criterion of worth and one more likely to lead to a search for publicity than for truth.

A second symptom of harmful conservatism is the figures published by the National Science Foundation on the distribution of funds for research. In the years between 1940 and 1954—a period in which sums allocated for research skyrocketed—the funds available for basic research (i.e., research not bound to any immediate application) increased ten times. But in this same period the *percentage* of funds allocated for basic, as opposed to applied, research decreased by half.

Moreover, applied research has become increasingly important in the universities which have traditionally remained free to support new ideas and their testing. Recently, in order to maintain themselves against rising costs (or so they rationalize, perhaps), universities have accepted more and more contracts for applied research. According to a report prepared by Dr. Vannevar Bush in 1945, basic research received 70 per cent of all the funds devoted to research by universities before World War II. This contrasts sadly with a recent estimate derived from the report of the National Science Foundation that basic research now accounts for only 35 per cent of universities' research funds.

One remedy would be to give more money directly to scientists for themselves, rather than for special projects. The federal government has already begun this on a small scale, although we apparently lag far behind the Russians. Such a system would have its weaknesses in this country, as it undoubtedly has in Russia. Its mistakes would be more obvious and perhaps more wasteful than those of the present system. But if we had more failures, we might also have more new knowledge. Certainly we will have no new knowledge at all unless we continue to foster ideas which shake present beliefs. Prophets have warned us. John Dewey told us "every great advance of science has issued from a new audacity of imagination." And Whitehead wrote that "every great idea sounds like nonsense when first propounded."

During the planning of the Rockefeller Institute for Medical Research, someone asked Dr. Simon Flexner, who was one of the chief architects of modern medicine: "Are you going to allow your men to make fools of themselves at your Institute?" As it turned out the Rockefeller Institute made many more discoveries than fools, but the freedom to make a fool surely contributed to its extraordinary success. Scientists at the Rockefeller Institute were given full support to pursue their own work in their own ways. Unfortunately, this system had almost no imitators (except in

Russia) and even the Rockefeller Institute departed in later years from its original principle. Today we badly need not only new institutes of the kind it was, but new freedom to pursue strange ideas. And scientists themselves must encourage each other to think brazenly and experiment boldly.

When I read about the now-primitive treatments practiced by our predecessors in medicine a hundred years ago, I cannot refrain from smiling at some of their fatuous remedies. My smile includes a little pity for them because they knew so little and some pleasure for us because we have come so far. Then I hope that a hundred years from now, some medical descendant will read our books with similar pleasure for similar reasons. If he does, this supposes that we in our time have remained humble about our knowledge and receptive to the new ideas which will furnish the justification for his pity. May it not be said of us: "No man having drunk old wine, straightway desireth new; for he saith 'The old is better'."

NOTES

1. Reprinted from *Harper's Magazine*, November 1958.—Ed.
2. All italicized introductions to Ian's papers in this volume are the original introductions to the paper by the journal editor (as in this paper) or Ian's own abstract of the paper.—Ed.
3. This statement, made in 1958, might be altered today to "excessively influenced by the theories of psychopharmacology." The point remains the same.—Ed.

THREE

What Are the Irreducible Components of the Scientific Enterprise?

1999[1]

In this essay Dr. Stevenson argues that many scientists (and laymen also) have come to take a narrow view of what constitutes science. They would exclude as "unscientific" observations that do not include a falsifiable theory with predictions testable and repeatable in laboratory experiments. In contrast, Dr. Stevenson contends that science is more an attitude than a method. The attitude is one of testing interpretations of observed phenomena against further observations until one interpretation emerges as the best. Unfortunately, judgments about the best interpretation vary greatly, and scientists with new ideas and new observations must often overcome biases in their colleagues before their work becomes accepted as scientific.

Perhaps I am unqualified to address the topic of this paper. The philosopher Hobbes "was wont to say that if he had read as much as other men, he should have known no more than other men" (Aubrey, 1949, p. 154). I have read so many papers and books on the philosophy of science that I surely know no more than other men. Therefore, in emulation of Hobbes, of whom Aubrey said that "his contemplation was much more than his reading" (p. 154), I have sought to neutralize my extensive reading by contemplation. This paper derives from my contemplations. In it I ask whether we can eliminate certain components that some experts describe as essential to scientific research. If we can do this, we would then expose an indispensable remainder. I will offer a list of what I reject as inessential and then describe the residue.

Before offering my list of eliminable features I wish to disclaim asserting that what is inessential is necessarily undesirable; in saying that we can do scientific research without some particular feature, I do not mean to disparage its inclusion when we find this feasible. I am searching for features without which we would not say that we are doing scientific research.

Perhaps the least essential feature is the location of our endeavors. We cannot conduct scientific research anywhere and everywhere; but we do not require a special room like a laboratory for its conduct. We can do it in a jungle, in a desert, and in many other places.

We can also dispense with experiments. These are of two types: those in which we make observations in a controlled setting and those in which, while maintaining all other features constant, we change one feature and record the result. Neither type of experiment seems essential. Astronomers would be unemployed if they were.

Observations do not have to be repeatable to qualify as scientific. The observations of paleontology and many of those of geology and astronomy are not repeatable, but we do not value them less for that. Indeed, it seems to be true that few reported observations are ever exactly repeated, even in laboratory experiments. Partly from additional curiosity and partly from a desire to be original, scientists repeating earlier observations frequently vary the details of their observations from what a predecessor has described.

I come next to the claim that we can only assert negatives (falsifiability) (Popper, 1959). Several factors warrant our rejection of falsifiability. First, scientists may disagree about whether a particular observation constitutes an adequate refutation of a theory (Lakatos, 1970; Naess, 1972). Second, a negative instance refuting a generalization may itself be trivial and the remainder much more important. For example, in the often cited example of black swans in Australia it is still the case that, so far as we know, all swans except the black ones in Australia are white. Mere falsifiability or actual falsification therefore tells us nothing about the importance of our observations, let alone what is important to investigate. Third, correlations may suggest causal relationships in which we can have confidence even when we cannot falsify our conclusion. No one who has examined the evidence can doubt that tobacco smoking is an important cause of lung cancer; the incidence of this disease clearly correlates with the duration and amount of tobacco smoking. Fourth, some of the most fruitful theories of science, such as that of evolution, are not falsifiable. Fifth, the belief that only falsifiable ideas are scientific may snuff out innovative ideas before they have had a chance to survive testing (Bohm & Peat, 1987).

I also believe that prediction is not an essential feature of scientific research. I include here predictions both of what exists but has not yet been "discovered" and of what will happen in the future. Three well-known examples will help me to justify my rejection of prediction as indispensable to scientific research.

Edmund Halley predicted in 1705 the return in 1758 of the comet later named after him. He based his prediction on his analysis of the orbits of comets reported in 1531, 1607, and 1682 (which latter appearance he had himself observed) and concluded that the same comet had been observed on each occasion and would return. Its return in 1758, however, added only a fourth observation to the three of which Halley took account before he made his prediction. This, in my view, made it only a little more likely that the comet would come back a fifth time. To this it may be replied that Halley had studied the orbits of the appearing comets and therefore had more data than their simple appearance at intervals of 75 years. Even so, how many of us would bet that an event observed four times would occur a fifth time? We would probably wish to have more instances before predicting a recurrence. Since the return of the comet in 1758 it has appeared in 1835, 1910, and 1986. Moreover, examination of earlier records, many of them Chinese, suggest that the comet has been observed at least 30 times altogether (Tattersfield, 1984). A person skeptical about predicting a recurrence after 4 instances would probably accept the likelihood of another recurrence after 30 instances. I go into these details in order to emphasize that Halley's prediction showed his confidence in the physics and cosmology of his friend Isaac Newton, but the predicted return of the comet in 1758 added little to the evidence justifying belief (at that time) that it would return after the appearance of 1758–59.

A second example occurred in the case of the discovery of Neptune in 1846. In that year Urbain Leverrier in France and John Couch Adams in England almost simultaneously predicted the existence of an outer planet whose gravitational force would account for the observed anomalies in the motion of Uranus. Each then tried to persuade his country's astronomers to search for the planet and told them where to look. Neither was successful with their own seniors, who controlled the observatories. Leverrier then appealed to the German astronomer Johann Gottfried Galle, who searched for the conjectured planet and found it. The predictions of Neptune's existence and location are widely regarded as the most important confirmation of Newton's scheme of the universe up to that time. I contend, however, that the predictions of Leverrier and Adams showed their confidence in Newtonian cosmology, but it was the existence of Neptune and its orbital behavior, not the predictions of them that provided a confirmation of the cosmology.[2] Neptune and its behavior like a planet might have been found without having been predicted. Indeed, it very nearly was. Later examinations showed that the French astronomer Joseph Lalande had observed Neptune's movement in 1795; he made two observations of what he thought was a star but that were different, and because of the discrepancy between them, he concluded that they were both wrong or doubtful. If he had made a third observation, he would have discovered Neptune 50 years before Galle did (Grosser, 1962).

My third example is that of Mendeleev's description of the periodic table of the elements. In this table Mendeleev arranged the 60 elements known at his time (1869) in the order of their atomic weights. He left four gaps in the table for elements whose discovery he predicted; he even described the properties that three of these would have, and these were identified within 20 years of the publication of his table (Asimov,1964; Kelman & Stone, 1970). I again say that the prediction added little evidence to what was already available. Three elements added to 60 are not many. Mendeleev's greater accomplishment was ordering the 60 elements in a system far superior to previous ones. His predictions of elements not yet known showed his confidence in his system as did his correction of some of the experimentally derived atomic weights. Mendeleev's theory exemplifies Eddington's (1935) aphorism according to which one should not "put overmuch confidence in the observational results that are put forward until they have been confirmed by theory" (p. 211).

I will make two more remarks about predictions in science. First, a reading of the statements and correspondence of Halley, Leverrier, Adams, and Mendeleev concerning their predictions and the theories from which they made them shows the great confidence they had in the theories from which the predictions derived. Second, although I contend that predictions are not a necessary part of science I think they are part of the joy in doing science.

Some readers may think I have belabored prediction. It is not difficult, however, to find writers who assert the indispensability of prediction for scientific research. One of Whewell's aphorisms states: "It is a test of true theories not only to account for, but to predict phenomena" (Butts, 1968, p. 138). Carnap (1966) wrote that "The supreme value of a new theory is its power to predict new empirical laws" (p. 231). Claude Bernard asserted that "real science is not being conducted until one can accurately predict the occurrence of phenomena and control them" (Bernard, 1865/1952, pp. 199–200; my translation). More recently, Ayala (1996) has made an even stronger statement: ". . . being predictive of unknown facts is essential to the process of empirical testing of hypotheses, the most distinctive feature of the scientific enterprise" (p. 442). On the other hand, I have good company for my position. John Stuart Mill (1846), differing from Whewell, stated:

> It seems to be thought that an hypothesis . . . is entitled to a more favorable reception if, besides accounting for all the facts previously known, it has led . . . to the prediction of others which experience afterwards verified. . . . Such predictions and their fulfilment are, indeed, well calculated to strike the ignorant vulgar. . . . But it is strange that any particular stress should be laid upon such a coincidence by scientific thinkers. (p. 296)

Albert Einstein (1930) believed the predictions made by the general theory of relativity are less important than the "simplicity of its foundation and . . . its logical consistency" (p. 183). Eddington, whose measurement in 1919 of gravitational light bending did much to arouse interest in the general theory of relativity, believed that "the observational predictions form only a minor part of the subject" [relativity] (Eddington, 1924, p. v; Brush, 1989). Bauer (1992) cited the example of the concept of phlogiston, which, although fecund with predictions, some of them correct, became overthrown by a better theory of combustion.

If, as I believe, prediction is not an essential feature of science, why have so many scientists asserted that it is? The answer may be that predictions prevent theorists from elastically adapting their theories to include new ill-fitting observations. Predictions add to the discipline of science.

Resuming my list of dispensable features I come to quantification, either in measurement or in counting. I know that some notable scientists believe these features essential for science. Kelvin (1891), for example, wrote that "when you cannot measure it [what you are speaking about], when you cannot express it in numbers . . . you have scarcely . . . advanced to the stage of science" (p. 80). Nevertheless, measurement had no part in a small number of significant observations that no one would exclude from a history of advances in science. I count as examples: Jenner's discovery of the effect of cowpox in preventing smallpox (1798); William Beaumont's observation that gastric juice could "digest" food not only in the stomach, but when removed from the stomach and added to food placed in a vial (Beaumont, 1833); and Pasteur's experiments that refuted the idea of spontaneous generation (Vallery-Radot, 1920).

The seventh and last feature that I believe dispensable is a control group. One can certainly engage in medical science without one. A single patient may be studied over a period of time by observations of what modifies a disease and what does not. Much of clinical medicine has to follow this method of trial, disappointment (or perhaps error), and a new trial of something different. Furthermore, such a process can produce results applicable to other patients, and we should not withhold the name of scientific research from it (Berwick, 1996; 1998).

In sum, I believe that seven features frequently mentioned as essential to scientific investigations are not (they are listed in Table 1). By eliminating them I am trying to reach a core of features that I believe are indispensable. As I cautioned earlier, however, some of the features that I have excluded from this core are frequently important—even essential—to certain kinds of research. In particular, repeatability is always desirable, and measurement and control groups are often essential, even though not always.

Table 3.1. Features That Are Inessential to the Scientific Enterprise

1. Location
2. Experimental control of conditions
3. Repeatability
4. We can only assert negatives (falsifiability)
5. Prediction
6. Quantification (as measurement or counting)
7. Control groups

What then remains of the core components that I consider essential to the scientific enterprise?

First, it is a public process. The methods of observing and analyzing the results must be openly described so that, in principle, another qualified person could duplicate the observations and obtain the same results.

Second, the events and objects of observation must also be public and capable of being observed by others. This excludes subjective states, although not a person's report of his or her internal thoughts and feelings. This requirement distinguishes scientific research both from philosophy and from religious inspiration. Private knowledge occurs and may be extremely important; but so long as it remains private it is not within my definition of science.

Third, the observer's beliefs and expectations should not modify his observations. Darwin wisely wrote that "there was much talk that geologists ought only to observe and not theorise; and I well remember someone saying that at this rate a man might as well go into a gravel-pit and count the pebbles and describe the colors. How odd it is that anyone should not see that all observation must be for or against some view if it is to be of any service!" (Darwin, 1903, vol. 1, p. 195). True enough, but the view should not interfere with the observation. This is a counsel of perfection, because our hopes and expectations can easily influence what we see and hear. We can strive toward objectivity by exposing as fully as possible all observations that tend to weaken our own preferred interpretation of the data. If adversaries fire at us, let them use ammunition that we have given them. (How we achieve, or even approach, objectivity is a major problem in science to which I shall return later.)

Fourth, scientific research should be an advance on simple observation and common sense. It should provide a comparison between some property (or it may be a group of properties) that seems unknown with what is already known, or thought to be known. Thus if I wish to say that reincarnation is the best explanation for a group of observations that I have recorded, I must name and disqualify rival explanations. Reincarnation is an unknown, at least in current science. For fraud, cryptomnesia, distorted memories on the part of informants, and even—some would say—for extrasensory perception, as well as for several other explanations of the data, we have independent evidence, and therefore they are known, or thought to be known.

Fifth, the new observations should generate a theory of greater explanatory power for both new and old observations. I do not satisfy my concept of scientific research by giving a new name to a group of familiar observations. I must also show that the interpretation that I favor can explain all related observations better than the alternative explanations that I should exclude before asking other scientists to accept mine. For example, the concept that the earth is a sphere can explain observations that the concept of a flat earth cannot. It explains the round shape of the earth's shadow on the moon during eclipses; why when a ship moves away from us on the sea its hull disappears from our view before its mast does; why when we continue to sail or fly in a westward direction, for example, we come back to our starting place; why different stars are seen in the sky as one travels north or south from the equator; and why if two travelers, one in Spain and one in Greece, are 1500 kilometers apart and then begin to travel north, they will find themselves at the level of England and Poland, only 900 kilometers apart.

The greatness of Kepler's accomplishment lay not especially in his finding—after 19 previous conjectures—that the different positions of Mars fitted an ellipse; instead, it was in the colligation that all the other planets also move in elliptical orbits.

There is, however, a hazard in explanatory power. The history of science, especially of medicine, offers numerous instances of concepts for which their adherents claimed great explanatory power.. Phrenology, homeopathy, and psychoanalysis are three examples, among many, of such theories. Later observations showed the claims made for them to be largely or entirely baseless. Mere explanatory value is unconvincing to most scientists (Stevenson, 1977).[3]

What was missing from the work of the proponents of superseded concepts? They were unable or unwilling to continue testing their theories against observations. My sixth essential element of scientific research is, therefore, the repeated testing of theory against later observations. Equally important is the continued testing of one's preferred theory against theories that other scientists may propose. This repeated testing of a theory against observations distinguishes scientific research from the dogmatic claims of cranks and pseudoscientists (Feyerabend, 1964). They assert their conclusions without testing them against observations.

I have already said that a scientist should publicly describe his or her methods so that another scientist can replicate them. We can rarely trust the observations of a single person in scientific matters. "All men are liable to error, and most men are, in many points, by passion or interest, under temptation to it" (Locke, 1690/1824, vol. 2, p. 235). Given the difficulty of making observations devoid of distortion due to the observer's expectations, replication by other investigators provides our best corrective of such distortion. Every scientist with confidence in his work and conclusions should welcome replication by other investigators. This is indeed the only way by which a scientist can win acceptance of his observations and ideas. Independent replication is therefore my seventh essential element in scientific research.

Table 2 lists the seven features of research that I consider essential. It also lists, separately, an eighth feature that I believe necessary for success in any scientific enterprise: the persuasion of other scientists to accept the validity and importance of one's observations.

This task brings us back to the problem of objectivity. We need to ask what its criteria are. I believe it is nothing more than the acceptance of a scientist's views by a sufficient number of other scientists. Ziman (1968) has written that "the objective of science . . . is a consensus of rational opinion over the widest possible field" (p. 9). Elsewhere Ziman (1978) wrote that the goal of science "is to achieve the maximum degree of consensuality. Ideally the general body of scientific knowledge should consist of facts and knowledge that are firmly established and accepted without serious doubt" (p. 6).

Ziman's idea of what we may call a majority vote that is needed to authenticate new observations or theories leads to the question of authority in science. Who is to say what facts "are firmly established and accepted without serious doubt"? Ziman's answer to this question is, continuing the quotation just cited, "an overwhelming majority of competent well-informed scientists" (p. 6). In practice these scientists, or other persons of authority, who control appointments, promotions, funding, and

Table 3.2. Features That Are Essential to the Scientific Enterprise

1. Methods must be public and publicly reported
2. The observed events must be public
3. Objectivity in observations, that is, investigator's beliefs and expectations should not influence the observations and reports of them
4. Comparison of one observation or set of observations (usually new ones) with another observation or set of observations (usually what is known or thought to be known)
5. Superior explanatory power of theory derived from the new observations
6. Repeated testing of theory against new observations and alternative theories
7. Independent replication of observations

****

8. Persuasion of a majority of scientists of the accuracy of the observations and the usefulness of the derived theory

access to publication in journals and books make judgments about objectivity.

Unfortunately, even the most experienced scientists may be found lacking in objectivity (Arp, 1987; Hetherington, 1988[4] ; Marshall, 1990). Moreover, they too often believe that current knowledge will endure forever. What we now teach, they tell us, will not be changed in any substantial way. In recent years two scientists have published confident assertions of the immutability of current knowledge (Cromer, 1993; Wilson, 1998). Such certitude has been given the name of a disease called "kelvinitis." The name derives from Lord Kelvin's statement, at the end of the 19th century, that "all the discoveries in physics had been made and . . . it remained only to adjust the last decimal point in a few measurements" (Asimov, 1964, p. 306)[5] . Another term for the same condition is "presentism," whose advocates assure us that present, reliable knowledge has finally replaced long periods of bleak ignorance (Micale & Porter, 1994). "They live under perpetual illusion of fundamental understanding" (Bauer, 1992, p. 75).

Persons afflicted with kelvinitis or presentism are usually unaware of the social and economic forces that facilitated the development of scientific ideas in one direction instead of in another. To them the way things are seems natural, immutable, and just the way they should be.

They are terribly wrong. The history of science offers us many examples of the supersession of one theory and the rise to dominance of a successor. Personal decisions and motives different from the search for truth frequently influence the succession of currently favored theories. To take only one example, the history of the ascent of genetics to its current hegemony in biology cogently demonstrates the influence of social and political forces in the evolution of one branch of scientific research. T. H. Morgan (1866–1945) began his professional career as an embryologist. Later, he became interested in the inheritance of traits. Considering that Darwin's *The Origin of Species* was published in 1859 and that Mendel's discoveries concerning inheritance were brought to the attention of a wider scientific readership in 1900, Morgan was slow to convert to the idea of evolution and to embrace genetics as a legitimate field of scientific research (Bowler, 1988; Shine & Wrobel, 1976). When he did convert in 1910, however, he, with his students and colleagues, established a scientific society and a journal of genetics; they trained graduate students who took teaching positions and propagated other students until their view of what is important in biology came to dominate the field and still does. Early in his enthusiasm for genetics Morgan separated it from embryology, and in the ensuing development of biology, embryology and the problems of morphology became neglected, almost overlooked (Bowler, 1988; Sapp, 1987). The few biologists who tried to draw more attention to morphology and its problems (Russell, 1916/1982; Thompson, 1917) were respected but largely ignored.

The history of science shows that today's facts may become tomorrow's falsehoods. At different times the following were regarded as facts: the earth stands still and the stars move; the sun goes around the earth; the earth is flat; stones cannot fall out of the sky because there are none there; atoms are indivisible; atoms may break up, but this can never be exploited as a source of energy; space is filled with ether; machines heavier than air can never fly; continents cannot split and the parts move away from each other.

Let me now list some of the current "facts" accepted by most of today's scientists: natural selection fully explains evolution; the mind is only the behavior of a physical object called the brain; a human mind cannot communicate with another mind without the mediation of the currently known sensory organs; personality derives entirely from genetic inheritance and postnatal environmental experiences. Research now under way, some of it by members of the Society for Scientific Exploration, is already producing observations that challenge the status of these assertions as "facts." I predict that at least some of them will cease to be regarded as "facts" by the middle of the next century.

Theories, like living organisms, have life histories. They are born, mature, grow old, and die. Like humans, they are often repaired, in their case with subsidiary explanations; but eventually unfitting anomalies lead to their demise. In saying this I adhere to Kuhn's idea of scientific revolutions (Kuhn, 1962). (I do, however, believe—contrary to Kuhn—that much scientific knowledge is cumulative.) Even before Kuhn, Polanyi had exploded the myths of detached observation and impersonal knowledge (Polanyi, 1958). Both of them, however, had a predecessor, Ludwik Fleck, who in 1935 published a book (in German) with the remarkable title (in English) of "Genesis and Development of a Scientific Fact: Introduction to the Concept of Thoughtstyle and Thoughtcollective" (Fleck, 1935/1979). By "thoughtcollective" Fleck meant the beliefs held by the majority of scientists at any one time. In order for new observations to achieve the status of fact they must become sufficiently persuasive to convince a majority of scientists that they deserve that promotion. The thoughtcollective, however, does not change easily. Lakatos (1970) put this more bluntly when he wrote that "the history of science cannot be fully understood without mob-psychology" (p. 140).

I believe it is more difficult now than formerly to introduce new ideas and concepts and have them accepted by scientists. I attribute this to the larger number of practicing scientists compared with former times. This larger number of scientists increases the likelihood that one or more of them will make important discoveries. Unfortunately, it also has the disadvantage of presenting a larger mass of scientists resistant to change. "A new scientific truth does not triumph by convincing its opponents and making them see the light, but rather because its opponents eventually die and a new generation grows up that is familiar with it" (Planck, 1950, pp.

33–34). To this we may add that death is often not a sufficient facilitator of the acceptance of new ideas.

How did science arrive at this condition? It sometimes seems that little has changed since Francis Bacon, who, surveying the world of learning in his time, remarked that "the last thing anyone would be likely to entertain is an unfamiliar thought" (1607/1964, p. 79).

Nevertheless, scientists have not been deprived of exhortations to open their minds to new ideas. Heraclitus (c. 500 B.C.) warned: "If you do not expect the unexpected, you will not find it" (Kahn, 1979, p. 31). Other notable scientists have urged their colleagues to examine every observation without prejudice. Bacon—justly regarded as the instigator, if not the practical founder of modern science—wrote "that rarities and reports that seem incredible are not to be suppressed or denied to the memory of men" (Bacon, 1605/1962, p. 29). Herschel, one of the first writers on the philosophy of science, told his readers "A perfect observer . . . will have his eyes opened, as it were, that they may be struck at once with any occurrence which, according to received theories, ought not to happen; for these are the facts which serve as clews to new discoveries" (Herschel, 1830/1840, p. 132). A little later, Claude Bernard, one of the founders of modern physiology, warned that "if one sees only facts congruent with one's formed ideas, one will often miss making discoveries" (Bernard, 1865/1952, p. 215; my translation).

One of the most subtle writers of advice for scientists was Laplace, who added to his admonition to be unprejudiced a further, neutralizing, phrase. He first wrote: "We are so far from knowing all the forces of nature and their processes that it would show little wisdom to deny phenomena just because we cannot explain them in the present state of our knowledge" (Laplace, 1814/1840, p. 133; my translation). To this, however, he added: ". . . we ought to examine them [inexplicable phenomena] as much the more scrupulously as it appears the more difficult to admit them." The Swiss psychologist Theodore Flournoy called this aphorism "Laplace's Principle," and stated it as: "The strength of the evidence must be proportional to the strangeness of the facts" (Flournoy, 1899, p. 345; my translation). Flournoy then goes on to ask who is to be the judge of the "strangeness of the facts" and reaches the obvious conclusion that such judgments are subjective. The credulous ignore Laplace's principle, but the skeptic can use it to demand evidence stronger than anything offered to him or her. Then, when given some stronger evidence, he or she may demand something yet stronger. Such a person can always protect a prior belief from erosion.

Scientists who think for themselves have few defenses against the thought-collective. In principle, peer review of research grant applications and articles submitted to scientific journals should boost their chances of escaping the vigilance of thwarting conservatives. That it does not do so is not news. In 1793 the Royal Society rejected Jenner's paper on vaccination (Magner, 1992); he published it privately five years later (Jenner, 1798). In the next century anonymous reviewers for the *Annalen der Physik* refused to publish Helmholtz's paper on the conservation of energy (Graneau & Graneau, 1993). Readers who wish experimental evidence of the imperfections of peer review can find it in Mahoney's (1977) study of the influence of personal bias on referee's judgments of the quality (and hence suitability for publication) of manuscripts submitted to a journal. Horrobin (1990) has gone so far as to stigmatize peer review as a suppressor of innovation.

Remedies have been proposed. I suggested that a portion of funds granted for research be trickled down through administrators who, at each level would be obliged to divide most of what they receive to those at a lower level; thus even a beginner in research would receive some funding with which he could do research as he wished (Stevenson, 1966). Wessely (1998) has reviewed other suggestions for improvement that have been suggested. Perhaps Horrobin (1996) has made the boldest recommendation. He proposed that the entire sum available for, say, medical research in the United Kingdom, should be divided among all (British) researchers with academic medical positions. By his calculations each investigator would thus receive about U.S. $85,000 per year. There would be no research grant applications, no reviewing committees, no required reports. Research administrators would disappear. The grants would be good for ten years. Renewal for another decade of support would require evidence of productivity in research. Horrobin predicted that his plan would lead immediately to increased productivity—and more innovation—on the part of scientists.

The Society for Scientific Exploration was founded to combat the problem presented by the resistance to new ideas on the part of scientists. The founders of the Society hoped that it would prize open the half-closed minds of other scientists so that deviant ideas could find more receptive audiences among their colleagues. A friend, whom I exhorted to join the Society when it was newly founded, declined and warned me that the new society could have an effect opposite to that intended. Editors of conventional journals, he believed, could say "We do not have to publish this wild paper. Let it go to the *Journal of Scientific Exploration.*" Thus the isolation of dissidents would continue without more than trivial discomfort to the authorities who were keeping them in exile. The Society and its members, he predicted, would become isolated and considered harmless, like an encysted foreign body in a living organism. I have to say that he may have been right. In this respect the Society has not succeeded. It has not, however, failed; and it can yet succeed. I am sure it will.

Some readers may reproach me for wandering away from the methodology of science into its sociology. I agree that persuading one's colleagues to take one's research seriously is not part of the research itself, but it definitely has to be part of the scientific enterprise. No scientist has completed his or her work until other scientists have been persuaded to continue the research he or she has initiated.

NOTES

1. Reprinted from the *Journal of Scientific Exploration, 13,* 257–270, 1999. This essay is an expanded version of the Dinsdale Prize Lecture presented by Dr. Stevenson at the 17th Annual Meeting of the Society for Scientific Exploration.—Ed.

2. One reader of a draft of this paper strongly disagreed with me regarding the discovery of Neptune. He pointed out that the computations of Adams and Leverrier based on Newton's cosmology permitted the prediction and discovery of a hitherto unknown planet.

3. In the paper cited I described the explanatory value of the idea of reincarnation for six important unsolved problems in biology and medicine. The paper drew considerable attention at the time, judging by an immense number of requests for reprints and considerable attention from the media. Nevertheless, no independent investigator undertook to replicate my observations about children who claim to remember previous lives for more than a decade (Mills, 1989).

4. Hetherington took his examples of lack of objectivity from astronomy. In an endnote on bibliography he gives references to lack of objectivity among scientists in other disciplines.

5. About a decade later, Michelson (1902) repeated the same assertion in different words. Three years after that, in 1905, Einstein published his special theory of relativity.

REFERENCES

Arp, H. (1987). *Quasars, Redshifts, and Controversies.* Berkeley, CA: Interstellar Media.

Asimov, I. (1964). *Asimov's Biographical Encyclopedia of Science and Technology.* Garden City, NY: Doubleday.

Aubrey, J. (1949). *Brief Lives.* O. L. Dick (Ed.). London: Secker and Warburg. (First published in 1813)

Ayala, F. J. (1996). The candle and the darkness (review of C. Sagan, *The Demon-Haunted World: Science as a Candle in the Dark*). *Science, 273,* 442–443.

Bacon, F. (1964). *Cogitata et Visa (Thoughts and Conclusions).* In B. Farrington (Trans.), *The Philosophy of Francis Bacon* (pp. 73–102). Liverpool: Liverpool University Press. (Written c. 1607)

Bacon, R. (1962). *The Advancement of Learning.* London: J. M. Dent. (First published in 1605)

Bauer, H. H. (1992). *Scientific Literacy and the Myth of the Scientific Method.* Urbana, IL: University of Illinois Press.

Beaumont, W. (1833). *Experiments and Observations on the Gastric Juice and the Physiology of Digestion.* Plattsburgh, NY: F. P. Allen.

Bernard, C. (1952). *Introduction à l'étude de la médecine expérimentale.* Paris: Flammarion. (First published in 1865)

Berwick, D. M. (1996). Harvesting knowledge from improvement. *Journal of the American Medical Association, 275,* 877–878.

Berwick, D. M. (1998). Developing and testing changes in delivery of care. *Annals of Internal Medicine, 128,* 651–656.

Bohm, D., & Peat, F. D. (1987). *Science, Order, and Creativity.* New York: Bantam Books.

Bowler, P. J. (1988). *The Non-Darwinian Revolution: Reinterpreting a Historical Myth.* Baltimore: The Johns Hopkins University Press.

Brush, S. G. (1989). Prediction and theory evaluation: The case of light bending. *Science, 246*, 1124–1129.
Butts, R. E. (ed.). (1968). *William Whewell's Theory of Scientific Method*. Pittsburgh: University of Pittsburgh Press.
Carnap, R. (1966). *Philosophical Foundations of Physics*. New York: Basic Books.
Cromer, A. (1993). *Uncommon Sense. The Heretical Nature of Science*. New York: Oxford University Press.
Darwin, C. (1903). *More Letters of Charles Darwin: A Record of his Work in a Series of Hitherto Unpublished Letters* (2 vols.) (F. Darwin & A. C. Seward, Eds.). New York: D. Appleton.
Eddington, A. S. (1924). *The Mathematical Theory of Relativity*. London: Cambridge University Press.
Eddington, A. S. (1935). *New Pathways in Science*. Cambridge: Cambridge University Press.
Einstein, A. (1930). Space, ether and field in physics. *Forum Philosophicum, 1*, 180–184.
Feyerabend, P. K. (1964). Realism and instrumentalism: Comments on the logic of factual support. In M. Bunge (Ed.), *The Critical Approach to Science and Philosophy* (pp. 280–308). London: Collier-Macmillan.
Fleck, L. (1979). *Genesis and Development of a Scientific Fact*. Chicago: University of Chicago Press. (First published in German in 1935)
Flournoy, T. (1899). *Des Indes à la Planète Mars*. Geneva: Edition Atar.
Graneau, P., & Graneau, N. (1993). *Newton versus Einstein: How Matter Interacts with Matter*. New York: Carlton Press.
Grosser, M. (1962). *The Discovery of Neptune*. Cambridge, MA: Harvard University Press.
Herschel, J. F. W. (1840). *Preliminary Discourse on the Study of Natural Philosophy*. New York: Harper and Brothers. (First published in 1830)
Hetherington, N. S. (1988). *Science and Objectivity: Episodes in the History of Astronomy*. Ames, IA: Iowa State University Press.
Horrobin, D. F (1990). The philosophical basis of peer review and the suppression of innovation. *Journal of the American Medical Association, 263*, 1438–1441.
Horrobin, D. F. (1996). Peer review of grant applications: A harbinger for mediocrity in clinical research? *The Lancet, 348*, 1293–1295.
Jenner, W. (1798). *An Inquiry into the Causes and Effects of Variolae Vaccinae*. London: Sampson Low.
Kahn, C. H. (1979). *The Art and Thought of Heraclitus*. Cambridge: Cambridge University Press.
Kelman, P., & Stone, A. H. (1970). *Mendeleyev: Prophet of Chemical Elements*. Englewood Cliffs, NJ: Prentice-Hall.
Kelvin, Lord. [Thomson, W.] (1891). *Popular Lectures and Addresses. Vol. 1. Constitution of Matter*. London: Macmillan.
Kuhn, T. S. (1962). *The Structure of Scientific Revolutions*. Chicago: University of Chicago Press.
Lakatos, I. (1970). Falsification and the methodology of scientific research programmes. In I. Lakatos and A. Musgrave (Eds.), *Criticism and the Growth of Knowledge* (pp. 91–196). Cambridge: Cambridge University Press.
Laplace, P.-S. de. (1840). *Essai Philosophique sur les Probabilités* (6th ed.). Paris: Bachelier. (First published in 1814)
Locke, J. (1824). *Essay Concerning Human Understanding* (2 vols.). New York: Valentine Seaman. (First published in 1690)
Magner, L. N. (1992). *A History of Medicine*. New York: Marcel Dekker.
Mahoney, M. J. (1977). Publication prejudices: An experimental study of confirmatory bias in the peer review system. *Cognitive Therapy and Research, 1*, 161–175.
Marshall, E. (1990). Science beyond the pale. *Science, 249*, 14–16.
Micale, M. S., & Porter, R. (1994). *Discovering the History of Psychiatry*. New York: Oxford University Press.

Michelson, A. A. (1902). *Light Waves and Their Uses.* Chicago: University of Chicago Press.

Mill, J. S. (1846). *A System of Logic, Ratiocinative and Inductive.* New York: Harper and Brothers. (First published in 1843)

Mills, A. (1989). A replication study: Three cases of children in northern India who are said to remember a previous life. *Journal of Scientific Exploration, 3,* 133–184.

Naess, A. (1972). *The Pluralist and Possibilist Aspect of the Scientific Enterprise.* London: Allen and Unwin.

Planck, M. (1950). *Scientific Autobiography and Other Papers.* London: Williams and Norgate.

Polanyi, M. (1958). *Personal Knowledge: Toward a Post-Critical Philosophy.* London: Routledge and Kegan Paul.

Popper, K. R. (1959). *The Logic of Scientific Discovery.* London: Hutchinson. (First published in 1934)

Russell, E. S. (1982). *Form and Function: A Contribution to the History of Animal Morphology.* Chicago: University of Chicago Press. (First published in 1916)

Sapp, J. (1987). *Beyond the Gene: Cytoplasmic Inheritance and the Struggle for Authority in Genetics.* Oxford: Oxford University Press.

Shine, I., & Wrobel, S. (1976). *Thomas Hunt Morgan: Pioneer of Genetics.* Lexington, KY: University Press of Kentucky.

Stevenson, I. (1966). New channels for grants [letter to editor]. *Science, 153,* 816–817.

Stevenson, I. (1977). The explanatory value of the idea of reincarnation. *Journal of Nervous and Mental Disease, 164,* 305–326.

Tattersfield, D. (1984). *Halley's Comet.* Oxford: Blackwell.

Thompson, D. W. (1917). *On Growth and Form.* Cambridge: Cambridge University Press.

Wessely, S. (1998). Peer review of grant applications: What do we know? *The Lancet, 352,* 301–305.

Wilson, E. O. (1998). Integrated science and the coming century of the environment. *Science, 279,* 2048–2049.

Vallery-Radot, R. (1920). *The Life of Pasteur.* Garden City, NY: Garden City Publishing Company.

Ziman, J. M. (1968). *Public Knowledge: An Essay Concerning the Social Dimension of Science.* Cambridge: Cambridge University Press.

Ziman, J. M. (1978). *Reliable Knowledge: An Exploration of the Grounds for Belief in Science.* Cambridge: Cambridge University Press.

2

The Nature of Human Personality

EWK

One major "new" idea in science is not really new at all—we just need to keep being reminded of it. This "new" idea, which played a major role in Ian's thinking from his earliest days in medicine, is that *understanding*, whether in science or anything else, comes from looking, to the extent possible, at wholes rather than parts. Thus, whether it is looking at science through the lens of history or looking at patients through the lens of their life histories and not just their symptoms, the broader the scope of one's view is, the truer one's understanding will be.

Another major idea that is similarly not new, and that stems directly from the first, is one that caused the vast majority of scientists and philosophers to resist, repudiate, ridicule, or—most frequently—ignore Ian's work, particularly in psychical research. Again from his earliest days in medicine, Ian held that human beings are not bodies alone but bodies *and* minds that interact—an observation that may seem simple, even trite, to most ordinary people but one that has aroused more contentious disputes in modern science and philosophy than any other issue.

All aspects of Ian's career were dominated by his dissatisfaction with the picture of human personality that in the last century has overwhelmingly come to dominate neuroscience, medicine, psychiatry, and psychology—that human personality is the product solely of physical processes, namely, the brain and its body, as well as its physical environment. Taking the two ideas described above—not, I repeat, new, but certainly unpopular in much of contemporary thinking—Ian sought a better view. Long before the recent upsurge of "holistic" medicine, when medical schools are even beginning to offer courses on spirituality, Ian was arguing for a medicine that treats the patient not as a malfunctioning machine that needs fixing but as a whole person whose emotions and life situations, especially stress and problems in relationships, play a central role in the onset, course, and prognosis of disease. Most of his first 50 papers, from 1941 to 1954, deal with this issue in one way or another.

When the patient is seen in this way, it becomes clear that there is no sharp dividing line between structural and functional diseases, that is, between physical diseases caused by organic factors and psychiatric or psychosomatic diseases caused by emotional or mental factors (see, e.g., Graham & Stevenson, 1963; Stevenson, 1952a, 1952b, 1954a).

One consequence of this view about the inseparability of physical and emotional factors in health and disease is the importance of having a physician who knows the patient over a long period of time and who thus knows the patient's life situation as well as physical condition. Ian wrote a series of papers in the 1950s in which he called for "A New Day for the General Practitioner" (the title of 1951a; see also 1951b, 1951c), a physician who can take a larger view of the patient, evaluate the interplay of emotional and organic factors, and manage the treatment accordingly. To this end Ian also published several papers on the basic principles of interviewing and psychotherapy for the general practitioner to use in eliciting information from the patient about emotional factors (e.g., Stevenson, 1952c, 1953, 1954b, 1956; Stevenson & Matthews, 1950[1]), papers which culminated in larger works for professional psychiatrists (Stevenson, 1960/1971, 1969, 1974; Stevenson & Sheppe, 1974).

It may seem that we have come a long way since the 1950s, in that the "holistic" approach to medicine has now become fashionable. In basic respects, however, the changes in medicine have really been only superficial. Psychological factors such as stress may now be accepted as major contributors to disease; but the basic assumption that human personality is a product of the physical organism not only has *not* changed but has, if anything, become even more entrenched and widespread. What has changed is that "psychological" factors have increasingly come to be regarded as states of the brain. The narrowly materialistic view of human personality that so dissatisfied Ian in the 1940s and 1950s remains.[2] But there are other, more serious challenges to this view than the psychosomatic nature of "ordinary" health and disease, and it was to these that Ian increasingly turned his attention after the 1950s. Ian's interest in the phenomena of psychical research, including telepathy, clairvoyance, psychokinesis (mind over matter), and experiences suggesting the survival of human personality after death—called collectively "psi" experiences—stemmed precisely from what they suggest about the power of mind to surpass the body's biological limitations. We will turn to these phenomena in Parts 3 and 4, but here I wish to emphasize Ian's interest in phenomena more closely related to medicine, namely, phenomena in which emotional or other psychological factors seem to have produced unusual and dramatic physical effects, usually on the person's own body, but sometimes even on the body of another person. Examples of the former include wounds such as stigmata and hypnotically produced blisters or analgesia (see, e.g., Stevenson, 1997b, Chapter 2 [reprinted below]; see also Kelly et al., 2007, Chapter 3). Examples of the latter include cases of maternal impression, in which a pregnant woman sees a person with an unusual birthmark, wound, or other disfigurement, and her child is subsequently born with a similar disfigurement (see, e.g., Stevenson, 1992 [reprinted in Part 4], 1997b, Chapter 3, [reprinted below]; see also Kelly et al., 2007, Chapter 3).

Phenomena such as these, from the most common and simple to the most rare and dramatic of psychosomatic effects—defined by Ian as "physical changes [that] accompany emotion" (1961, p. 12)—convinced him that a view of the relationship of mind and body radically different from the prevailing physicalist one is needed. He declined for the most part to enter into philosophical debates about the mind-body problem, preferring to keep his focus on the empirical phenomena that he thought must inform those debates. Nonetheless, he did on occasion express views that suggest his sympathy with a "filter" model of mind. Some psychologists and philosophers have recognized that the undeniable correlation of mind and brain does not entail the view that the brain *causes* consciousness. An alternative view is that the brain restricts, limits, or filters consciousness in accordance with evolutionary demands, a view of the brain's function that James called "transmissive" or "permissive", rather than "productive" (James, 1898/1900, p. 15).[3] Similarly, Ian suggested that "our bodies may act for our minds as a corset acts for some bodies. Removal of the corset allows the body to expand—but the body remains what it was, even though it has changed scope" (1980, p. 414).

Moreover, Ian firmly took the position that this broader perspective on the mind/body problem supports the view that the physical body is a temporary vehicle for mind, or human personality, and that the latter may find a new vehicle when the former dies. Rather than refer to this hypothetical vehicle in one of the many existing but vexed terms, such as "astral," "subtle," or "spiritual" body, that come from a variety of religious or occult traditions, Ian proposed calling it the "psychophore." The word means simply "soul-bearing" and is meant to convey only the idea that the new vehicle, whatever it is, carries at least some memories, behavioral characteristics, and physical features of the person (1987/2001, p. 234; 1997a, ii:2083–2092). Because "a disembodied existence is difficult to conceive, and for me the task has proven close to impossible," Ian insisted that the psychophore "must be made of some substance." This substance might take the form of a kind of field, but this field, like those proposed in biology and embryology, "seem[s] to require some feature not included in our present concepts of matter" (1997a, ii:2083, 2086).

This larger view of human personality, as something that interacts with but is neither identical with nor wholly dependent on the biological body, provided Ian with an avenue to understanding the problem that he called the "leitmotif" of his career—namely, the source of individual differences, both in character and in susceptibility to particular diseases. The view that the physical body is simply a temporary vehicle for mind suggests that those differences are not simply the result of "chance" combinations of genes or environmental influences, but that the person had earlier (premortem) experiences that contributed to producing those differences. In the rest of part 2, I have included selections in which Ian described his views on medicine, the influence of mind on body, and the relationship of mind and brain.

NOTES

1. In his 1952 book *A Manual for Psychiatric Case Study* the psychiatrist Karl Menninger referred frequently to this paper, and in a copy of the book that he sent to Ian, he wrote an inscription in which he thanked Ian, among other things, for "an expressed attitude of *feeling* for the patient which I would like all my residents to acquire."

2. As late as the mid-1980s, Ian published two papers arguing that medicine is still dominated by "the almost unchallenged concept that most doctors today have" of humans as biological machines and medicine as a technology for fixing those machines (Stevenson, 1984, 1985 [excerpts reprinted below]). These papers were written as a consequence not only of Ian's professional observations, but of his personal observations as he and his first wife went through her long and difficult final illness.

3. Others who have argued for a similar view are Bergson (1913), Broad (1953), Burt (1968, pp. 58–59), Huxley (1954/1990, p. 23), and Schiller (1891/1894, pp. 293–295). See also Kelly et al. (2007, pp. 28–29, 72–73, 603–607).

REFERENCES

Bergson, H. (1913). Presidential address. (H. W. Carr, Trans.). *Proceedings of the Society for Psychical Research, 27*, 157–175.

Broad, C. D. (1953). *Religion, Philosophy and Psychical Research*. New York: Harcourt, Brace.

Burt, C. (1968). *Psychology and Psychical Research*. London: Society for Psychical Research.

Graham, D. T., & Stevenson, I. (1963). Disease as response to life stress. I. The nature of the evidence. In H. I. Lief, V. F. Lief, & N. R. Lief (Eds.), *The Psychological Basis of Medical Practice* (pp. 115–136). New York: Harper & Row.

Huxley, A. (1990). *The Doors of Perception*. In A. Huxley, *The Doors of Perception and Heaven and Hell* (pp. 7–79). New York: Perennial Library. (Original work published 1954)

James, W. (1900). *Human Immortality: Two Supposed Objections to the Doctrine* (2nd ed.). Boston & New York: Houghton, Mifflin. (Original work published 1898)

Kelly, E. F., Kelly, E. W., Crabtree, A., Gauld, A., Grosso, M., & Greyson, B. (2007). *Irreducible Mind: Toward a Psychology for the 21st Century*. Lanham, MD: Rowman & Littlefield.

Schiller, F. C. S. (1894). *Riddles of the Sphinx: A Study in the Philosophy of Evolution* (2nd ed.). London: Swan Sonnenschein; New York: Macmillan. (Original work published 1891)

Stevenson, I. (1951a). Guest editorial: A new day for the general practitioner. *G.P., 4*(2), 29–31.

Stevenson, I. (1951b). Evaluating psychosomatic disorders. *G.P., 4*(5), 1–5.

Stevenson, I. (1951c). Analyzing psychosomatic relationships. *G.P., 4*(6), 6–16.

Stevenson, I. (1952a). Illness from the inside. *Harper's Magazine, 204*, 61–67.

Stevenson, I. (1952b). Observations on illness from the inside (bronchiectasis). In M. Pinner & B. F. Miller (Eds.), *When Doctors Are Patients* (pp. 223–235). New York: W. W. Norton.

Stevenson, I. (1952c). Psychotherapy: How to begin. *G.P., 6*(6), 57–63.

Stevenson, I. (1953). Psychotherapy: How to guide interviews. *G.P., 7*(1), 69–79.

Stevenson, I. (1954a). The diagnosis of cardiac disturbances of emotional origin. *Medical Clinics of North America, 38*, 1535–1545.

Stevenson, I. (1954b). Management of common psychiatric problems. *G.P., 9*(1), 69–75.

Stevenson, I. (1956). Psychotherapy by the general practitioner. *Journal of the Louisiana State Medical Society, 108*, 129–134.

Stevenson, I. (1961). A western view of karma. *Vedanta and the West, 147*, 11–22.

Stevenson, I. (1969). *The Psychiatric Examination*. Boston: Little, Brown & Co.

Stevenson, I. (1971). *The Diagnostic Interview* (2nd ed.). New York: Harper & Row. (Original work published in 1960 as *Medical History-Taking*. New York: Paul B. Hoeber)

Stevenson, I. (1974). The psychiatric interview. In S. Arieti (Ed.), *American Handbook of Psychiatry* (2nd ed., Vol. 1, pp. 1138–1156). New York: Basic Books.

Stevenson, I. (1980). The possible nature of post-mortem states: A discussion. *Journal of the American Society for Psychical Research, 74*, 413–418.

Stevenson, I. (1984). On preserving the healing power of hope. *Pharos, 47*, 20–22.

Stevenson, I. (1985). The end of patient abuse in medical care. *Virginia Quarterly Review, 61*, 565–583.

Stevenson, I. (1997a). *Reincarnation and Biology: A Contribution to the Etiology of Birthmarks and Birth Defects* (2 Vols.). Westport, CT: Praeger.

Stevenson, I. (1997b). *Where Reincarnation and Biology Intersect*. Westport, CT: Praeger.

Stevenson, I., & Matthews, R. A. (1950). The art of interviewing. *G.P., 2*(4), 59–69.

Stevenson, I., & Sheppe, W. M., Jr. (1974). The psychiatric examination. In S. Arieti (Ed.), *American Handbook of Psychiatry* (2nd ed., Vol. 1, pp. 1157–1180). New York: Basic Books.

FOUR

Why Medicine Is Not a Science

1949[1]

Most of us are probably under the impression that the medical profession has arrived at a zenith of scientific achievement, from which it will go on from triumph to triumph. But medicine suffers today from a defect which, unless remedied, may halt its future progress.

The defect is that medicine is not now a science, in the sense in which mathematics, chemistry, and physics are sciences. What makes a science is not the collection of facts, but the organization and generalization of those facts and the formulation and understanding of the general laws which govern them. As President Conant of Harvard has pointed out, the great advances in science have come, not from the collection of new data, but from the development of new concepts. Chemistry, for example, gained more impetus from Dalton's atomic theory than Priestley's discovery of oxygen. The discovery of the periodic table by Mendelyeev enabled him not only to organize the available knowledge of the elements, but to predict the behavior and even the existence of others; it freed him from servitude to a host of isolated and apparently unrelated facts. Medicine will not achieve the stature of a science until the basic laws of health and disease have been disclosed. But the search for these laws has hardly begun. No discipline can claim a greater array of equipment by which its research is carried on, yet none is inferior to medicine in organizing its knowledge into coherent principles.

That there do exist underlying principles of medicine, if only we could discover and formulate them, has been a haunting thought with great physicians for centuries. Among the Greeks it was particularly common, and the greatest of Greek physicians, Hippocrates, wrote that "in order to cure the human body it is necessary to have a knowledge of the whole of things." Jerome Cardan, the leading Italian physician of the sixteenth century, wrote that he had discovered "how from a comparison of cures of one member and another, some understanding of the causes of disease and methods of treatment may be deduced." And only twenty-five years ago one of the greatest of modern physicians, Sir James Mackenzie, returned to the same theme.

> For the intelligent practice of medicine [wrote Mackenzie] and the understanding of disease, the simplification of medicine is necessary. . . . I hold that the phenomena which are at present so difficult of comprehension, on account of their number and diversity, are all produced in a few simple ways, and that with their recognition what is now so complex and difficult will become simplified and easy to understand. This means a recognition of principles and a knowledge of their application.

Yet what is the situation in medicine today? Each bodily system—if not each individual disease—is handled by specialists ignorant of other fields. The leading textbooks of our time are mere catalogues of disease states; they rarely offer a generalizing statement which might enable a student to apply the experience he has gained in one disease to the management of other diseases. Even such a standard modern textbook as Osler's *Principles and Practice of Medicine* is essentially an inventory of diseases neatly arranged and classified with the skill of a nurseryman's catalogue. More understanding of the general principles of medicine was shown in the works of Hippocrates written two thousand years ago. Teachers of medicine, almost without exception, are innocent of any hint that their subjects might be amenable to broad principles. At medical meetings and among medical editors the presentation of papers dealing with medical theory is frankly discouraged, and hypotheses are often rejected as "unscientific speculation."

If the principles of medicine are today unknown, or known to only a slight extent, this is a direct result of the fact that they are no longer sought. Medicine, in short, has succumbed to the twentieth-century habit of concentrating upon techniques rather than upon the quest for understanding; of thinking that when phenomena have been described they have been explained.

This defect tends to be self-perpetuating for the amount of medical knowledge that has been accumulated is so vast as to be far beyond the capacity of any one man to grasp and use. Each year two large and closely-printed volumes of the *Quarterly Cumulative Index Medicus* display to the alarmed and ignorant physician the titles alone of medical books and articles published throughout the world. Only the exceptionally talented and indefatigable specialist can "keep abreast of the times" even in his own field, to say nothing of doing any reflective thinking about the facts he has consumed, or of obtaining knowledge of what is happening in other fields. The judgment of Sir Charles Singer, the English medical historian, is apt: "If from the facts no laws emerge, the facts themselves become an obstacle, not an aid, to scientific advance."

Most of this vast and unmanageable array of facts has been produced, not through the development of medicine itself, but through the application to medicine of physics and chemistry. Furthermore, most of it has been produced by means of laboratory experiments, many of them upon animals. These experiments have helped physicians to glimpse the intermediate pathways of disease, but have thrown little light upon the true nature of disease. The pancreas of a dog is removed; the dog thereupon shows symptoms much like those of *diabetes mellitus*; and that fact leads to the isolation of the pancreatic hormone, insulin, which can thereupon be used to control diabetes. Certainly a great discovery; yet few diabetics develop diabetes as a result of having their pancreas removed; and though we are now able to control the disease with considerable effectiveness, we cannot claim to be much closer to understanding the cause of it than we were fifty years ago.

Hundreds of other examples could be cited of laboratory experiments which have taught us much about the intermediate mechanisms of the morbid process, but almost nothing about its primary cause. For whenever man, by experimenting, interferes with nature, he removes himself from nature, whose own experiments are delicate and prolonged, revealing themselves only to the most patient observer. It is only by observing the experiments of nature that we shall learn the secrets of biological life—its success in health and its failure in disease and death. "Man who is the servant of nature," wrote Bacon, "can act and understand no further than he has observed, either in operation or contemplation, of the method and order of nature."

Not only have we fallen victim to the fallacies involved in artificial experimentation; we have also become so entranced with technical procedures that we have lost sight of the patient himself, the individual person who is subjected to so many of these laboratory tests. He becomes a "case" of a certain disease. We say that we have seen so many "cases" of pneumonia, forgetting that we have merely seen so many superficially similar, but profoundly different, febrile pulmonary reactions in as many different persons. We have come to consider disease not as "life in altered form," but as a mysterious parasitic entity growing on man like mistletoe on an oak. It is fashionable to smile at the seventeenth-century physician who might record in his account book that he had "seen Peter's wife who lay abed of a fever." We are proud that we have broken down the term "fever" into a great number of entities and can distinguish readily between scarlet fever and typhoid fever. Yet we have well nigh lost sight of the most important item in the seventeenth-century physician's diagnosis, which was "Peter's wife." We have forgotten that the actual number of differential diagnoses is no less than the number of people upon this planet.

Thus we have neglected both the similarities among different disease states and the differences among patients with apparently similar diseases. This is because modern medicine, particularly in its research phases, is almost wholly in the hands of specialists, each treating or investigating one organ or system of organs, and necessarily neglecting the others. One may make great progress in studying the liver by restricting one's attention to that organ alone. But in the human body the liver is not alone; and it cannot be studied completely without knowing about the forces which act upon it from other parts of the body. A study of the liver alone eventually becomes no study of the liver at all. Nor is this the only trouble with such specialization. It overlooks also the fact that the person as a whole is something different from a collection of viscera; the wholeness gives some extra, if indefinable, quality to the individual organs. Today we pay for our knowledge of the parts in ignorance of the whole.

By this approach, specialism perpetuates itself in medicine. We have different doctors for asthma, diabetes, cancer, and brain tumors because the knowledge of the specialist in one of these diseases has no bearing on another. Had we a grasp of underlying principles in medicine a physician would feel equally at ease with any of these conditions. Yet the specialist studying one organ or one disease is unable to liberate himself by the detection of principles common to all organs and all diseases. Specialism is a necessary evil of modern medicine but is not a necessary accompaniment of the good medicine of the future.

How can we return to a study of the patient as a whole? In the first place, our knowledge of patients must be greatly extended in depth. The physician must know them and their environment hardly less thoroughly than he knows himself and his family. Attempts to do this are frequently discouraged as too time-consuming, but for the student of biological medicine they are essential.

Our study must also be prolonged. Physicians of a former generation were able to follow their patients for twenty or thirty years, and in rural areas this is still possible. But in the cities it is more unusual; and in the large urban clinics where medical research is mostly conducted today, patients are rarely followed by one physician for more than a few months or a year. A patient may come back later to the same hospital, but even then he will probably be seen by different specialists in different clinics, and his identity will be dissolved in a large "series" of similar cases.

There are three states of ill health. The first is a functional impairment or misuse which is often impossible to detect and may not be noticed by the patient or his physician; the second brings definite symptoms of illness; the third brings structural changes. At present, patients are rarely seen before the second stage has been reached; more often, not before the third stage. To try to learn about an ailment under such circumstances is something like trying to learn about chess by watching only the last moves of a game between two experts, unaware that the outcome is frequently decided in the first moves.

Only if individual physicians can study individual patients over a long period of time, and through all the gradations from health to death, observing carefully the similarities between different disease states and also the dissimilarities between different "cases" of the same disease, will we stand a chance of discovering the laws of medicine.

Two British experiments point the way. At the zenith of his career as a consulting cardiologist, Sir James Mackenzie gave up his London practice, went to the small university town of St. Andrews in Scotland, and founded an institute for clinical research. He deliberately chose a small town with a relatively stable population, for he wanted to make a long-term study of disease from its beginnings. When Mackenzie died the project withered without his inspiration, but it had already proved the worth of his ideas.

The other British enterprise is the Peckham Experiment,[2] a large health center in London which provides facilities for many kinds of sport and recreation. The only stipulations of membership are that entire families join and that every member must submit to annual health examinations. The medical observers have plentiful chances to watch the members under everyday conditions.

The success of these and similar studies lies in the fact, common to all, that they have brought the observers to the people and have not awaited the arrival of the latter at large hospitals. Since the large medical centers are manifestly unsuited for such a study by outlook and location, opportunities for its development must be sought elsewhere. It may be that this research can be accomplished only by the one person who sees his patients in their natural habitat, the general practitioner. "People who have spent their lives observing nature," said Aristotle, "are best qualified to make hypotheses as to the principles that bring great numbers of facts together."

But if I point to the general practitioner as the key to our problem, I do not mean the general practitioner as we have usually known him. The public today tends to regard him as the admirable menial of the profession, the genial and beloved drudge who may be roused in the middle of the night to allay some trivial anxiety but is hardly to be trusted with a serious disease. And it is true that he seldom has a chance to be very useful in the study of disease. For even if he has the inclination for research—which in many cases he lacks—he has neither the time nor the money for it. And he is likely to be out of touch with the university centers of research and training. Some way must be found to combine the general practitioner's breadth of experience with the facilities and influence of the medical schools.

Why not a system of fellowships and subsidies to enable young physicians to establish themselves in small towns, with sufficient means to combine medical practice with a far more thorough study of their patients than is now possible? Groups of such doctors could in time take over the entire medical practice in certain communities. They should also have appointments on the staffs of neighboring medical schools, in order to keep these schools in touch with the general problems of ill health.

Such an experiment would take time. Meanwhile is it too much to hope that our medical schools and medical journals might awake to the need for actively encouraging inductive thought about medicine, and the search for hypotheses? Indeed there is need for a new medical journal dedicated not to the competitive publication of isolated chips of information, but to the broad understanding of disease.

Furthermore, the training required of physicians must be broadened and liberalized. In the past thirty years it has become more and more technical, though not necessarily more scientific. Studies which might humanize the students are jostled aside to make room for courses so restricted in content as to make him, frequently, a sort of scientific barbarian, unaware of the truth of Professor Clark Kennedy's dictum: "In medicine we are bound to deal with human life and experience as a whole, and half the art of medicine is to adopt a reasonable and practical attitude to the unknown."

In ancient Greece the doctor was primarily a philosopher and secondarily a physician. He was first a student of nature, and secondly a student of nature perverted by disease. Despite the great technical advances of our day, the future of medicine may well depend upon the training of physicians who will be once more humanists and biologists, as well as chemists and physicists.

NOTES

1. Reprinted from *Harper's Magazine*, April 1949.—Ed.
2. Described by Mary Palmer in *Harper's*, May 1947.

FIVE

The End of Patient Abuse in Medical Care

1985[1]

If you were to take your automobile to a garage for an adjustment of the carburetor and have it returned with the carburetor working better but with heavy stains on the upholstery, several new dents in the body, and the paint badly marred, you would, I think, be vexed. If you then grumbled about these damages to the garage manager, and he said that was what you should expect when you have your carburetor fixed, your annoyance might well get out of control. Yet something comparable to this can happen to many patients admitted to hospitals today. People have come to tolerate mishandling of themselves in hospitals that they would not allow to happen to their cars in a garage. A patient admitted to a hospital—especially a university or a teaching one—may undergo a variety of extremely noxious experiences; no single one of these may be grave in itself, but taken together—as they must be—they often amount to a serious personal injury. We are gradually learning to check child abuse and wife-beating; now we are also beginning to check neglect and mistreatment in hospitals, the extreme forms of which may fairly be described as patient abuse. . . .

Here I should introduce the distinction now commonly used in medicine between "curing" and "caring." In the 16th century the great French physician Ambroise Paré said (of a soldier): "I dressed his wounds; God healed him." Until as recently as one or two generations ago, Paré's epigram summarized the little that doctors could contribute by drugs and surgery toward a patient's recovery from most illnesses. They could relieve pain and modify the symptoms of some illnesses, but when a patient recovered he could nearly always attribute this to his own natural processes of healing instead of to the drugs or other visible treatments of his doctor. The curing side of medicine was negligible, its caring side almost everything. Now this has changed. Medicine has made important advances in the understanding of disease during the past two generations; and, although we still do not have cures for many diseases, we have developed measures for stabilizing and arresting some of them, so that patients who would formerly have died can now usually continue to live, often productively and happily. With other diseases, however, the technological advances have been far from satisfactory. The life that they sustain may be so miserable as to be not worth living. With more than a few diseases we can say without exaggerating that modern technological devices do not prolong life so much as they prolong dying. Meanwhile, our population is growing older, and old people are particularly liable to the multiple small disorders that can be patched up but rarely fully healed. An increasing number of patients cannot be cured but do need continuing care. Unfortunately, while we have been improving the curing side of medicine, we have been neglecting its caring side. Indeed, a patient needing only care is in some respects worse off today than one was with a similar illness 50 years ago. How can this be true?

In the first place, a patient today is not nearly so likely to have a doctor as was one 50 years ago. This may seem strange to say when hospitals swarm with doctors and patients can expect to see ten or more of them within the first three days of a hospital stay. I am not talking about all these doctors; I am referring to one single doctor who assumes overall responsibility for the coordination of what all the others do or recommend; a doctor, moreover, who continues to exercise that responsibility whether the patient is in the hospital, staying in his home, or back at his work. Nearly every elderly patient, and many younger patients with serious illnesses, have disorders in several organs. In much of current medicine, different doctors handle each of these organs, and most of them have or show no interest in any of the others. What is worse, in hospital care each of them has usually only a transient position in the patient's treatment. After a few days, or at most a few weeks, the doctors assigned to one group of patients are "rotated" to other patients; or (less frequently) they go off for weekends or on vacations. Other doctors succeed them only to be replaced, in their turn, a few weeks later by other new doctors. Still other doctors take over when the patient leaves the hospital. A patient whose course I followed closely had contact—on a modest reckoning—with more than one hundred different doctors during a ten-month period of illness. . . .

I now come to the aspect of hospital practice that I consider most baneful. I said earlier that up until as recently as one or two generations ago doctors could claim almost no credit for the drugs or other visible treatments that they could offer their patients. In saying this, however, I did not mean that doctors had no effect on the course of an illness. On the contrary, they often profoundly influenced the outcome of one. This influence, however, came from their conveyance of faith, hope, and love to the patient. These are powerful healing forces, and we are only now beginning to learn just how powerful they are.

One evidence of the healing effect of these positive emotions comes from studies of the markedly increased incidence of illness and mortality among widows and widowers during the first year or two after they have lost a spouse. The increased ill-health of those in a state of bereavement probably has several causes. For example, after the death of a partner, they may eat less nutritious food and otherwise neglect themselves. It seems likely, however, that the main factor in their increased susceptibility to illness comes from the survivor of a good marriage no longer having the opportunity to give and receive love in an intimate relationship. Numerous observations—both in the laboratory and in everyday life—show that negative emotions, such as fear and anger, adversely affect the functioning of our bodies. It follows that maintenance of the positive emotions, such as love and hope, helps to sustain and improve our health; and widows and widowers are, for a time, without these healing forces.

Studies of the pharmacologically inert tablets or capsules known as placebos have given us further information about the healing effect of faith, hope, and love. A placebo has no chemical activity on the body; its effect depends entirely on the patient's belief that he has been given an effective remedy. Placebos frequently produce startling improvements in patients. These are often substantial enough to have forced off the market drugs of marginal value that could not produce in competition a benefit equal to that evoked by the suggestive effect of a placebo. Unfortunately, many members of the medical professions have interpreted the effects of placebos to discredit patients. They say that if a patient responds to a placebo this proves that he needs less pharmacologically active medication than he thought he needed. They fail to see that what it really shows is that patients need less medication when we give them faith, hope, and love. This brings me back to the role the doctor had in former times—one that he will resume in the improved medical climate of the future.

The effect of a placebo is not automatic; it depends on the person who gives it to the patient and on the trust the patient has in this person. The stronger the bond of trust between the giver and receiver the greater the effect. Strong emotional links, however, can only develop with time. We are not born, it seems, with automatic trust of other people; if anything, we may have an innate distrust of them until they have gained our confidence. The doctor of former times usually had this confidence. He had earned it by knowing a patient throughout many years and by staying with him when he was ill for many hours at a time. . . .

My contentions may receive more support by comparing the results of treating patients with the same diseases in a hospital and in their homes. It is not easy to be sure that the groups in such comparisons are otherwise similar and properly matched. Nevertheless, two studies of this type give cause for concern, if not alarm. One investigation compared treatment at home and in the hospital for patients suffering [from] severe kidney disease requiring dialysis; the other compared patients who had had heart attacks. In both studies the patients treated at home did as well as those admitted to the hospital. In comparisons of this type the hospital has the great advantage of equipment and staff that are not available in a home; this being so, any adverse change in the patient's condition can be more quickly detected and remedied in a hospital than in a home. It follows, therefore, that the hospital—in these comparisons—must have had some harmful effect that canceled the advantage it had in technological facilities. . . .

[One source of the present conditions of medical care in hospitals] derives from the almost unchallenged concept that most doctors today have of the nature of man and his diseases. This is that human beings consist only of their physical bodies; these are machines, and when they become diseased they need to be repaired like other machines. I deliberately opened this essay with the metaphor of an automobile needing repair because the concept of the human body as a machine dominates modern medicine, and the automobile is our most familiar machine. The analogy has its merits; the human body has numerous organs just as an automobile has different parts. Some mechanics know more about transmissions than others, who, in turn, know more about cylinders; similarly, some doctors know more about hearts, others more about kidneys. Nor is the analogy of a human body to a machine without some value in treatment. If you can get a stone out of the urinary tract, the urine will again flow just as water will flow again through a drain that was blocked and then unstuck. Nevertheless, you can quickly reach the limit of usefulness of this analogy, for two reasons. First, automobiles and other machines have no reparative processes of their own that a mechanic's efforts can help or hinder; and second, they have no central self that provides control and coordination for the different parts as our brains do for the different organs of our bodies. A doctor adopting a purely mechanical approach to medicine can fail to help a patient use his natural healing processes; indeed, he can seriously interfere with these. The theme of this essay is that much of what patients experience in hospitals can have such an adverse effect and thus works against both the patient's self-healing and the intended effects of a doctor's treatment.

Some of my colleagues may think that I and the increasing number of doctors who share my concern about these matters are a new type of Luddite wanting to discard the technological advances of modern medicine. That is far from being my stance. I think we can have a medicine that is both technologically advanced and attentive to the needs of the individual patient as a person. These two aspects of medicine need not be rivalrous. They only seem so to a generation of hospital staffs that has become overawed by the technical side of medicine.

NOTE

1. Excerpts from paper originally published in *The Virginia Quarterly Review, 61,* 565–583, 1985.—Ed.

SIX

Psychosomatic Medicine Part I: What We Know about Illness and the Emotions

1954[1]

Both a teacher of medicine and a psychiatrist, Dr. Stevenson explores the ways in which the mind can damage the body—or help to heal it.

I wish the word psychosomatic had never been invented. It has aroused new interest in an old subject, but at the same time—as so many words do—it has blocked the growth of wider concepts. A belief has spread that the psychosomatic disorders form a special kind of illness—that a disease either is psychosomatic or it is not. But the psychological element is universal in illness and must be considered in every patient.

The knowledge that mind and body interact is scarcely new. Some twenty-five hundred years ago Aristotle observed that "The soul is the essence of the whole living body." That truth is undergoing a new examination and elaboration today—but though we have advanced considerably in our knowledge of both body and mind, we know no more of how they actually interact than Aristotle did.

Many authorities even doubt the independent existence of the mind and soul. They use the word "mind" only to refer to the collective functions of the brain. Much evidence supports this plausible view. Certainly the mind expresses itself through the brain, and disturbances of the brain disturb the functions of the mind. Anyone can prove this to himself with an ounce or two of whisky. These facts, however, do not prove the identity of mind and brain, or prove that the brain secretes thoughts the way the liver secretes bile. When we squeeze a sponge, water runs out, but this does not make water a product of the sponge. Our current knowledge of the brain does not account for all the known attributes of the mind. Moreover, if we accept the possibility of telepathy—for which increasing evidence is accumulating—then we must acknowledge that the mind can sometimes express itself independently of the known functions of the brain. To express a personal bias, I do not believe science has heard the last of the mind or the soul.

We must acknowledge, too, that the influence of the mind on health has been known for centuries. Able physicians of Greece, Rome, and the medieval Arab world exploited this knowledge skillfully. So have many of their successors. As a minor hobby, I enjoy collecting passages from writers of former ages illustrating knowledge of what we now call psychosomatic medicine. In my note books, for example, I have this from Martin Luther: "Heavy thoughts bring on physical maladies; when the soul is oppressed, so is the body."

And this from John Wesley's Journal:

> Reflecting today on the case of a poor woman who had continual pain in her stomach, I could not but remark the inexcusable negligence of most physicians in cases of this nature. They prescribe drug upon drug, without knowing a jot of the matter concerning the root of the disorder. Whence came this woman's pain? (which she would never have told, had she never been questioned about it)—from fretting for the death of her son. And what availed medicine, while that fretting continued?

. . . A good many people of other generations would have thought our new-found wisdom in this area rather commonplace.

WHAT EMOTION DOES TO THE BODY

. . . An emotion is a private feeling which reflects an attitude toward something in the environment. But emotions also modify our physical states, as if to prepare us for coping physically with that something. For example, when we are afraid, our bodies act as if we were going to run away, even though we have no such intention. The lungs breathe rapidly to furnish more oxygen to the blood. The heart pumps more blood to muscles, which tense up as if for a struggle or a flight. And anger, gluttony, lust, grief, and all the other emotions cause other appropriate changes in the body. Or, rather, the changes would be appropriate if we followed our impulses and turned thoughts into action. This actually happens probably less than once in a thousand times. So much of the rest of the time we live in a state somewhat resembling that of a ship tied up at a dock with steam up and propellers racing. In the human body, the physical changes associated with emotional disturbance lead first to poor function and then—if the stress continues—to structural damage of the tissues.

This does not happen to everyone. Our poor ability to concentrate saves most of us. Our thoughts wander here and there, and happily our emotions go with them. First a passing grief knots the intestines; and then, before colitis starts, some new annoyance pours acid into the stomach. But before the acid eats out an ulcer there, a new joy quiets all organs for a time. We do not usually remain preoccupied with any of our problems for long enough to damage or kill ourselves. But sometimes we do, and then the psychosomatic disorders follow.

One of the significant achievements of our generation has been the detailed study and accurate measurement of the physical changes which occur during emotional disturbances. Some of the most extensive contributions to this study have come from Dr. Harold G. Wolff and his colleagues at Cornell University Medical College, but other groups of workers, too numerous to cite, have contributed no less. Although this work has discovered nothing fundamentally new, it has established a firm relationship between specific emotions and physical changes. It has, in other words, quantified the relationship.

A great many physicians have somewhat vaguely known of a connection between emotions, thoughts, and physical health. But since they lacked positive evidence, or perhaps had only a few isolated personal observations, they could—if they wished—dismiss the subject from their minds. The careful, quantitative work of such men as Dr. Wolff and his associates now forbids any physician to ignore the subject, unless he wishes to incur the epithet "unscientific." . . .

CREATING ILLNESSES

This by no means completes the list of ways in which mental functions influence the body. Some persons have, by training or talent, achieved remarkable skill in influencing the body by thoughts. The performances of Hindu Yoga, for instance, deserve more attention than they have received. We have well authenticated accounts of such feats as rendering the body insensitive to pain, slowing the heart almost to a standstill, and achieving a state amounting to suspended animation.

Some of the feats of Hindu yogis can be duplicated in the state of hypnotism and a few by simple training. Many are repeated involuntarily by a special group of afflicted people called hysterics. These people have an aptitude for the translating of ideas into physical changes. An hysteric believes that her arm is paralyzed, and so it becomes. Such ideas often seize the mind and hold on with the tenacity of a barnacle. Hysteria is a malady chiefly of the uneducated and the uncritical, for hysterics are notoriously simple, suggestible folk. Other people are protected from believing that their limbs are paralyzed—or from other such beliefs—by the learning, which tells them that it just cannot be so without some organic disease of brain or limb. The hysteric, innocent of such learning, knows that it can be so. And it is.

The limbs and skeletal musculature are the chief sites of hysterical phenomena. But ideas about the body also influence the functioning of internal organs. For example, there is the extraordinary, but not really uncommon illness called pseudocyesis, which is medical neo-Hellenic for "false pregnancy." The patient—whether through fear of pregnancy or a wish for it—believes herself to be pregnant. She ceases menstruating, her abdomen enlarges (although her uterus does not), and her breasts undergo changes similar to those of pregnant women. The hormones of the pituitary glands and ovaries of such patients show changes which closely resemble in kind, but not in degree, the hormonal changes in women who are really pregnant. Unless the pseudo-mother can be persuaded to surrender belief in her pregnancy, this serio-comic physical fantasy may be culminated after nine months by efforts to deliver an imaginary baby.

Let no man laugh at this strange disorder, for men, too, sometimes imagine themselves pregnant and suffer from vomiting and labor pains, which is, to say the least, even more bizarre.

Other equally striking connections between ideas and physical function are found in many patients. A few years ago I saw a young man who had great difficulty breathing. A physical examination showed no disease of his heart or lungs which could account for his symptom. His father also had difficulty in breathing, but his father had serious heart trouble. When the patient saw, or even thought of his father's heavy breathing, he himself began to pant imitatively.

Another young man watched over his father carefully during the latter's final illness and death from heart disease. He used to feel his father's pulse solicitously and often noticed a disturbance in the rhythm. Not long after his father's death he sought medical help, complaining of palpitations. His heart-beat was indeed irregular—but the cause appeared to be entirely mental and emotional.

A middle-aged woman complained of an intractable pain in her right chest. Exhaustive examinations failed to uncover any structural disease which could account for her pain. Then it was learned that her son at the time lay dying of cancer. His cancer and his pain were in the right chest. After he died—and she became reconciled—her pain went away.

For reasons which are not relevant here, these patients wished (mostly unconsciously) to be like their respective relatives. But they did not merely imagine their illnesses; more accurately, they first imagined and then created the illnesses; but the symptoms resulted from genuine physical changes.

I do not mean to make too sharp a distinction between hysterics (including the suggestible patients mentioned above) and other people.

Thoughts markedly influence the bodily functions of everyone. I have had the opportunity of recording large variations in the rate and rhythms of the breathing evoked by simple thoughts. One enterprising physician, during a routine inspection of the bronchial tubes of a patient through a bronchoscope, asked the patient a few questions. When he asked how the patient would feel if he were deprived of his pension, the bronchial tubes constricted. When he asked how the patient felt when his party won an important election, the bronchial tubes relaxed and widened broadly. In other words, the patient expressed with his bronchi what he might have said with his lips if he could have spoken.

These examples may sufficiently demonstrate that everyone, to some extent, molds his body by his thoughts. We know that the extent of such molding varies widely among different people; we do not understand why these variations occur, and we hardly understand the mechanism of the molding at all. But we do know that ideas can have an immense influence on the body.

The disorders which have been chiefly studied and labeled psychosomatic—for example asthma, hypertension, peptic ulcer, hay fever, colitis, and others—have episodic courses. Their symptoms come and go like the tides, except that they fluctuate with the emotional state of the patient rather than with the phases of the moon. Their many fluctuations have simplified the study of the relationships between emotions and physical changes in these illnesses.

But emotions are no less important in conditions which pursue a steadier course. Recent work has demonstrated the great significance of emotional factors in heart failure and in diabetes. Indeed there now remains no organ of the body in which physical changes related to emotions have not been proved of major importance. The modern physician—free from doubt over whether or not emotional factors are important in his patients' illnesses—knows now that they are always important to some degree and spends his time discovering in each individual case the magnitude of that degree, and applying treatment accordingly.

NOTE

1. Excerpts from *Harper's Magazine, 209*, 34–37, 1954.—Ed.

SEVEN

Bodily Changes Corresponding to Mental Images in the Person Affected

1997[1]

The bleeding wounds known as stigmata on the hands, feet, chest, and (sometimes) other parts of the body are among the best known and least understood of abnormal bodily changes. Different writers have attributed them all to sanctity, to hysteria, and to malingering (that is, self-inflicted wounding). As generalizations, these opinions are all incorrect. A few instances of persons wounding themselves, usually from zealous identification with Jesus, have been exposed. In the great majority of cases, however, we can confidently exclude artifactual wounding; many of the subjects have been under close surveillance, and in a few cases observers have actually watched stigmata (or at least the bleeding) develop before their eyes.

St. Francis of Assisi was the first notable person to develop stigmata. His wounds came on toward the end of a long period of about 40 days that he spent by himself, during which he was entirely absorbed in contemplating the Passion of Jesus. (His stigmata were also among the most unusual ever observed in that protrusions somewhat in the form of clenched nails were said to have come out of his wounds.) In the seven and a half centuries following St. Francis's death, about 350 cases of stigmatists have been recorded. The stigmatists were nearly all religious persons, such as nuns, and a few were saints; St. Catherine of Siena and St. Gemma Galgani were two of these. St. Catherine of Siena had a vision of Jesus with his wounds and with rays of light running from them to her body. Her stigmata then occurred at the sites of her body where the rays seen coming from Jesus impinged on her.

Until the second half of the 19th century nearly all writers about stigmata believed them to be the result of a special grace bestowed on saints or saintlike persons. The attribution of saintliness thus might be given retrospectively to someone who developed stigmata; whoever had stigmata must be saintly.

In the second half of the 19th century, some early psychologists began to study what we now call psychosomatic relationships and came to view stigmata as illustrating these. They were in the first instance encouraged in this interpretation because nearly all the authenticated cases of stigmata had occurred in women. Women were notoriously more liable than men to develop what was then called hysteria, which was being understood with increasing clarity as a psychosomatic disorder in which beliefs about the body become expressed in changes in bodily functions. (Young women of child-bearing age are more hypnotizable—therefore more suggestible—than men or than women of other ages.) Then it was noted that some stigmatists, although pious in their ways, were far from being saints. Furthermore, the stigmata varied greatly in form, size, appearance, and even location. Nearly all stigmatists showed wounds at the feet, hands, and lower chest. Three stigmatists were credibly reported to have developed marks and deep indentations around the wrists as they relived the scene when Jesus was arrested and bound with ropes; the marks on the stigmatists' wrists seemed to reproduce the marks that binding ropes would make. (I ask readers also to remember these last cases when I describe in later chapters [of *Reincarnation and Biology* and *Where Reincarnation and Biology Intersect*] children who had ropelike birthmarks that informants attributed to ropes binding the previous personalities shortly before they died.) Readers should also note the case described later in this chapter, the ropelike marks of which are shown in Figure 7.1.

The stigmatists' chest wounds showed important variations. Some of them had the chest wound on the left side and some had it on the right. The Bible does not say into which side of Jesus a Roman soldier thrust his spear; and because there was only one spear thrust recorded, right or left may be correct, but both cannot be. Such variations strongly suggested that stigmata were bodily changes produced by the mental images of the stigmatist.

There was other pertinent evidence. Some of the stigmata bore a close relationship to the wounds on the representation—for example, a statuette—of Jesus before which the stigmatist was accustomed to worship. An early 19th-century stigmatist had on her chest a Y-shaped lesion that matched an unusual Y-shaped crucifix in the church where she worshipped. And the biographer of another stigmatist (of the late 19th century) remarked on the close correspondence between the stigmatist's wounds and those on the statuette of Jesus before which this saint worshipped. In the 1920s, a German physician had the good fortune to find a young girl—a Protestant—who easily went into deep hypnosis. This girl (Elisabeth K.) had a high degree of impressionability. She attended a slide show that vividly depicted the sufferings of Jesus as he was led to the cross and crucified. On the following day the girl complained of severe pain in her hands and feet (at the sites of the nails driven into Jesus' limbs). The physician, seizing this opportunity, hypnotized the girl and told her to imagine that nails were being driven deeply into her hands and feet. The next day the girl had open wounds at these places. Subsequently, the physician readily induced in this girl simulacra of Jesus' other wounds, including those of a crown of thorns complete with triangle-shaped lesions, similar to wounds that thorns might make.

None of this newer evidence or revised appraisal of old evidence need detract from the reputation for sanctity that the great majority of stigmatists had and deserved. It does, however, undermine the idea that stigmata are a grace vouchsafed only to the elect. What then is the role of sanctity in the occurrence of stigmata? I suggest that the connection occurs through the concentration of the mind on particular parts of the body. Many saintly persons are almost fully absorbed in the life and death of Jesus and determined to be as much like him as they possibly can. It is difficult for the ordinary person to understand the intense identification with Jesus that some of them have achieved. In doing so, their concentration on his wounds acts to produce similar lesions in themselves. I do not mean to say that concentration is the only factor of importance in the occurrence of stigmata; but before returning to this topic I shall describe some other examples of the effects mental images may have on local bodily functions.

A mother sometimes develops imitative or "sympathetic" pains at the same location as her child has a pain, say from a toothache. Sometimes the imitative effects go beyond pain and include visible changes in the tissues affected. For example, one mother watching her little son at play saw a heavy window sash fall on his hand and crush three of his fingers. She immediately felt severe pain in the same fingers that had been injured in her son; and afterward her fingers became swollen and inflamed so that pus developed in them and had to be evacuated.

Hypnosis is not a state that I wish or need to define. It depends, in the first place, on the replacement of ideas in the mind of the subject with ideas in the mind of the hypnotist. This is what we mean by suggestion. Once the subject accepts the initial ideas of the hypnotist, he or she enters a state of increasing susceptibility to further suggestions offered by the hypnotist. In this way the hypnosis can be "deepened" and the subject also enabled to go into hypnosis more readily at the next occasion. Another important feature of hypnosis is heightened concentration of the mind. Hypnosis also facilitates the links between mental images and bodily functions that the images may influence. It greatly lubricates, so to say, the psychophysiological processes of the body.

We have no understanding at present of the mind's ability to select and influence the right processes in order to carry out a suggestion given during hypnosis. Consider our physical experience when we become thirsty. A dryness of the mouth leads us to describe ourselves as thirsty and needing more fluid. Already, however, the body will have made its own adjustments by reducing the excretion of water in the urine. This entails modifying the release of a certain hormone from the pituitary gland, the one that controls water excretion. Now let a person who is not dehydrated and not thirsty be hypnotized and told that he or she is thirsty. Soon his or her kidneys will diminish the excretion of urine just as they would if he or she had been dehydrated. Somehow the body has picked out the right hormone (or perhaps some other link in the process of urine formation) and implemented a decrease in the excretion of urine.

Hypnosis has been used to modify a wide variety of bodily functions through the offering of appropriate instructions to a hypnotized person. The heart rate can be slowed or speeded up. Bleeding can be stopped and menstruation started at certain times. Breasts can be enlarged. Anesthesia can be induced, including an unusual type of anesthesia known as "glove and stocking anesthesia." This phrase refers to the abrupt line of demarcation at the upper end of the induced anesthesia, a line that does not correspond to the distribution of the nerves serving the arms and legs, but corresponds instead to the idea implanted in the subject's mind. (Glove and stocking anesthesia may also occur spontaneously in persons who give themselves this idea of what an area of anesthesia is like.) There is a rare condition called *oedème bleu* in which an arm becomes swollen, painful, bluish, and of little use. It may follow some relatively minor injury to the arm that concentrates the patient's attention on it. In the 19th century *oedème bleu* was induced and removed with hypnosis.

Between about 1880 and 1930 a large number of experiments were conducted to study the induction of blisters on the skin of hypnotized subjects. To indicate the proposed site for the blister, the hypnotist would sometimes touch the subject at the place with some object, usually a cold one. The subject was told, or led to believe, that he or she was being burned. Many subjects responded with a blister at the indicated site, as if they had been burned. Some of the early experiments were insufficiently rigorous in that the patient was not kept under surveillance, so that he or she might have scratched the indicated site in an effort to comply with the hypnotist's suggestion. Most experiments have avoided this mistake, however, and I believe that the evidence is strong enough to convince all but the most resolute skeptics that the phenomenon is genuine.

Most of the experimenters who induced blisters during hypnosis used a small stimulus of no unusual form—such as the tip of the finger—with which to touch the subject at the site where the blister was to occur. A few, however, applied stimuli in the form of letters of the alphabet (or some other unusual form), and the ensuing marks reproduced the recognizable form of the stimulus.

One experimenter thought that blisters induced during hypnosis might occur only if the subject had previously been burned at the site where blisters were to appear. I do not believe that any evidence supports this assertion as a generalization, although a previous burn at a particular site may facilitate the occurrence of inflammation and blisters suggested at the same site.

The examples I have given of bodily changes induced with hypnosis are largely derived from experimental demonstrations of the range and power of hypnosis. The changes in bodily function during hypnosis that I have mentioned cannot be induced in everyone. For many of the effects demonstrated, we now have other and quicker means of bringing about the results obtained, if we want them. For example, chemical anesthesia is superior to hypnosis for surgical operations.

Hypnosis, however, still has an important role to play in relieving pain. It may also be of great value in some intractable skin diseases. For example, warts have been successfully removed with hypnosis. Moreover, they may be removed from one area at a time, another demonstration of how the mind somehow finds the right part of the body for executing the instructions given. A particularly impressive improvement in a skin disease occurred when a hypnotist successfully treated a patient with intractable ichthyosis ("fish-scale disease"). He treated his patient limb by limb with improvements occurring successively in each limb as it was indicated by the suggestions offered.

The intense revival of memories of some earlier physical trauma may be accompanied by the appearance of wounds that closely resemble the original wounds. (It may be difficult to be precise about the resemblance if no firsthand observer of the original wounds is available to compare them to the later wounds accompanying the revived memories.) In the 1950s, several examples of this phenomenon were published. In one of the most impressive, the subject relived (with the help of ether) an occasion when, being in a hospital and requiring restraint, his arms had been tied with a rope. When the patient relived this experience, deep curved depressions appeared on his lower arms. They were exactly like those that occur on the flesh of a person tied with a rope (Figure 7.1). (I ask readers also to remember this case when I present, later in this work [of *Reincarnation and Biology* and *Where Reincarnation and Biology Intersect*], the cases of persons with birthmarks that informants attributed to marks made by ropes that had tied the previous personality before he or she was killed.) In another published case a patient relived a severe caning inflicted on her by a sadistic father. He had used a carved cane, and the unusual pattern of the carving on the cane appeared on the skin of the patient as she relived being beaten with this cane.

No case of this kind has come under my direct observation. Two psychiatric colleagues of mine, however, sent me written accounts of cases they had observed. In both instances, the patients relived—one with LSD and one with hypnosis—memories of severe beatings. And in both cases, during the reliving, clearly visible marks—actual wheals in one case—appeared at the places where the patients said they had been beaten.

A rare type of physical change corresponding to a mental image sometimes occurs in the experiences of persons in India who come close to death and survive. After regaining consciousness, some of them say that they were mistakenly seized by messengers of the King of the Dead and taken to the "realm of the dead." With discovery of the mistake, they were sent back. Upon recovery, some of these subjects state that they were burned while in the realm of the dead, and they show areas of inflammation or scarring at the sites of the burning. The subject (Durga Jatav) of one of the most bizarre cases of this kind that I have encountered

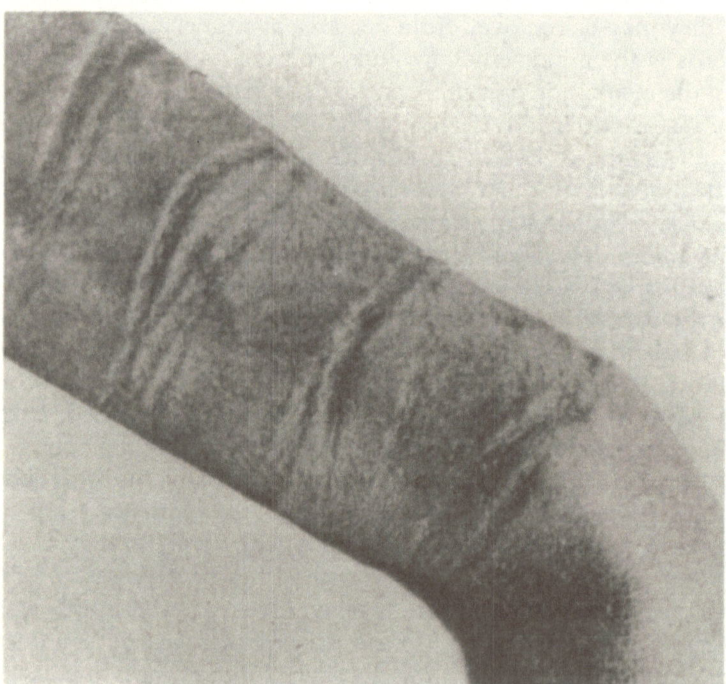

Figure 7.1. Wheals in the form of rope marks that developed after a patient relived an episode in which he had had his arms tied behind his back 9 years earlier. In some of the depressed areas one can notice smaller patterns corresponding to the strands of which the binding rope was made. (Patient of Dr. R. L. Moody.) Reprinted from *The Lancet* (28 December, 1946), Robert L. Moody, "Bodily Changes during Abreaction," 934–935, with permission from Elsevier.

said that he resisted being dragged from life by the messengers of the King of the Dead. He struggled so much that in desperation the messengers cut off his legs at the knees. When the registrar (in the place to which he had been taken) exposed their mistake, they said that he could return; but he then asked to have his legs replaced. Somehow he was refitted with legs and sent back to terrestrial life. He regained consciousness in the bed where his family believed he had died. The remarkable feature of the case was the presence on this man's knees of large scar-like lines closely resembling scars that might occur after horizontal cuts with a knife. We obtained X-ray photographs of the patient's knees, but these showed no abnormality.

I shall now discuss what I consider the common factors underlying most, if not all, of the bodily changes that I have described in this chapter. Violence is the first of these. Readers will have noticed the prominent part that violence and physical injury have played in the spontaneously occurring cases. This is certainly true of stigmatism, in which the subject's attention becomes closely focused on the ordeal of Jesus' crucifixion. Physical injury is also prominent in the cases of the recurrence of wounds with the revival of memories of traumatic beatings or restraint. It also enters into the experiments with blisters induced during hypnosis, in which the subject believes he or she is being burned. Violence and the threat of injury are concentrators of attention. I wish to bring them forward here because of the high frequency of violent death, which I mentioned in Chapter 1 [of *Reincarnation and Biology* and *Where Reincarnation and Biology Intersect*], among the cases with birthmarks and birth defects related to previous lives. Violence is not, however, the only concentrator of attention. Indeed, stigmatists concentrate on Jesus out of love for him and only secondarily become involved in the violence of his death.

At least two other important factors must enter into the production of physical changes corresponding to mental images. One is a factor of impressionability, now often called absorption. Highly impressionable subjects quickly "lose" themselves in a scene viewed or imagined. If someone calls their name, they seem not to hear and do not respond. Many persons would have seen the slide show of Jesus' crucifixion without being affected as was Elisabeth K., who so readily developed stigmata at the site of Jesus' wounds; they lacked her capacity for absorption.

The third factor we must consider is the reactivity of the tissues of the skin. Persons vary widely in the sensitivity of their skins to stimuli. For example, 25% of persons who are firmly stroked on the skin with a blunt instrument will develop a definite flare around the area stroked, and 5% will show a wheal where the stroking instrument passed over the skin; but the rest will show nothing. It is sometimes possible to write letters on the skin (of the back, for example) of the sensitive patients; this condition is called dermographism, and I will describe an example of paranormal dermographism in the next chapter [the next paper reprinted in this section].

Another example of varying reactivity of the skin occurs in the formation of the dense, indurated scars known as keloids. These occur much more often in some persons than in others and more often in some races, such as Africans, than in others.

I do not mean this list of factors to be exhaustive; there may, for example, be subtle differences in the central and autonomic nervous systems that mediate control of the blood vessels of the skin, and these may play an important part in the changes with which we are here concerned.

A formula that might represent the principal factors would be:

$$CA+DI+PF=CS$$

where CA stands for Concentrated Attention or Absorption, DI for Duration of the Imagery, PF for the hypothetical Physiological Factor (or Factors), and CS for the resultant Changes in the Skin. Although this formula looks simple, I intend it to underscore the complexity of the subject and the deficiencies in our understanding of how physical changes corresponding to mental images occur.

I wish to emphasize that many of the physical changes I have described do not correspond to known configurations of nerves or blood vessels of the skin. I already mentioned this discrepancy in connection with glove and stocking anesthesia. It is equally true of the lesions of stigmatists and of blisters induced by hypnotic suggestion. Concerning the last-named phenomenon, some years ago a leading expert on hypnosis carefully reviewed the literature on such experiments and came near to concluding that the phenomenon must be genuine. He pulled himself back, however, because, he wrote, the occurrence of such blisters makes no sense in relation to the known distribution of the nerves and blood vessels of the skin. He is not the first scientist to deny facts discordant with his assumptions, but he does deserve credit for his candor. The term *paranormal* seems to fit phenomena such as stigmata and hypnotically induced physiological changes. It explains nothing, but has the merit of not denying the occurrence of phenomena for which we have as yet no satisfying explanation.

NOTE

1. Chapter 2 of *Where Reincarnation and Biology Intersect*, Ian Stevenson, M.D. Copyright © 1997 by Ian Stevenson. Reproduced with permission of ABC-CLIO, LLC, Santa Barbara, CA. This is a synopsis of a much larger treatment of the subject in Chapter 2 of *Reincarnation and Biology: A Contribution to the Etiology of Birthmarks and Birth Defects*, Westport, CT: Praeger, 1997. In the larger work readers may find references, not included here.—Ed.

EIGHT

Bodily Changes Corresponding to Another Person's Mental Images

1997[1]

In the preceding [paper] I concluded that some paranormal process must occur between the mental images in a person's mind and the production on his or her body of wounds, such as stigmata or blisters induced during hypnosis, the shapes of which have no relationship to the anatomical distribution of the blood vessels or nerves of the skin. Future research may someday show presently undiscovered patterns of nerves and blood vessels that could account for the correspondence between mental images and local bodily changes in the person having the images. Even so, we should still need the word *paranormal* in trying to understand how mental images in one person's mind may affect changes in another person's body. This chapter is about such changes.

The simplest examples occur as variants of what I call telepathic impressions. The word *telepathy* means communication between minds without the known sensory organs. In many instances of telepathy the percipient obtains substantial information, perhaps in the form of a visual representation, about the circumstances of another person, called the target person or agent. (The word *sender*, sometimes used for this person, is not so helpful, because the agent often plays no conscious active role in the communication.) In the variant of telepathy called telepathic impressions, almost no content is conveyed, only an impression that, say, someone known to the percipient needs help. Occasionally, a little more detail may be included, such as that the agent is in a hospital; and sometimes less detail is included. For example, a traveler away from home may feel unexpectedly impelled to turn around and go back because something is "wrong at home"; but the percipient does not know what is wrong there or who needs help. In a variant of the telepathic impression the percipient has a pain (or sometimes another physical symptom) that corresponds to a pain (or other symptom) in the agent. Here are three examples, the first from the 19th century, the second and third from my own investigations. I give more details of these three cases in my book *Telepathic Impressions*.

A woman awakened one morning with the impression of having received a sharp blow on the mouth. Without understanding this she dressed and went down to breakfast. Her husband, who had been out sailing, joined her. She noticed that he kept dabbing at his mouth with a handkerchief and asked him what he was doing. He then explained that while he had been sailing a gust of wind had suddenly come up, and before he could get out of the way the tiller struck him on the mouth, causing his lip to bleed. This had happened at almost the exact time his wife had awakened with the sense of being struck in the mouth.

In a case that I investigated, an American housewife and mother one morning suddenly experienced a sharp pain in her right leg and buttocks. She was startled and, although she was alone, she said "Oh." Somehow she identified her pain with some trouble to one of her children, who were then away at school. When they came home, she asked them whether anything unusual had happened to them at school. Her 10-year-old daughter then said that while she was playing in the school yard, a boy on a bicycle had run into her and hit her on the backside. She had cried "Oh." As nearly as they could tell, the daughter had been hit at the same time that her mother had had her unexpected pain at the same location.

My third example involved twin sisters. One was in Pennsylvania and known to be pregnant; but she was thought to be in good health, and her delivery was not imminent. Her twin sister was in Naples, Italy, with her husband, a physician. The sister in Italy suddenly developed severe pain in her chest and upper abdomen, with shortness of breath. Her husband could find no signs of physical illness to account for these symptoms. They later learned that her sister in Pennsylvania had gone into labor prematurely and had developed serious complications at the time she was having her symptoms. The twin in Pennsylvania suffered from pain in her chest and shortness of breath, apparently due to a clot in a vein that had broken loose and lodged in her lungs (pulmonary embolus).

Cases of this type require careful appraisal of their details. If we are to consider seriously the interpretation of such a case as an instance of telepathic impression, the temporal coincidence between the symptoms of the two participants must be exact or extremely close; the symptoms must be identical or closely similar and in the same organs or regions of the body; and finally, we must be confident that the percipient had no normal means of learning about or inferring the agent's symptoms before his or hers occurred. I believe the three cases I described meet these criteria.

Mediums, who are persons apparently able to communicate with discarnate personalities, occasionally take on the symptoms of a communicator's fatal illness. In one published case of this kind, the medium began to choke and cough as she described the death of a communicator from heart disease. (Patients with what is called congestive heart failure frequently cough.) The medium had no normal knowledge of the communicator's mode of death. In another case, a medium developed symptoms in a knee when she handled a glove that belonged to a young woman who had injured her knee in a bicycle accident and continued to have pain there. The sensitive knew nothing of this accident or symptom.

Olga Kahl, a Russian clairvoyant living in France during the 1920s, provided some of the most impressive evidence of the representation of mental images in one person by bodily changes in another. Before describing the standard experiments involving her, I should mention that she showed extreme impressionability, even as a child and young adult. On one occasion she misplaced a string of pearls; the loss preoccupied her, and while the pearls were missing, she developed round areas of redness on the skin of her arms which suggested the form of the missing pearls. On another occasion, when living in Istanbul, she watched a group of dervishes, one of whom pushed a skewer through his cheek; the next day she developed an abscess of the cheek at the corresponding site where the dervish had pushed the skewer through.

Olga Kahl's experimental routine provided for a visitor or experimenter to write (hidden from her) a name or perhaps a design on a small piece of paper. The visitor rolled the piece of paper into a ball, which he kept in his hand without showing it to Olga Kahl. After a short interval, the name or design would appear on the skin of Olga Kahl's arm (sometimes on her upper chest). The letters would stand out in red, evidently from extremely localized changes in the superficial blood vessels. Sometimes a letter of a name was omitted, but then a space would be left for it, as if at some level Olga Kahl was aware of the entire word. Olga Kahl sometimes facilitated the process of her kind of dermographism by rubbing the part of her body where the letters were to appear; but such rubbing covered the entire area affected, and no one ever observed Olga Kahl in any endeavor to scratch the words on her skin. (In the last chapter I described dermographism, but that of Olga Kahl involved no actual tracing of letters on her skin.)

Some of the leading French and English scientists who studied such phenomena during the 1920s investigated Olga Kahl. All expressed themselves fully satisfied that her dermographism was genuine. I am not asserting that the mental image in the mind of the experimenter (who wrote the word or design on a piece of paper) directly influenced Olga Kahl's skin. Perhaps her mind obtained a copy, so to speak, of the experimenter's mental image and reproduced that on her skin. At times, she seemed to know what the target word was before it appeared on her skin, but at other times she did not.

The most widespread evidence of the effect of one person's mental images on the body of another living person occurs in cases of what are generally called maternal impressions. This is the phrase used to designate the supposed causal connection between some event that shocks or frightens a pregnant woman and a defect in her later-born baby. A typical case—a published one—is that of a pregnant woman who happened to see on the street a man with partly amputated feet. She became distressed and began to fear that her baby would be born with similar defects. In fact, it was; parts of its feet were absent, and the defects in its feet corresponded to the ones on the man its mother had seen.

The reality of maternal impressions is accepted in most parts of the world today. It was accepted without challenge in the West until the early 18th century. Advances in anatomy and physiology then showed that there is no physical connection between a pregnant woman and her gestating baby through the placenta or otherwise that could mediate the expression in the baby of a mental image in the mother-to-be. The skepticism that these observations stimulated spread slowly. In the 19th century and through the first two decades of this one, the leading medical journals of the United States, Great Britain, and Europe published numerous reports of maternal impressions. Occasionally, a dissident voice would draw attention to the fact that some or many women were frightened when pregnant, expected to have a malformed baby, but then delivered a normal one. On the other side, one 19th-century author pointed out that the absence of any nervous or other known connection between the mother and child signified nothing, because of the possibility that "mind does in some mysterious way operate across matter." (This admirable refusal to deny phenomena because we cannot explain them foreshadowed the beginnings in 1882 of the scientific study of paranormal phenomena by more than 30 years.)

In 1890 a pediatrician of the University of Virginia reviewed 90 cases of maternal impressions that had been published between 1853 and 1886. He concluded that in 69 (77%) of the 90 cases there was "quite a close correspondence" between the impression upon the mother and her baby's defect. He, too, was aware of the growing skepticism about such cases and commented that "thinking men came to doubt the truth of those things which they could not understand."

I decided to review the evidence for maternal impressions.[2] In doing this, I read reports of approximately 300 cases in medical journals, books, and other publications of the United States, Great Britain, France, Germany, Italy, Holland, and Belgium. From these I selected 50 cases for a detailed analysis. I chose cases in which the correspondence between the stimulus to the pregnant woman and the baby's defect was close. I also chose cases in which both the stimulus to the mother and the defect were unusual. As an example of the latter I mention the case of a woman whose brother had to have his penis amputated for removal of a cancer. While she was pregnant, her curiosity impelled her to have a look at the site of her brother's amputation; she afterward gave birth to a male baby without a penis. I have obtained figures for the incidence of some birth defects in the general population, and that for congenital absence of the penis is 1 in 30,000,000. Other birth defects figuring in these cases are more common, but most are rare or even extremely rare.

An unexpected finding of my analysis of these cases was the discovery that the seemingly causative stimulus to the mother occurred much more often than would be expected by chance in the 1st trimester than in the 2nd and 3rd ones. It seems likely that pregnant women would be equally liable to be exposed to some frightening stimulus at any month of a pregnancy; this observation therefore suggests that susceptibility of the embryo is one important factor in maternal impressions. The 1st trimester is also the one during which the embryo is most sensitive to noxious drugs, such as thalidomide, and to viral infections, such as rubella (German measles).

Some further useful information emerged from my analysis. In more than half the cases, the woman was closely involved with the wounding of another person—an eyewitness, perhaps—or was wounded herself. These woundings acted as the stimulus for the maternal impression. The duration of the woman's exposure to the stimulus seems to have had little effect on the occurrence of a maternal impression. In at least two cases, a woman's fear did not quite match her curiosity about some wound, so she just peeked for an instant at the wound; but that sufficed. Most of the women became "shocked" or "frightened" by the stimulus. Some forgot about it quickly, others became obsessively preoccupied with it and could not stop thinking about it. Some of the women were afraid their babies would be affected, others were not, and a few were (mistakenly) confident that their babies would be normal. The beliefs of the women concerned about the effect on the baby had almost no predictive value.

I have been able to investigate seven cases of maternal impressions of different types and will summarize two of them here.

The mother of the first subject (Calvin Ewing) was a Tlingit of Alaska named Sylvia Ewing. She was born with a small hole—in medical terms, a sinus—near the inner corner of her right eye. This was immediately recognized as a defect corresponding to a chronic stye at the same place from which a deceased relative had suffered. On the basis of this correspondence, an announcing dream, and some evidence from Sylvia's behavior, she was identified as the reincarnation of this relative. Hers was a straightforward case of the reincarnation type, although a somewhat weak one with regard to the strength of the evidence. (I give a detailed report of her case in *Reincarnation and Biology* [1997].) In childhood, Sylvia suffered a certain amount of discomfort from the sinus, which discharged fluid, especially if she had a cold. She also underwent cruel teasing about the defect from her schoolmates.

In due course Sylvia grew up and married. When she became pregnant, she began to fear that her baby would have a defect like hers. She told me: "I was afraid he would look like me. That is all I thought about—whether he would look like me." Her husband confirmed her statement by saying: "She was always worrying about whether the baby would have a hole in the eye like hers."

After the baby was born and brought to Sylvia, the first place she examined was his eye "to see if he had a hole." He had, and it was at exactly the site of her own—near the inner end of the right eye.

Unlike his mother, this baby boy was not identified as the reincarnation of a deceased relative or of anyone else. There were no identifiable causative factors other than the mother's fear of the reproduction of her defect in her child.

The correspondence between the two defects in this case was exceedingly close both in location and size. . . .[3]

In the second case, a male baby (Sampath Priyasantha) was born in Sri Lanka without any arms and with severely deformed legs.[4] One of my assistants learned about these unusual defects and sent me a photograph of the baby. I decided to investigate the case as soon as I could, but by the time I was able to reach Sampath Priyasantha's village he had died. He had been able to crawl about a little and was just beginning to speak when he died at the age of about 20 months. He had said nothing about a previous life.

The village was somewhat remote, and having taken the trouble to reach it I decided to ask a few questions. From other cases that I had studied—and that I describe later in this book [*Where Reincarnation and Biology Intersect*]—it occurred to me that Sampath might have been the reincarnation of someone known to his family who had died after having his arms badly injured, perhaps in an industrial accident. I therefore asked the baby's father whether he knew of anyone who had died after having his arms injured. "Yes," he replied. "There was a man I killed by cutting off his arms and legs with a sword." He then went on to tell me how this had happened. The murdered man was a young ruffian of the village, a notorious bully, and a member of a family given to violence. (The brother of this man told me that he had personally killed three of the family's enemies; they had lost their father when a bomb that he was preparing dropped from his hands and blew him to pieces.) A quarrel broke out over a dog belonging to the bully's family that had come onto the property of Sampath's father and eaten some food. Sampath's father decided to finish with the offensive young man. Without much difficulty, he and his brother got him drunk and lured him over to their side of the village. They then cut off his arms and legs and left him to die. (I obtained a postmortem report in this case, and, with some discrepancies, it confirmed the murderer's account of what he had done; limbs were described as "dangling," not totally severed.)

The murdered man's mother was enraged at her son's death. She repeatedly cursed the murderer and his family, saying that they would be punished for killing her son by having a defective child. (Informants differed as to exactly what she said in cursing the family, but the baby's mother definitely thought the angry mother had specified that she would have a defective child.)

The murderers were arrested and sentenced to imprisonment. The father could come home sometimes on leave, and his wife had another baby, a normal female. The parents thought they had perhaps neutralized the curse. Then the dreadfully malformed Sampath Priyasantha was born, and they realized that perhaps they had not.

The villagers we interviewed for this case were divided between those who believed that Sampath Priyasantha was the reincarnation of the murdered man and those who believed he was simply sent to the murderer's family as punishment for the murder they had committed. In particular, the murdered man's mother could not accept the possibility that her son, who had "done nothing" in her view, should be condemned, if reborn, to a life in a defective body. In view of her curse of the murderer's family, a maternal impression remains a plausible interpretation of the case, but it is unlikely that we shall ever be able to reach a firm conclusion on the matter.

I have devoted more than half of this chapter to maternal impressions because readers should remember this phenomenon as they consider the best interpretation for the cases in succeeding chapters [of *Where Reincarnation and Biology Intersect* and *Reincarnation and Biology*]. In most of them, the child's mother knew about or had even seen the wounds on the deceased person whose life the child (usually) claimed to remember when it could speak. So we need to ask whether the correspondences in these cases could have arisen from maternal impressions instead of through some other paranormal process, including reincarnation. This explanation could not apply in some 25 cases in which the mother did not see or know about the wounds on the deceased person; but it could certainly be relevant in many other cases.

NOTES

1. Chapter 3 of *Where Reincarnation and Biology Intersect*, Ian Stevenson, M.D. Copyright © 1997 by Ian Stevenson. Reproduced with permission of ABC-CLIO, LLC, Santa Barbara, CA. This is a synopsis of a much larger treatment of the subject in Chapter 3 of *Reincarnation and Biology: A Contribution to the Etiology of Birthmarks and Birth Defects*, Westport, CT: Praeger, 1997. In the larger work readers may find references, not included here.—Ed.

2. This review paper is included in Part 4.—Ed.

3. Photographs of both Sylvia's and Calvin's affected eye are published in *Where Reincarnation and Biology Intersect*.—Ed.

4. The full report of this case is included in Part 4.—Ed.

NINE

Comments on the Psychological Effects of Mescaline and Allied Drugs

1957[1]

Most reports of the therapeutic value of these agents [mescaline and LSD] have stressed their role in freeing the expression of thoughts and emotions connected with events of the past. . . . Other psychological effects of these drugs which have not yet received the attention they deserve are the changes in the perception of present experiences. . . . If I put on my glasses and see the details of the distance more sharply, no one could say that I am hallucinating! But if under the influence of mescaline I see color and forms which I did not see before, they say I am hallucinating. But is this necessarily so? It may be that I really have achieved a new and better vision of external reality.

The brain has been compared to a great filter which screens many stimuli from the mind. Mescaline may reduce the filtration powers of the brain and let in some of the beauty which our brains ordinarily hide from our awareness. Gastaut (Gastaut, Feuer, & Castells, 1953), from a neurophysiological point of view, seems to have meant something similar when he suggested that the fundamental action of LSD consists in decreasing the "filtering" activity of the central nervous system and thus increasing the number of stimuli reaching awareness. Although I will not deny that some and perhaps many false perceptions may occur under the influence of these drugs, I think it is a mistake to overlook the possibility that these drugs may bring us, at least partially, into contact with a world of which we know little and should know a great deal more. . . . The significance of this aspect of the mescaline experience is that the subject may come to have a different attitude towards perception. Most persons who have thought much about perception have discarded the theory of naive realism. That is, they know intellectually that the sense data they perceive differ from the real object which is the source of the stimuli for these sense data. I say they know this, but they, nevertheless, do not know it with conviction. Such conviction can come during and after a mescaline experience. The difference resembles that between reading a play and seeing a play performed or, better still, performing in one. The ultimate truth about perception still evades us. It may be that our every day perceptions do indeed present to us one aspect of reality (Moncrieff, 1954), and that in other mental states (such as that induced by mescaline) we experience another aspect of reality. What matters is that we should avoid identifying our sense data with the totality of the objects perceived. After the mescaline experience, the subject may have a heightened realization that his every day sense data only present (and most imperfectly) a part of the real world around him. This may bring him further along the path of detachment from sense data, towards the non-attachment (and accompanying peace) of which mystics tell me.

Another relevant experience is the subject's realization of the instability of his own perceptions and of his own thought images. He may have acquired a strengthened awareness of his own Self. Some subjects become temporarily lost in the imagery evoked by the drugs. They cease to distinguish observing Self from images and, losing sight, enter a state which may be indistinguishable from dream states, deliria or schizophrenic reactions. Other subjects experience something which I compare to a spectator's remembrance of himself in a theater. Sometimes the playgoer becomes lost in a play. We say that he identifies himself with the actors and the stage. But then for a moment or longer, he may remember that he is sitting in his seat watching the actors. Something like this may also explain what happens during the mescaline experience. Watching the images pass before the observing Self, the subject may suddenly have a realization of the separateness of that Self from the images. Thus, he may come to distinguish what Jung (Fordham, 1951) has called the objective psyche and the Self. In this respect, his experiences may resemble mystical states. It reminds one of the Hindu's distinction between Atman and non-Atman.

I have emphasized that the experiences and effects, mentioned above, do not come to all subjects. Much of modern psychotherapy seems excessively preoccupied with the past to the exclusion of techniques which will change the patient's experience of the present and his way of viewing his existence. Mescaline and similar drugs may offer means of helping patients to such changes. . . .

NOTES

1. Excerpts from *The Journal of Nervous and Mental Disease, 125*, 438–442, 1957. For a more recent discussion of the potential contribution of research on psychedelic drugs to an understanding of mind and brain, see Kelly et al., 2007, pp. 542–553.

This paper is one of more than a dozen in which Ian reported his research at the University of Virginia with psychedelic drugs (for references, see the Appendix). He and other psychiatrists in the 1950s and 1960s became interested in such drugs because they seemed to offer an avenue both for eliciting important emotional responses from patients and for understanding the biochemistry and mechanisms of psychosis. As he mentioned in his autobiographical lecture (reprinted in the Introduction of this volume), in the course of this research and particularly as a result of his own experiences with mescaline and LSD, he also became aware of the potential they offer to understanding perception and hallucination. The insight he gained from the experiences of himself and others with these drugs provided yet another piece of evidence for him that the brain and body limit, and do not generate, mind.—Ed.

REFERENCES

Fordham, M. (1951). The concept of the objective psyche. *British Journal of Medical Psychology, 24*, 221–231.

Gastaut, H., Feuer, S., & Castells, C. (1953). Action de la diéthylamide de l'acide d-lysergique (LSD_{25}) sur les fonctions psychiques et 1'électroéncephalogramme. *Confinia Neurologica, 13*, 103–120.

Kelly, E. F., Kelly, E. W., Crabtree, A., Gauld, A., Grosso, M., & Greyson, B. (2007). *Irreducible Mind: Toward a Psychology for the 21st Century*. Lanham, MD: Rowman & Littlefield.

Moncrieff, M. M. (1954). *The Clairvoyant Theory of Perception*. London: Faber & Faber.

TEN

Can We Describe the Mind?

1980[1]

The founders of psychical research, predecessor of parapsychology, had as one of their principal motives the hope of obtaining support through scientific investigation for a view of man different from the materialist one that late-nineteenth-century scientists developed rapidly and aggressively. The part of man previously identified as a soul had no place in the new understanding of man's nature that post-Darwinian biologists fashioned, usually with the open alliance of the fledgling branch of science known as psychology. Psychical researchers attended, participated, and met other psychologists on equal terms in the early congresses (now called conventions) of psychologists that were held at the end of the nineteenth century, but they were soon extruded from the company they were keeping when nearly all other psychologists closed ranks around the materialist outlook. Parapsychologists have persisted as a tiny, but fortunately hardy, minority convinced (for the most part) that man has an important component not adequately accounted for by present orthodox knowledge of his physical body, a component that we say has the capacity at times to communicate and obtain information by means other than the known sensory organs of our physical bodies. This belief is, I think, almost all that parapsychologists have in common, apart from their commitment to the scientific method for testing it; in other respects we have different allegiances, or at least different professional boundaries. Our shared belief in a nonphysical element in man gives us, despite our diversity, a unity that the awareness of Jewishness gave to the Jewish people before the founding of the political state of Israel. (We parapsychologists, however, are rather more like the Kurds, a people still without a recognized nation to call our own.)

If I am correct in saying that belief about the incompleteness of the prevailing scientific view of man unites parapsychologists, it is puzzling that we have not done more to describe or even conjecture the qualities of the component of ourselves to whose existence we have dedicated our professional lives. I must immediately add that a small number of philosophers and parapsychologists have written important papers on the nature of mind from the perspective of someone willing to take account of the data of parapsychology; and some of these writers have even boldly speculated about the life we may live after death. My extensive obligations to these authors have deprived me of all claim to originality, except where I have made errors or deviations of which they would not approve.[2] Yet I think it fair to say that the majority of parapsychologists have concerned themselves little with the attributes of the mind that they believe, at least implicitly, may exist independently of the body, although associated with it during our familiar life. This failure may derive from intimidation by neurophysiologists, who, having made great advances in their field, sometimes proclaim that they will soon resolve all residues of difficulty concerning the relationship of mind and brain; and some of them claim to have done this already by asserting, dogmatically, the identity of brain and mind, which, if true, would make the mind-brain problem a pseudo-problem. Yet surrender to orthodoxy at this time seems particularly ill-advised, because several neuroscientists have recently declared bankruptcy, in effect, with regard to the ability of neurophysiology alone to solve the mind-brain problem. . . .

You will naturally wish to know first how I define "mind" and "mental." By "mental" I mean all those processes and contents that I can attend to that are inherently private, that is, those that I and I alone can observe by introspection. (Here I must add the qualification—with regard to this feature of privateness—that it pertains only under some circumstances; a parapsychologist could not deny that minds sometimes invade each other's privacy.) By a "mind" I mean that part of a person in which the processes called "mental" occur. By a living "person," I mean a mind and its associated physical body. (For me the word "personality" has a more restricted definition than the word "person," but this need not detain us here.) By "physical," I mean whatever is not mental. Since I can conceive of minds having a structure, I must also suppose this structure to be of something, that is, of some "substance." This may be some type of material—a mental material, if you like—that our methods have not yet detected. And here I introduce another topic to which I shall return later.

I have already acknowledged—albeit quite inadequately—the debt I owe to philosophers and parapsychologists who have preceded me in considering these questions. Readers will also surely wish to know from what other sources of information I draw the data for my description of the mind. Consistent with the definition of "mental" that I have just given, much of that information comes from my observations of my own mental contents and processes. I have widened the range of my experiences, compared with that of most persons, by paying more than average attention to my dreams, by some practice of meditation, by five personal excursions with hallucinogenic drugs, and by observations of many other persons to whom I gave such drugs when this was still legal. I have also drawn data for my concepts from spontaneous cases in parapsychology. Spontaneous cases occur to people in abnormal states of mind. This is not to say that they occur to abnormal people in the psychopathological sense, but only that they show properties of minds, and relationships between minds, that are not usually discernible when people are in their normal states.

I must here acknowledge that I have not so far learned much about minds, or the processes of their paranormal communications, from parapsychological experiments. The common factor of successful experiments appears to be emotion, or what I prefer to call the intensity of an experience; but we can observe the effects of strong emotion much better in spontaneous cases than in laboratory experiments. The important events of life that generate strong emotions do not happen in laboratories, or not often. I am referring here to such events as serious illnesses, accidents, other stresses, and—above all—death. Almost any type of spontaneous case, from the faintest telepathic impression to the most tornado-like poltergeist, may tell us something about the mental processes that generate it. I think, however, that we learn more about minds from some types of spontaneous cases than from others. I refer to those in which we have reports of mental activity that seems to be slightly or not at all associated with a physical body. I have therefore found it particularly helpful to study: apparitions; near-death experiences and other types of out-of-the-body experiences; and cases of the reincarnation type. . . .

I believe that at some level all minds are united, just as all the islands and continents on our planet are attached to each other beneath the surface of the oceans. A few persons become aware of this underlying unity at special moments or even for longer periods. We often refer to such experiences of the unity of all things as mystical, but this need not mean that they are unreal. Skeptics sometimes use the word "mystical" pejoratively in order to dismiss claims of glimpsing a truth that is hidden from persons unfortunate enough not to have such an experience.

The mystic enjoys a sense of general unity with everything else in the universe. Other persons who cannot have such a widely encompassing experience may nevertheless become aware of the underlying unity of minds in a more restricted fashion. I mean here persons who have what we call paranormal perceptions. Many of their experiences seem to be of unity, not with the universe, but with a particular person at a particular time. Typically, paranormal communications—at least those of which we become aware—occur between persons who have shared many intense experiences, such as members of the same family; and they occur especially at times when one concerned person is in distress and another is asleep, somnolent, or otherwise giving diminished attention to the events in his physical vicinity.

If all minds are united and form part of one whole mind, the union is either stronger or rendered more readily observable in certain groupings of persons than in others. I referred above to the occurrence of paranormal communications between members of the same family. Studies of spontaneous cases show that the effective link is not biological but emotional; paranormal communications occur as commonly between husbands and wives as between parents and their children. I think Whately Carington was right in assuming that all minds are one. But his application of the laws of association to paranormal communications omitted the important contribution that the intensity of feelings makes toward the strength of associational bondings; paranormal experiences occur mostly when the ties are strongest and when one person urgently needs another to whom he is already strongly attached.

We who claim that paranormal communications occur often should ask ourselves why they do not occur more often. One answer may be that although we have calamities enough, we do not love each other enough; and another may be that normal means of communication in the West make paranormal communication there less necessary than it was in earlier periods, and than it still is in some parts of the world today, where it may still be the only means of sending information over long distances. . . .

Now I shall turn back in the direction of the mind-brain relationship, not to show how brain and mind relate—I have already denied any capacity to describe this—but to offer some conjectures about the mind that reasonably derive, I believe, from the improbability of explaining it in purely neural terms. Up to the present, neuroanatomists have failed to account for the differences in sensory modalities by detecting differences in the structure or function of neurones in the different regions of the brain that are concerned with sensation. They may in the future find such differences, but this does not now seem likely. (It seems even less likely that neuroscientists will ever tell us, in their vocabulary, what it is like to experience orangeness, to say nothing of a sunset by Turner or a sunset in the sky.) We do, however, experience different sensory modalities, and different qualities within a particular modality (for example, we can discriminate between the sound of a rock falling on a tin roof and that of a chord played on a piano), and these different types of experience probably occur because the various parts of the mind respond differently to stimuli they receive from the brain. The mind must somehow fit the brain, perhaps somewhat in the way a football player's helmet fits his head. The activities of neurones in different parts of the brain may then cause different mental experiences by influencing the different parts of the mind with which they interact. The retina of the eye responds to light waves and passes signals to the visual sensory cortex and its association areas; but the retina does not respond to sound waves. I suppose, similarly, that the part of the mind interacting during life with the visual cortex and its association areas responds to changes in the neurones there, but not to those occurring in neurones elsewhere, such as in the auditory cortex. (Some exceptions apparently occur during the abnormal experiences of synesthesiae, which suggest a kind of reverberation within the mind from one sensory modality to another; I believe that next to parapsychology and the study of dreams, a better understanding of synesthesiae will contribute most to the coming anatomy of the mind.) Brain events, therefore, do not constitute mental events, but are one cause of them, although not the only one. Similarly, on the motor side, mental events may cause brain events and thus initiate and execute the various physical activities of which we are capable.

I conjecture further that the mind has a somewhat variable attachment to the brain, rather as the connection between the engine and wheels of an automobile may vary with changes in the clutch. In the conditions I mentioned earlier—in dreams, when we are under the influence of hallucinogenic drugs, and as death approaches—the mind is more detached from the brain than it normally is. In these states, it becomes freer of the usual restrictions that its association with a physical body imposes on it during the life that we now have. In these freer conditions we notice a greater tendency for the presentation in consciousness of ordinarily unconscious memories, for synesthesiae to occur, and also for the occurrence of direct (non-sensory) communication between one person and another.

This type of communication—directly from mind to mind—provides perhaps the greatest single obstacle (and there are others) to our ever understanding mental processes exclusively in terms of brain states. It may be misleading and retarding of our progress to describe such communication as "extrasensory." Perhaps the process is not sensory at all. We usually refer to the person receiving the information as a percipient, but the more neutral word "experient" may prove more helpful when we try to describe a process that often suggests knowing more than perception; to be sure, the knower's new knowledge may be cast into the form of a perception that resembles his ordinary ones, but we cannot account for it by any of the physical stimuli that initiate normal perceptions.

Many persons have claimed that they could at certain times perceive their own physical bodies from a position other than that of their physical eyes. It is possible to explain away a substantial number of such claims on the grounds that the person had a hallucination of seeing his own body. This interpretation, however, becomes strained in certain cases, especially those in which the subject not only claimed to see his supine physical body, but also provided evidence of having had some paranormal cognition at the time he thought he was out of his physical body. It also fails to account adequately for cases in which the subject provided a stimulus for other persons to have had simultaneous paranormal experiences in which he figured, such as his being seen as an apparition at a distant place. If cases of this type—few though they be—are accepted as authentic, as I think some of them should be, they may throw light on all processes of perception. It is a feature of such experiences that the subject, when he is out of his body, goes on "seeing" the people around him, such as, for example, a medical staff struggling to revive his body, just as he sees them (although from a different position, that of his eyes) after he returns to his normal state of consciousness.[3] The small number of subjects who claim to remember events that they observed during an intermediate existence between death and presumed rebirth report similar visual observations. In short, persons of both the groups I have just mentioned claim to have had visual experiences (or vision-like experiences) without the use of their physical eyes and other parts of their body's neural equipment. This raises the question of whether all vision is not in one sense eyeless, that is, clairvoyant. (I am not the first person to suggest that all our physical apparatus of vision from the cornea back to the visual cortex may merely canalize most of our visual experiences without being necessary for them.)

I have already said that minds have spatial properties and a structure that one can, in principle, anatomize; and this structure must be of something. I have also emphasized the persistence of our memories during years when our physical bodies change. What persists, I maintain, are the patterns of our imaged and behavioral memories, not the unstable physical body with which they are associated during this life. I believe that our mental patterns—not just of our memories, but of our purposes also—will persist after our deaths. Then, however, we shall have no physical body, so the patterns must also exist in something else. I call this a mental "substance" without being able to define it further, except negatively by saying that it must differ markedly from the known ingredients of our physical bodies.[4] I am aware of the hazards of using a word like "substance," and concerned about the rashness of conjecturing the existence of something I cannot describe.[5] Yet I do not see any way of avoiding such a further step after reaching the point at which I have arrived.

The special conditions—dreams, intoxication with hallucinogenic drugs, and the approach of death—to which I referred above provide, I believe, some preview of our probable condition after death. If I am correct in believing that they show what happens when the mind becomes partly loosened from its physical body, studying them may help us to prepare ourselves for what we shall experience when the separation becomes complete — when we shall see face to face and no longer through a glass darkly. . . .

This concludes my speculations about the nature of the mind. It remains only for me to make a few remarks to justify my offering these rash conjectures to you. I believe in the value of the scientific method, and some readers may wonder why I have not framed my speculations in the form of testable hypotheses. They may even reproach me with leaving science and wandering in the realm of metaphysics. This objection would both mistake my intention and contradict my view of how science proceeds. I think that many advances in science come from an intuition about a truth that precedes the obtaining of evidence for it. Yet I believe also that we should keep speculation only slightly ahead of data. This introduces the subject of the nature of evidence and its variable acceptance by different persons. With the advantage of working in the medical school of a university, I have never been as isolated from scientists in other disciplines as some other parapsychologists—through no fault of theirs—have been. I may therefore appreciate better than they can that facts established for me are not so for many other parapsychologists, and are so for an even smaller proportion of scientists outside our field. Perhaps those who do not think my remarks adequately supported by sufficiently acknowledged facts may nevertheless accept them as expressions of intuitions in search of facts.

NOTES

1. Excerpts from "Can We Describe the Mind?," Presidential Address to the Parapsychological Association. In W. G. Roll & J. Beloff (eds.), *Research in Parapsychology 1980* (pp. 130–142). Metuchen, NJ: Scarecrow Press, 1981.—Ed.
2. I have written this address without giving references either to support my assertions or acknowledge my debts. The latter are, however, so great and so obvious that readers will easily recognize my creditors.

   In order to avoid excessive length I have left the address dense, although I realize that some matters to which I have alluded in a sentence—or even a phrase—deserve paragraphs, and perhaps chapters, for their proper development.
3. Some of these experients later claim to have seen much more than their physical bodies and the people around them while they were seemingly dead or nearly so. They sometimes claim to have traveled deeply into mental space and met there deceased relatives and saintly guides. However, I wish here to emphasize only the essential sameness—as it seems to these persons—of their visual experiences when viewed from within the physical body, so to speak, and from without it.
4. As I mentioned in the Introduction to Part 2, Ian later called this "substance" the "psychophore." He often expressed his belief that survival after death must entail "some kind of entity . . . which has some kind of form. . . . Is this the astral body theory? If so, I espouse it, although I dislike the word 'astral,' which tends to force commitment to a folklore about which I have serious reservations" (Stevenson, 1972, pp. 155, 158).—Ed.
5. In using the word "substance" I feel the reproach of David Hume, who (in the Appendix to *A Treatise of Human Nature*) wrote: "When we talk of self or substance, we must have an idea annexed to these terms, otherwise they are altogether unintelligible."

REFERENCE

Stevenson, I. (1972). Survival and embodiment. *Journal of the American Society for Psychical Research, 66,* 154–161.

3

Psychical Research—Principles and Methods

EWK

All the themes in Ian's work that we have discussed so far come together most completely in psychical research. The field of psychical research was founded in 1882 in England by a group of people whose aims were precisely those of Ian—to broaden our understanding of the nature of human personality and the nature of the scientific enterprise, in particular by examining phenomena and experiences that suggest the power of mind to surpass physical limitations and that thus fall outside the current scope of accepted scientific knowledge.[1] These phenomena included telepathy, clairvoyance, premonitions or precognition, apparitions of the living as well as of the dying or dead, hauntings and poltergeists, mediumship and multiple personality (now called dissociative identity disorder), hypnosis and mesmerism, near-death and death-bed experiences, and unusual healings. Ian himself, at one time or another, studied cases of, and published papers on, all these phenomena. It is important to recognize, however, that these phenomena were most definitely *not* studied by Ian or by the founders of the field simply because they are "anomalous," a word much in vogue in present-day parapsychology. They were studied because they suggest strongly the need for a better understanding of the relationship of mind and brain than that provided by a physicalist philosophy of science.

An important corollary to this belief in studying the phenomena of psychical research, not because they are isolated "anomalies" but because of their potential to expand our understanding of human personality, is that we must search in them for underlying principles that can lead to the development of a comprehensive theory. This in turn requires that we investigate in depth large numbers of cases and look for patterns in them. For Ian, therefore, it is not only important *what* we study but *how* we study it. Just as he had emphasized in medicine the importance of looking at the whole person rather than isolated symptoms, Ian emphasized (as early as 1949 ["Why Medicine Is Not a Science," reprinted in Part 2]) the importance of studying phenomena in their natural settings, with all the factors contributing to them, rather than under the artificial conditions of the lab, where the factors are limited, controlled, and altered. Although he never denied the importance of laboratory experimentation—just as he would never deny the importance of having a detailed description of a patient's symptoms—he argued that the isolated findings of the lab will never alone lead to the understanding that comes from the broader picture that nature itself provides.

For much of the duration of his career in psychical research, Ian was nearly alone in pursuing the study of spontaneous cases, that is, experiences occurring to people in everyday life rather than in the lab. Ian understood that those "imprisoned in laboratories" (Stevenson, 1995, p. 75) had retreated there in an attempt to emulate other sciences, particularly physics and psychology, and thereby win the approval of mainstream scientists. But he also understood that this strategy has not worked. The number of eminent scientists who take psychical research seriously has in fact shrunk since its early days. Critics attack modern experiments with as much vigor and venom as they attacked earlier reports of spontaneous phenomena—and often with similarly uninformed (and sometimes even dishonest) remarks.

Moreover, as Ian discusses more fully in his paper "Changing Fashions in the Study of Spontaneous Cases" (1987, reprinted below), the undeniable potential weaknesses in reports of spontaneous cases have been largely overcome by the methods that the early psychical researchers, and then Ian, used to investigate them. These weaknesses include inadequate observation, failures of memory, the unreliability of eyewitness testimony, and the possible influence of expectation or suggestion on the occurrence as well as the reporting of experiences. Psychical researchers, however, far from being unaware of such problems, led the way, even before lawyers and psychologists, in systematically describing them and developing methods to overcome them (see, e.g., Gurney, Myers, & Podmore, 1886, Chapter 4). These methods include interviewing firsthand witnesses, obtaining independent corroboration from other persons or relevant documents, and analyzing recurrent features in large numbers of cases.

The patterns that Ian observed provided another strong argument for the limitations of laboratory research. Just as psychological factors such as emotion and belief play an important role in both disease and healing, so do they play an important role in both generating and suppressing spontaneous psi phenomena. Furthermore, just as the intensity of emotion displayed during a medical interview is often a signpost to the psychological issues contributing to the patient's ill health, so the vividness and emotional intensity of dreams or intuitions may be a marker of their paranormality (e.g., Stevenson, 1963).

Another observed pattern in psi experiences—a corollary of the important role of emotion—is that such experiences usually involve two or more people who have a strong bond or relationship: "One aspect of telepathy recurs so frequently, one can almost say invariably, in both spontaneous cases and experimental investigations that I think we can refer to a 'law' in connection with this aspect. I refer to the dominant importance in telepathy (and other types of paranormal experiences) of emotional relationships and conditions" (Stevenson, 1969, p. 25). As Ian said about his friend Rosalind Heywood, who reported having many paranormal and intuitive experiences, "the common factor in nearly all her experiences was: someone of whom she was fond needed her at that time" (Stevenson, 1981, p. 269). Ian's first paper in psychical research was, in fact, "A Proposal for Studying Rapport Which Increases Extrasensory Perception" (Stevenson, 1959).

Nowhere do strong emotions and strong bonds come together more compellingly than in the context of death. Not surprisingly, therefore, many psi experiences occur at or near the time of death, or of a threat of death, whether to oneself or to loved ones. People often see apparitions—hallucinations that are *not* pathological in origin[2]—or have other telepathic impressions at or near the time of a distant loved one's death or other crisis (e.g., Gurney, Myers, & Podmore, 1886; Stevenson, 1970). People who are close to death often have apparitions of already deceased loved ones (e.g., Barrett, 1926/1986). Out-of-body experiences and apparitions of deceased loved ones often occur when a person is threatened with death, but survives (e.g., Cook [Kelly], Greyson, & Stevenson, 1998; Kelly, 2001). Even the bizarre poltergeist-like case that provided the basis for the book and movie *The Exorcist* seems to have been precipitated by the death of the subject's aunt, which had "devastated" him (Stevenson, 1995).

Finally, Ian emphasized the role of belief and faith in psi experiences—that is, the relationship between belief in what is possible and the occurrence of a phenomenon. Belief may allow an experience to occur, disbelief inhibit it. Because of this, "not all periods in history are equally suited to the bringing forth of certain types of evidence" (Stevenson, 1969, p. 20). Similar processes may manifest differently in different times and places, and some phenomena may disappear altogether, although perhaps temporarily. Ian had long noted the importance of faith in healing, whether faith in a doctor or in a treatment. Phenomena ranging from the commonly observed effects of a placebo pill to the rare and dramatic effects at places such as Lourdes (e.g., Stevenson, 1954; see also Kelly et al., 2007, Chapter 3) attest to this factor. Similarly, the belief of many people that hallucinations are always pathological may inhibit not only the reporting of an apparition but even the experience of one (e.g., Stevenson, 1983).

It is clear that strong emotion, love, faith, and death are not often found in the artificial setting of a lab experiment. But it is equally clear that these factors are not the whole story—they are neither necessary nor sufficient. Some psi experiences involve strangers, not loved ones. Ian suggested (Stevenson, 1963) that perhaps in such cases the bonds may not be of shared affection or experiences, but of shared interests. Conversely, the vast majority of situations involving strong emotion, death, love, and faith, do *not* result in psi experiences. Our understanding of how, when, why, and to whom psi experiences occur has only *begun* with observations of these patterns; it most certainly does not end there.

NOTES

1. For an excellent account of the origins of psychical research, see Gauld (1968).
2. As had many of his predecessors in psychical research, Ian emphasized that many "hallucinations" occur to people who are physically and emotionally healthy. Because the word "hallucination" has become so entangled with the idea of pathology, however, he proposed that we adopt a new word, "ideophany," for nonsensory induced perceptions (Stevenson, 1983). Unfortunately, the word has never caught on, and the association of hallucinations with pathology persists.

REFERENCES

Barrett, W. (1986). *Death-Bed Visions*. London: Methuen. (Original work published 1926)

Cook [Kelly], E. W., Greyson, B., & Stevenson, I. (1998). Do any near-death experiences provide evidence for the survival of human personality after death? Relevant features and illustrative case reports. *Journal of Scientific Exploration, 12*, 377–406.

Gauld, A. (1968). *The Founders of Psychical Research*. London: Routledge & Kegan Paul.

Gurney, E., Myers, F. W. H., & Podmore, F. (1886). *Phantasms of the Living* (2 Vols.). London: Trübner.

Kelly, E. W. (2001). Near-death experiences with reports of meeting deceased people. *Death Studies, 25*, 229–249.

Kelly, E. F., Kelly, E. W., Crabtree, A., Gauld, A., Grosso, M., & Greyson, B. (2007). *Irreducible Mind: Toward a Psychology for the 21st Century*. Lanham, MD: Rowman & Littlefield.

Stevenson, I. (1954). As a man thinketh . . . psychosomatic medicine, Part II. *Harper's Magazine, 209*, 83–87.

Stevenson, I. (1959). A proposal for studying rapport which increases extrasensory perception. *Journal of the American Society for Psychical Research, 53*, 66–68.

Stevenson, I. (1963). A postcognitive dream illustrating some aspects of the pictographic process. *Journal of the American Society for Psychical Research, 57*, 182–202.

Stevenson, I. (1969). Some implications of parapsychological research on survival after death. *Proceedings of the American Society for Psychical Research, 28*, 18–35.

Stevenson, I. (1970). *Telepathic Impressions: A Review and Report of Thirty-five New Cases*. Charlottesville: University Press of Virginia.

Stevenson, I. (1981). Remembering Rosalind Heywood. *Journal of the American Society for Psychical Research, 75*, 267–271.

Stevenson, I. (1983). Do we need a new word to supplement "hallucination"? *American Journal of Psychiatry, 140*, 1609–1611.

Stevenson, I. (1995). Possession and exorcism: An essay review. *Journal of Parapsychology, 59,* 69–76.

ELEVEN

Changing Fashions in the Study of Spontaneous Cases

1987[1]

The scientific study of psychical phenomena began with spontaneous cases, and psychical researchers emphasized them for at least forty years. In the 1920s and 1930s interest in spontaneous cases decreased among psychical researchers, who turned increasingly to experimental work and—perhaps to emphasize the change—began calling themselves parapsychologists. Critics had pointed to the weaknesses of spontaneous cases during the early years of psychical research, but such criticisms did not lead to lessened interest in them. Economic factors may have made experiments less costly to conduct than cases were to investigate. A more important reason for the shift to experimental work may have been the desire to imitate experimental psychology and other branches of science amenable to experimental controls. However, experiments (so far) have not led to acceptance of parapsychology by other scientists; nor have they greatly increased understanding of paranormal processes. On the contrary, one-sided emphasis on experiments may have retarded our gaining the knowledge about paranormal processes that we can only obtain from the study of spontaneous cases. Biologists have discovered the importance of naturalistic observations in their field, and parapsychologists should follow their lead. The next generation of investigators should develop a more balanced program of research that will draw new information from both experiments and spontaneous cases.

Psychical research began with the study of spontaneous cases. This is well known, and it is also well known that within about 6 decades spontaneous cases fell into disrepute and were almost entirely replaced by experiments in the preoccupations of investigators. Although the change in emphasis from spontaneous cases to experiments took place over several decades, I think the years between 1925 and 1935 were the most important ones.[2] There are some signs now—5 decades later—that spontaneous cases are again coming into favor. I applaud this trend, but I would not wish to see the field move all the way back to the other extreme. A protoscience such as parapsychology cannot afford to neglect any method or the study of any phenomena that may advance it. It may be helpful, therefore, toward achieving a sound distribution of our future efforts to look back and ask ourselves why spontaneous cases fell into neglect. We should also ask why they should again receive more attention.

A standard explanation for their neglect—often heard and sometimes printed during the period of their eclipse—was that one cannot rely on informants' memories for accounts of events that happened before an investigator came to the scene of a case. It had been quickly learned that few percipients took the trouble to write down an account of their experience before they obtained normal knowledge of the related events; even for cases not over within a few seconds, it was rare—as it still is rare—for an investigator to be able to observe the phenomena directly. Whence, however, comes the evidence that informants' memories are inadequately reliable?

That some witnesses are unreliable has been known for a long time, and the early psychical researchers were fully aware of the fallibility of human observation and memory. It would be difficult to improve, even today, on the skepticism and precautions in this matter shown by the authors of *Phantasms of the Living* (Gurney, Myers, & Podmore, 1886). They quickly developed several defenses against the defects of individual witnesses: personal interviews and multiple informants (whenever possible), the checking of statements against each other and against any written sources available, and independent verification of events related to the percipient's experience. Their confidence in the authenticity of the reports given to them increased when they discerned recurrent features in large series of cases and began to identify distinctly different types of cases. New cases could then be appraised against the standard developed from the older cases (although they were not accepted or rejected only because of conformity or lack of it to a type).

The rigor of Gurney and his colleagues did not protect them from criticism. Far from it; almost immediately after the publication of their great work, Innes (1887) assailed the lack of written evidence supporting the witnesses' memories. To this, Gurney (1887) made a lengthy and—it seems to me—effective reply.[3] British and American psychical researchers continued to use the methods of the pioneers, although they always hoped to find cases earlier, to find better-documented ones, and to find ones amenable to direct observation by the investigators. At the same time some of them continued to interest themselves in problems of malobservation (Davey, 1887; Hodgson, 1887, 1892). Indeed, psychical researchers can claim priority over lawyers and psychologists in giving attention to malobservation by witnesses. In England, for example, lawyers did not become adequately aware of the possibilities for harm from malobservation until the case of Adolf Beck (Williams, 1963) forced it on their attention in the first decade of this century. Beck had been arrested, convicted, and imprisoned twice, solely on false recognitions of him by several women who all swore that he was the man who had swindled them. This dreadful injustice led to the establishment in 1907 of the Court of Appeal, Criminal Division, in England.

Psychologists were still further behind than lawyers in this matter, and their first substantial contribution to it was Münsterberg's (1908/1923) attack on the credibility of many witnesses in legal proceedings. Münsterberg cited one of the early experiments (by a psychologist) on eyewitness testimony. Numerous later experiments have also shown that eyewitness testimony is often flawed, sometimes badly.[4] One can appeal to the evidence in such experiments in different ways and according to what one would like to emphasize. Some persons have said that the deficiencies of witnesses in failing to observe or afterward remember the simplest details (of events staged in these experiments) discredit informants for spontaneous cases. However, the experiments may also support a different interpretation. Although the witnesses in the experiments got many details wrong, they also got many right (Crocker, 1930). Moreover, even though they may have gotten some details wrong, the main event they observed did in fact take place; therefore, one cannot use errors on the part of witnesses about details to deny that something fairly close to what they reported actually happened (Rollo, 1967).

If we leave abstract criticism and turn to actual cases, we find that—so far as I have been able to learn—only six cases (out of several thousand) published by the SPR (or in association with it) have had to be withdrawn because of later evidence about errors of testimony in them.[5] Moreover, five of these cases have one or another special feature that makes them atypical among standard cases. Two were cases of claimed phantom houses in which the percipients failed to search in the right place for the actual houses they had seen normally ("Case . . . ," 1942; Heywood, 1961; Lambert, 1963; Parsons, 1962). One was a hoax by a teenager (Gurney et al., 1886, vol. 2, pp. 671–675; "Note on a case . . . ," 1898). One was considered suspicious before publication, but was mentioned in a footnote (Sidgwick, 1885) and then fully exposed as a fraud two years later (Sidgwick, 1887). The fifth case (Balfour, 1884; Barrett et al., 1884; Gurney, 1885; Gurney & Myers, 1884; Hornby, 1884) may yet be rehabilitated by evidence that is still unpublished.[6] In the sixth case (Barrett et al., 1882), the informant was found to have made errors in dates and other important details to the extent that his credibility as a reporter became destroyed (Gurney, 1885).

In fairness, two further comments should be made about the paucity of published cases proven later to be inauthentic. First, barring some fortuitous confession or other revelation about the unreliability of the witnesses for a published case, about the only way of showing that it is in fact inauthentic is to investigate it again. This, however, is extremely difficult. The witnesses understandably do not wish to go over old ground with new interviewers, and we should not interpret their reluctance as evasiveness. Even when they agree to a second investigation, time has further elapsed since the original events of the case; discrepancies in testimony about details are almost inevitable and not necessarily discrediting to the case.

The second relevant point is that although only six published SPR cases are known to be inauthentic, many more may be inauthentic without this being known. West (1948, 1982) has been the leading spokesman for this suggestion. His first paper on this topic has never been surpassed with regard to its cogent criticisms of the evidence in many spontaneous cases. Because it is often cited in discussions of spontaneous cases, I shall make some additional comments about it. First, West's paper did not show for any case not already known to be inauthentic that a normal explanation was preferable to a paranormal one; he merely pointed out possible sources of errors in the testimony in some published cases. Second, West did not recommend abandoning the study of spontaneous cases. On the contrary, he called for further efforts to study them with improved vigilance to detect errors in testimony and a renewed search for stronger cases; his was not a counsel of despair, but one of perfection. Third, critiques like that of West were published some years after spontaneous cases had begun to fall out of favor; we should regard them more as expressions of the change that had taken place than as causes of it.

What then were these causes? I have tried to show that the study of spontaneous cases did not fall out of fashion because new criticisms about their weaknesses were raised or because a large number of them were shown to be inauthentic. We must look elsewhere for the understanding we seek. Economic changes may have played a part. The pioneer investigators in England were spared from domestic drudgery by servants, and some of them had enough money and enough free time for traveling around to interview witnesses as the adequate investigation of spontaneous cases always requires. In contrast, their successors have had to give more attention to the practicalities of earning a living and running a household. When experiments first came into high favor, they required no traveling and the equipment used cost almost nothing. During that phase, experiments were less costly to conduct than cases were to investigate—so far as we can make a comparison. (This situation has since changed somewhat; travel for the investigation of cases has become again somewhat easier; and, meanwhile, equipment for some experiments, such as those requiring complex computer systems and those requiring sleep laboratories, has become highly expensive.)

Perhaps other reasons may have influenced the falling off of interest in spontaneous cases among psychical researchers. They may have become discontented with the yield from spontaneous cases of useful information about how paranormal phenomena occur. Evidence that such phenomena do occur is rarely sufficient by itself to satisfy curiosity; a scientist always wants to learn how phenomena happen, not merely that they do happen. During the period when psychical researchers were losing interest in spontaneous cases, many of them developed a strong interest in mediumship, and this phase lasted for several decades. The absorption of psychical researchers in mediumship may have reflected an increasing wish to observe psychical phenomena under more controlled conditions, because a mediumistic séance provides a semiexperimental situation.

Although I would give some weight to the factors I have mentioned in hastening the decline in the study of spontaneous cases, I think another was more important. This is the hope that experiments offered of convincing other scientists about the reality of paranormal phenomena. It was abundantly clear by the 1920s that most other scientists had not become convinced of the existence even of telepathy—to say nothing of other paranormal phenomena of an apparently more extraordinary kind. Yet the persuasion of other scientists became increasingly important as scientists themselves came to control more of the financial resources of the whole enterprise of science. In the last quarter of the nineteenth century, experiments in physics and chemistry had begun to achieve enormous successes, and these have continued to the present day. Psychologists and biologists hoped to emulate the physicists' and chemists' success, and to some extent they have done so. Psychical researchers began to think that they must follow the same route or go out of business.

What most scientists of living things failed to realize was that many important phenomena within their fields are not amenable to repetition and experimental manipulation. They must be observed as they occur naturally or ignored altogether. Flammarion, who was both a distinguished astronomer and an outstanding psychical researcher, railed against the narrow definition of science that was becoming dominant at the end of his life. He wrote:

> Some criticisms end up by becoming exasperating. One is the claim that for an observation to be considered scientific you must be able to repeat it at will. You might as well say that a lightning strike did not occur because you could not make it happen again; or that a fall of meteorites is impossible because you cannot bring one on when you want; or that an eclipse is a fable because you have to wait for special circumstances of the sun and moon in order to see it again; or that an earthquake did not happen because you cannot repeat it. This is con-

> fusing two completely different orders of things: observation and experiment. One observes a spontaneous phenomenon; one makes experimentally a chemical compound. Nevertheless, it is not unusual to notice this mistake in reasoning even among persons who are familiar with scientific methods. (Flammarion, 1923, p. 52; my translation)

Biologists, ahead of psychologists (and parapsychologists), first recognized the limitations of investigations confined to laboratories. I think that advocates of the study of spontaneous cases owe many thanks to ethologists, who first awakened their fellow biologists to this fact. The award in 1973 of Nobel Prizes to Lorenz, Frisch, and Tinbergen did much to reinstate naturalistic observations to respectability in the life sciences. At about the same time, many psychologists became disenchanted with a purely experimental approach to their subject, and their secession led to the development of humanistic psychology. However, humanistic psychology ran out of steam, perhaps because it had no place for paranormal phenomena.

What should that place be? This question raises that of why parapsychology should now try to become better balanced by renewed investigations of spontaneous cases. I will give two reasons for this recommendation. First, experimental parapsychology has not brought us to the promised land of recognition by our fellow scientists with the increment of funding for further research that such recognition will eventually provide. It has failed to do this not only because the results from experiments are often of marginal significance and not repeatable on demand. An equally important point about experiments is that they have proven to have the same vulnerability to criticism that spontaneous cases have: namely, doubt about authenticity. Critics of parapsychology have accused experimenters of incompetence and even of fraud. These complaints are nearly always unjust, but they have tended to put experiments and spontaneous cases on a more equal footing: In the end, the credibility of both depends upon the persons making the reports.

Second—and I regard this as the more important of the two reasons—experimental parapsychology has failed to provide the basis of a satisfactory theory by which paranormal phenomena might be harmonized with other branches of knowledge. Nor can it ever do so; the data from cases tell us—almost shout at us—that paranormal phenomena are nearly always spontaneous and nearly always somehow related to strong emotions. This is why we see spontaneous cases so often associated with death and with love. And because these occur meagerly in laboratories, we can never dispense with spontaneous cases. Those who have thought they could do so have sawed off the branch of the tree on which they were sitting; and they should now pick themselves up and climb the tree again.

NOTES

1. Reprinted from *Journal of the American Society for Psychical Research, 81*, 1–10, 1987. Published with permission of the American Society for Psychical Research, Inc. (ASPR), 5 West 73rd Street, New York, New York 10023, Webpage: aspr.com, e-mail: aspr.com.—Ed.

2. Some historians might set a more precise date for the change in emphasis: that of the publication of J. B. Rhine's *Extra-Sensory Perception* (Rhine, 1934). It does not detract from Rhine's important contribution to insist that he was not the founder of experimental parapsychology. Numerous experiments had been published before he entered the field. Perhaps the best brief evidence on this matter can be found in the issue of the *Proceedings of the Society for Psychical Research* in which Thouless (1935) reviewed Rhine's book. That same issue includes a note inviting readers to volunteer for experiments then being conducted by members of the Society (Salter, 1935). See also Inglis (1984) and McVaugh and Mauskopf (1976).

3. Innes (1891) renewed his criticisms 4 years later. By this time Gurney had died (in 1888), but Podmore (1892) replied and even published some cases satisfying Innes's more stringent requirement of written records of the experience made before its verification. The founders of the SPR had always valued and sought such records, but percipients, as Podmore explained, rarely appreciate the value of these to scientists.

4. I reviewed all the experiments of this type about which I could learn up to 1968 (Stevenson, 1971). For accounts of more recent experiments, see Loftus (1979).

5. The search for withdrawn cases has included a careful examination of the indexes to the SPR publications under all words indicative of fraud, hoaxes, cases withdrawn, etc.

I have not counted in this inventory any case that was known to be fraudulent and that was published anyway, for the lesson it might give to investigators. An example of this type is the Brown case published in the SPR *Journal* ("A Fictitious Communicator," 1924).

6. From documents on file at the SPR, which I have been able to examine, it appears that the percipient of this case, Sir Edmund Hornby, may have made a false statement in order to protect the reputation of his third wife, who was perhaps living with him before they were married. Balfour (1884) stated correctly that although Hornby had referred to his wife as being in his house at the time Hornby saw the apparition, he had not married his third wife until 3 months after he had his apparitional experience. In Victorian England (and the foreign colony of Shanghai, where this case occurred) it would have seemed more honorable to pretend that one had made an error in dates and to withdraw a case than to disgrace a lady. It is important to note also that it was Gurney (1885) who withdrew the case, not Hornby. All Hornby (1884) said was that his memory might have been mistaken as to the date of his vision.

REFERENCES

Balfour, F. H. (1884). Note. *Nineteenth Century, 16*, 851.

Barrett, W. F., Keep, A. P. P., Massey, C. C., Wedgwood, H., Podmore, F., & Pease, E. R. (1882). First report of the Committee on Haunted Houses. *Proceedings of the Society for Psychical Research, 1*, 101–115.

Barrett, W. F., Massey, C. C., Moses, W. S., Podmore, F., Gurney, E., & Myers, F. W. H. (1884). Fourth report of the Literary Committee: A theory of apparitions, Part II. *Proceedings of the Society for Psychical Research, 2*, 157–186.

Case: A collective hallucination at Boscastle, 1933. (1942). *Journal of the Society for Psychical Research, 32*, 174–178.

Crocker, G. G. (1930). A significant experiment. *Bulletin of the Boston Society for Psychic Research, 12*, 88–98.

Davey, S. J. (1887). The possibilities of mal-observation and lapse of memory from a practical point of view: Experimental investigation. *Proceedings of the Society for Psychical Research, 4*, 405–495.

A fictitious communicator. (1924). *Journal of the Society for Psychical Research, 21*, 306–314.

Flammarion, C. (1923). *Les Maisons Hantées.* Paris: Ernest Flammarion. (Published in English in 1924 as *Haunted Houses*)

Gurney, E. (1885). Retractations and alterations of view. *Journal of the Society for Psychical Research, 2*, 2–4.

Gurney, E. (1887). Letters on phantasms: A reply. *Nineteenth Century, 22*, 522–533.

Gurney, E., & Myers, F. W. H. (1884). Visible apparitions. *Nineteenth Century, 16*, 68–95.

Gurney, E., Myers, F. W. H., & Podmore, F. (1886). *Phantasms of the Living* (2 Vols.). London: Trübner.

Heywood, R. (1961). Collective hallucinations of non-existent buildings. *Journal of the Society for Psychical Research, 41*, 198–201.

Hodgson, R. (1887). The possibilities of mal-observation and lapse of memory from a practical point of view: Introduction. *Proceedings of the Society for Psychical Research, 4*, 381–404.

Hodgson, R. (1892). Mr. Davey's imitations by conjuring of phenomena sometimes attributed to spirit agency. *Proceedings of the Society for Psychical Research, 8*, 253–310.

Hornby, E. (1884). Correspondence. *Nineteenth Century, 16*, 851–852.

Inglis, B. (1984). *Science and Parascience: A History of the Paranormal, 1914–1939*. London: Hodder & Stoughton.

Innes, A. T. (1887). Where are the letters? A cross-examination of certain phantasms. *Nineteenth Century, 22*, 174–194.

Innes, A. T. (1891). The psychical society's ghosts: A challenge renewed. *Nineteenth Century, 30*, 764–776.

Lambert, G. W. (1963). Phantom scenery. *Journal of the Society for Psychical Research, 42*, 1–6.

Loftus, E. (1979). *Eyewitness Testimony*. Cambridge: Harvard University Press.

McVaugh, M., & Mauskopf, S. H. (1976). J. B. Rhine's *Extra-Sensory Perception* and its background in psychical research. *Isis, 67*, 161–189.

Münsterberg, H. (1923). *On the Witness Stand: Essays on Psychology and Crime.* Garden City, NY: Doubleday. (Original work published 1908)

Note on a case in "Phantasms of the Living." (1898). *Proceedings of the Society for Psychical Research, 14*, 114.

Parsons, D. (1962). A non-existent building located. *Journal of the Society for Psychical Research, 41*, 292–295.

Podmore, F. (1892). In defence of phantasms. *National Review, 19*, 234–251.

Rhine, J. B. (1934). *Extra-Sensory Perception.* Boston: Boston Society for Psychic Research.

Rollo, C. (1967). Thomas Bayes and the bundle of sticks. *Proceedings of the Society for Psychical Research, 55*, 23–64.

S[alter], W. H. (1935). An appeal for co-operation in further experiments in extrasensory perception. *Proceedings of the Society for Psychical Research, 43*, 38–39.

Sidgwick, Mrs. H. [E. M.] (1885). Notes on the evidence, collected by the Society, for phantasms of the dead. *Proceedings of the Society for Psychical Research, 3*, 69–150.

Sidgwick, Mrs. H. [E. M.] (1887). Phantasms of the dead. *Journal of the Society for Psychical Research, 3*, 69–71.

Stevenson, I. (1971). The substantiality of spontaneous cases. *Proceedings of the Parapsychological Association, 1968*, No. 5 (91–128). Durham, NC: Parapsychological Association.

Thouless, R. H. (1935). Dr. Rhine's recent experiments on telepathy and clairvoyance and a reconsideration of J. E. Coover's conclusions on telepathy. *Proceedings of the Society for Psychical Research, 43*, 24–37.

West, D. J. (1948). The investigation of spontaneous cases. *Proceedings of the Society for Psychical Research, 48*, 264–300.

West, D. J. (1982). Thoughts on testimony to the paranormal. *Parapsychology Review, 13*(5), 1–8.

Williams, G. (1963). *The Proof of Guilt: A Study of the English Criminal Trial* (3rd ed.). London: Stevens and Sons.

TWELVE

Comments on Paper by Michael Scriven

1962[1]

As someone with a particular interest in the spontaneous phenomena of parapsychology, I should like to make some comments about Dr. Scriven's summary dismissal of these experiences. . . .

I think Dr. Scriven's error, as I take it to be, derives from a misunderstanding of what is ordinarily meant by the word "veridical." Dr. Scriven refers on page 307 to "alleged veridical phantasms." Now by "veridical" I think psychical researchers have meant verifiable by other persons as to the correspondence between events and perceptions. This is, after all, the fundamental difference between subjective and objective experiences. The hallucinations or illusory experiences which occur rather commonly . . . are mental images of persons and objects usually having emotional significance for the percipient. The percipient sometimes perceives these images as located in his ordinary sensory field, i.e., "projected" into the environment. The images may or may not happen to coincide with a verifiable external event. But if they are images of only a face or figure without accompanying action, it is extremely unlikely that they will correspond with an identifiable external event or that, if they do, anyone could detect the correspondence. They are then regarded as subjective only. Psychiatrists interest themselves in these experiences but I see no reason why parapsychologists should.

The case is different, however, when the perceived images match events which others can verify. The possibility of chance coincidence between the perceived images and the related events will then depend upon the singularity of the events. . . .

To have an image of one's dead sister's face signifies little, but what of an image of that face with a scratch exactly where the sister's face once had a scratch known to only one living person?[2] As matching details accumulate, we gain confidence that there has been a distant perception of a unique event that cannot be confounded with any other. To see at a long distance an image of one's brother, even an image of one's brother on a tug boat, signifies little. But when that image includes additional details of the brother falling forward over a bulwark, of his feet caught in a rope, and of his wearing no coat, a blue shirt, and trousers turned up so the lining shows,[3] and when such an image occurs on the day of the brother's drowning in the same manner, it becomes absurd to suggest that perception and events are related by chance. Surely actual events of this kind are not merely philosophically unique, but obviously unique beyond any possible confusion with other similar events, such as the brother diving into a swimming pool. Additional details matching between events and perception do not make the events "more unique," which is impossible. What they do is make us more certain that the perceptions match one particular group of unique events and no other.

The first recorded parapsychological experiment belonged to this type. Croesus, King of Lydia (according to Herodotus), asked various oracles to say what he was doing on a particular day. He then engaged in the most unusual activity he could think of, boiling a tortoise and a lamb in a cauldron of brass with a brass lid. The oracle of Delphi sent him the correct answer. Assuming the reliability of witnesses, should we call the correlation between the King's actions and the perceptions at Delphi a matter of chance? If the foregoing and my other illustrations derive from earlier days, recent examples are also at hand of the matching of several details between perceptions and events.[4] . . .

The problem with regard to chance in spontaneous cases is that of deciding the number and type of details that must match between perceptions and events in order that we can be sure of not confounding one set of unique events with another somewhat similar, but actually different set. The problem resembles that of deciding when a suspected criminal is actually the man of whom a description has been given by the victims or eye-witnesses of his crime. It is generally agreed that as the number and unusualness of matching details increase, the identity becomes more certain. Since the rarity, e.g., a scar under the left eye, as well as the number of matching details enter into the inferences, we cannot assign (or at least have at present no methods for assigning) a number to the probability that the suspect corresponds with the real criminal. And similarly, we cannot assign a number to the probability that the perception in a spontaneous case corresponds with one unique group of events and no other. But of the cases with abundant or unusual detail such as those I have cited, I do not believe one can argue on the point of correspondence between perceptions and events. In the words of Mr. W. H.

Salter arguments on this point with regard to the richer cases (in detail) require a "ludicrous straining of probability."[5]

Reports of detailed perceptions that match events at a distance must pass other tests besides those of correspondence in detail between perceptions and events before we can assign a paranormal explanation to them. But we should not discard them on the grounds that chance brought together events and perceptions. Rather, the task for the investigator is to decide how the percipient acquired information at a distance about this unique group of events. It is a task primarily for the parapsychologist and hardly at all, as yet, for the neurophysiologist.

That altered brain function may induce sensory phenomena of an illusory kind cannot invalidate the occurrence of genuinely veridical sensory experiences of the kind I have described. Advances in neurophysiology may eventually lead to the discovery of certain sites and conditions of the brain which favor such veridical experiences, but they will not explain them away as Dr. Striven supposes. And I doubt if neurophysiology will explain them at all until it reaches the stage where it has something useful to say about veridical "out-of-the-body" experiences. These cases surely must strain the empiricism of hardened monists who believe in obligatory correspondence of cerebral and mental events. They must either deny such cases out of hand or admit that (at least with regard to the mind-brain problem) neurophysiology is as young a science as parapsychology.

Some of Dr. Scriven's difficulties may arise from his apparent conviction that advances in one branch of science necessarily "squeeze" another branch. Hence the impression that neurophysiology is absorbing parapsychology or that, to quote Dr. Scriven, given a good ESP experiment, "goodbye physics." This kind of extravagant surrender of whole fields of scientific activity (or claims of surrender, as the case may be) will not advance either our subject or its respect among colleagues in other branches of science. Moreover, it encourages a timid abandonment of empiricism in the face of contradictory concepts, or data that are at first glance contradictory, but not really so.

In the present limited state of knowledge, it is easy and tempting to assume the posture of the tough-minded critic. But this role carries responsibilities also, one of which should be thoughtful respect for the work and ideas of predecessors. Dr. Scriven's handling of the spontaneous cases made me share Dr. Woodruff's opinion that he had not done his "homework" on this topic also. For if he had, he would surely have acknowledged (although he did not need to agree with) the many psychical researchers who have considered the question of chance in spontaneous cases. The published material on this matter starts (I believe) with an early attempt at a mathematical treatment reported in the *Proceedings* of the S. P. R.[6] and continues through the many years following. The subject was discussed at length and cogently in Tyrrell's *Apparitions* as recently as 1942. But that date lies before the bibliographic watershed of 1950 behind which, as Dr. Osis complains, few authors venture.[7]

NOTES

1. Excerpts from a Letter to the Editor (*Journal of Parapsychology, 26,* 59–64, 1962), commenting on a paper by a philosopher, Michael Scriven ("New frontiers of the brain." *Journal of Parapsychology, 25,* 305–318, 1961).—Ed.
2. See *Proceedings of the Society for Psychical Research, 6,* 17–18, 1889.
3. See *Proceedings of the Society for Psychical Research, 7,* 33, 1891.
4. For example: Rhine, L. E. (1954). Frequency of types of experience in spontaneous precognition. *Journal of Parapsychology, 18,* 93–123; and also Dale, L. A., White, R., and Murphy, G. (1962). A selection of cases from a recent survey of spontaneous ESP phenomena. *Journal of the American Society for Psychical Research, 56,* 3–47.
5. See p. 126 of his book *Zoar: The Evidence of Psychical Research Concerning Survival.* London: Sidgwick and Jackson, 1961.
6. See *Proceedings of the Society for Psychical Research, 2,* 53–55, 1882.
7. Ian was here referring to the tendency of too many scientists, then and now, to consider "outdated" any research that occurred earlier than the past decade. The historical myopia of many scientists was also noted and lamented nearly a century earlier by Thomas Huxley (1874), who urged the importance of studying one's history because "there is assuredly no more effectual method of clearing up one's own mind on any subject than by talking it over, so to speak, with men of real power and grasp, who have considered it from a totally different point of view" (p. 556).—Ed.

REFERENCE

Huxley, T. H. (1874). On the hypothesis that animals are automata, and its history. *Fortnightly Review* (n.s.), *16,* 555–580.

THIRTEEN

Thoughts on the Decline of Major Paranormal Phenomena

1989[1]

Major paranormal phenomena, defined as phenomena detectable by the senses alone without a need for statistics, have diminished in the contemporary publications of the Society [for Psychical Research] compared with the publications of its first several decades. The lack of reports of such major phenomena may reflect diminished interest in them on the part of investigators, most of whom have turned their attention to laboratory experiments that elicit marginal results requiring statistical analysis. However, it seems likely that the major phenomena occur less frequently in the West today than they did formerly. Skepticism derived from philosophical materialism may inhibit normally the occurrence of major paranormal phenomena. It may also inhibit them through paranormal processes. The most promising sources of major paranormal phenomena today may be in industrially undeveloped countries, among a few specially gifted individuals, and in certain unusual experiences, such as those of persons who come close to death and recover.

The daunting prospect of trying to deliver a Presidential Address in any way worthy of being placed on the same shelf as previous Addresses impelled me to read, in recent months, many of the Addresses that I had not previously studied. In doing this I paid particular attention to the speakers' appraisals of the Society's accomplishments. Although I made no attempt to rank the speakers on a scale of optimism versus pessimism in their judgments of the Society's work, I noted that several emphatically expressed optimism about the outcome of our labors. I am not referring to confidence in the worthiness of the enterprise, but to assertions of success in it. In the decades between 1910 and 1980 at least six Presidents asserted that telepathy had been proved or nearly so (Flammarion, 1923–1924; McDougall, 1920; Prince, 1930–1931; L. E. Rhine, 1982; Salter, 1946–1949; and Smith, 1910).[2]

One might ask why, if telepathy had been proved by 1910, later Presidents thought it necessary to reiterate the claim so often in subsequent years. I can think of two reasons why they might have felt a need for such renewed affirmation. First, each generation of investigators, perhaps each decade of them, has believed its methods superior to those of its predecessors. This has entailed the temptation to hint at, or even to say openly, something like: "Our forerunners thought they had solid evidence of paranormal phenomena, but their methods were crude compared with ours. We have finally proven the reality of these phenomena." Second, they knew that what they and the audiences listening to their Addresses—largely the members and friends of the Society—regarded as proof did not seem that to the majority of scientists. The rest of the world had not heard, or had not listened if it did hear. They needed to be told again. Unfortunately, the need still exists.

Our inability to persuade larger numbers of educated persons, especially scientists, to take seriously our endeavors and accomplishments seems more than a disappointment; it may now be a fatal weakness. Until the present generation new recruits in psychical research always seemed available to fill the places of investigators who died; and for a time it looked as if the study of paranormal phenomena was taking root in universities. However, we must admit that today psychical research has almost gone from the universities, at least on the continent of Europe and in North America. Even in the United Kingdom, psychical research is almost extinct in universities south of the Tweed. We are not gaining the interest of well-qualified younger investigators with new ideas in sufficient numbers to succeed those of us whose ideas need to be replaced by other insights and better methods.

The decline during recent decades in the acceptance of our achievements—even of the legitimacy of our endeavors—on the part of other scientists must have several causes. I have written elsewhere about what I believe to be one of the less important of these causes, namely the misguided effort to identify a separate discipline of science called parapsychology (Stevenson, 1988). However, that is not my theme in this Address. Instead, I wish to suggest other causes of the decline effect in psychical research. I think by far the most important of these causes is our inability to observe and report major paranormal phenomena. Here I emphasize the word *major*, by which I mean phenomena so gross that we require no statistics for their demonstration. In specifying further what I am thinking about, I shall say little about physical phenomena and consider mainly spontaneous (mental) cases, mental mediumship, and the feats of unusually gifted sensitives or clairvoyants. The volumes of the early and middle years of our Society's publications contain numerous reports of carefully investigated major phenomena subsumed under these categories, and I wish to address the question of why we publish little or nothing of this sort today.

Some of my listeners and readers may ask whether a return of such major phenomena would improve the fortunes of psychical research. After all, if these phenomena failed to carry conviction outside a fairly narrow circle[3] before, why should they do so today? The point is a good one, and to it I can only reply that the minor phenomena requiring statistics for their demonstration are certainly not exciting interest among modern scientists, and perhaps the major phenomena would. A survey by McClenon (1984) of "elite scientists" offers some support for this view. He found that 29 percent of the respondents said that they believed in extrasensory perception. However, as the basis for their belief, twice as many of the believers cited personal experience as cited reports in scientific journals. Moreover, among 351 scientists responding to McClenon's questionnaire only nine cited a journal in our field as a source of information on the subject. We are not justified in believing from the information available that the elite scientists surveyed by McClenon experienced what I think of as major phenomena, although some of them may have done so. We may, however, believe that they would be more impressed by such major phenomena, if we could report them, than they now are by the marginal results of most laboratory experiments that require statistics for their demonstration.

Next we come to the distinction between the reporting of phenomena and the occurrence of them. The paucity of reports of such major phenomena may reflect nothing more than lack of interest or lack of resources for investigations on the part of psychical researchers. Or there may have been a real decline in the occurrence of the phenomena. Or both these factors may be present.

We could argue that the preponderant attention given in our journals to experimental studies compared with reports of the major phenomena reflects a lack of interest in the latter on the part of investigators. A decline of interest in the major phenomena appears to have set in during the 1930s, when they were still more plentiful than they appear to be today. It is worth asking why this occurred.

Several causes may have contributed to investigators having less interest in the major phenomena than they earlier had. Changing economic conditions may have drawn them away from spontaneous cases, the study of which was more costly than experiments were, at least in the early days of the fashion for experiments.

Perhaps researchers became afraid of the phenomena. Eisenbud (1983), Tart (1984) and White (1985) have suggested that psychical researchers are afraid to acknowledge (and hence afraid to observe) the vast paranormal powers of which they assume at least some persons are capable. Who would want to believe that by thinking alone he could move mountains, kill a neighbor, or sink the *Titanic*? This argument seems based on assumptions instead of evidence. Moreover, it must include a discrediting judgment of ourselves compared with our predecessors, because certainly nineteenth-century investigators and some of those in the early years of this century did not hesitate to encounter tables and persons that levitated as well as the appearance or the reality of full-form materializations of the dead.

It seems to me that the psychical researchers of the last two generations have been less afraid of the major phenomena than they have been of the disapproval of colleagues in other branches of science. This led many of them to imitate psychologists, who, in their laboratories, were trying to imitate physicists and chemists in theirs. The unbalanced emphasis on laboratory experiments that has now prevailed among two generations of psychical researchers needs correction, as I have argued elsewhere (Stevenson, 1987). We are bound to have fewer reports of major paranormal phenomena if we have fewer investigators interested in studying and reporting them. Moreover, the paucity of scientists known to take an interest in these phenomena means that persons having paranormal experiences have little information about qualified professional persons to whom they might describe whatever experiences they have. Also, persons who have or think they may have special sensitivities or mediumistic abilities have almost no one qualified in psychical research to whom they can turn for encouragement and guidance.

Nevertheless, I do not believe that we can attribute the decline in the reporting of major phenomena entirely to lack of interest on the part of investigators, whatever factors may have contributed to that lack. Also, some of the decline in the interest of investigators may now result from a falling off in the amount and quality of the phenomena available for study. For judging the truth of this conjecture we have little reliable data. I can assure you that claims of the major phenomena that warrant investigation have not ceased altogether, because our unit at the University of Virginia continues to be notified of them from time to time. However, our informants are not a random sample, both because they have the initiative to telephone or write to us and because they know of our existence in the first place. Surveys conducted during recent decades (Haraldsson, 1985, 1988–1989; Kalish & Reynolds, 1973; Palmer, 1979) tell us that the proportion of the general population who *believe* that they have experienced some paranormal phenomenon has not declined from that found in earlier surveys (Sidgwick, H. & Committee, 1894; West, 1948). Unfortunately, the modern surveys have elicited reports of beliefs *about* paranormal experiences, not evidence that the reported experiences are paranormal. Haraldsson (1988–1989) is the only modern surveyor of psychical experiences who has also investigated some of the claims his respondents have made. In Iceland, at least, veridical and death-coinciding apparitions seem to be reported with a frequency not appreciably less than that observed in nineteenth-century England (Sidgwick, H. & Committee, 1894). However, I believe that Iceland may not be typical of Western countries, and I think—admittedly on insufficient evidence—that a real decline in major paranormal phenomena has occurred in the West during this century. In the remainder of this Address, I propose to accept this assumption and consider some of the possible reasons for this decline.

Physical theories about the nature of extrasensory perception have been proposed since the late nineteenth century (Barrett, Gurney, & Myers, 1882); they achieved some prominence from Berger's (1940) conjectures and in recent years have become fashionable. They have gained many adherents without winning universal acceptance among persons whose opinions we should respect. If we were to decide that some physical feature, such as extremely low frequency electromagnetic waves (Persinger, 1987), correlated reliably with manifestations of extrasensory perception, we might decide that the increase during recent decades of "electronic smog" (Fox, 1988) (at least in regions having much electronic equipment) has been an important cause of the decline in major paranormal phenomena. This would lead us to expect that manifestations of extrasensory perception would vary from region to region with differences in the amount of electronic smog. Unfortunately, with our present meager resources we cannot undertake a project of the magnitude required for adequately testing this hypothesis.

I recognize in myself a bias against physical theories of extrasensory perception, because I believe that we can understand it better by a dualist concept of brain and mind that permits minds, under certain circumstances, to communicate directly with each other (outside known physical means of communication). Accordingly, my search for causes in the decline of the major paranormal phenomena has concentrated on possible psychological explanations. I have tried to think of features in which life in the West now differs from what it was one hundred years ago and from what it is in other parts of the world today. I shall consider the changes that seem to me important under the two headings of normal processes and paranormal ones.

The normal processes I further divide into changes in our conditions and manner of living and changes in our attitudes. To take the former first, I think that we have learned from the study of spontaneous cases the importance for their occurrence of both love and death. The participants are nearly always persons having bonds of affection, and the event communicated is most often some peril endangering the agent. We can say that the percipient has a need to know what is happening to the agent and the agent a need to let the percipient know (Murphy, 1943).

When normal communication is infeasible, the need for paranormal communication increases. The authors of *Phantasms of the Living* (Gurney, Myers, & Podmore, 1886) may not have realized that violent death occurred frequently among the events communicated in the cases reported in their great work. At least they did not draw attention to the fact. Nevertheless, among 314 *Phantasms* cases involving death, it had occurred violently in 28 percent. Furthermore, among the approximately two-thirds of the cases in which death had occurred naturally we found that in one-third the death had occurred suddenly (Stevenson, 1982). (We defined a death as "sudden" if it occurred within 24 hours of the deceased person's being thought well or at least, if ill, in no danger of dying.) A violent death in the nineteenth century was nearly always also a sudden one, and, if this be agreed, then almost 53 percent of the deaths involved in the *Phantasms* cases occurred suddenly. Furthermore, the persons concerned were often physically separated by long distances and normal communications were, by modern standards, extremely crude. (The telegraph was not adequately developed until the second half of the nineteenth century, and the telephone not until its last quarter.) The slowness and sometimes the impossibility of a normal communication would, I believe, increase the need to have a paranormal one. In the hundred years since the founding of our Society normal long-distance communications have greatly improved. Advances in medical care and their better deployment have also resulted in delayed deaths from violence, so that although violent deaths still occur they are not so apt to be sudden as they once were. These changes, I suggest, have reduced the need for a person who dies violently, or is accidentally injured, to communicate paranormally with those who love him or her.

The *need* to communicate paranormally has therefore diminished. Can we say that the *desire* to communicate has declined also? I said above that percipients and agents in spontaneous cases are nearly always linked in a loving relationship. No one has found a way to measure love, but certain social indicators, such as the increased rate of divorce, of crime, and perhaps of child abuse, suggest to me that our society has become, on the whole, more selfish, that is, less loving than at least some societies of other times and places. If so, this may be another factor in the decline in paranormal communications.

A third normal feature of Western society that has changed markedly during the past one hundred years is the growth of philosophical materialism. Most scientists, for example, believe in materialism as unquestioningly as they believe in Copernican astronomy. A survey of the belief in life after death conducted in 1981 showed that in the United States 67 percent of the general population believe in life after death, whereas only 32 percent of leading physicians and only 16 percent of leading (nonmedical) scientists do (Gallup, 1982). Most of us are probably familiar with the prevalence of materialism among scientists. What is not sufficiently recognized is that, although about two-thirds of respondents among the general public believe in life after death, almost one-third do not. It is to that substantial minority that I wish to draw your attention. I am not familiar with any surveys of belief in life after death in the nineteenth century, and I think there were none. However, a question posed about the belief in life after death would have shocked nearly all respondents of that time. Galton's study of the efficacy of prayer assumed that most persons attended church, prayed when they were in church, and believed—some perhaps only perfunctorily—in the power of their prayers to preserve the life of the British sovereign (Galton, 1883). I think we may assume also that everyone who engaged in prayers for the sovereign believed that the sovereign had a soul that would survive physical death; and they believed the same of themselves.

Some persons can segregate beliefs about different aspects of nonmaterial existences and events. This would be particularly likely to be true of persons who have made a special study of psychical phenomena. We know that at least two (and probably more) former Presidents of our Society have believed in paranormal cognition but not in the survival of human personality after death (Dodds, 1934; Richet, 1922). However, I think that members of the general public do not usually make such a distinction. For most of them, a belief in life after death almost entails a belief in miracles, such as the phenomena described in the Bible, and also a belief in what we call paranormal cognition. Conversely, members of the general public who do not believe in life after death are also likely to be skeptical about all kinds of paranormal phenomena, the recognition of which would imply for them a soul that would survive bodily death. If these assumptions are justified, we can conclude that the belief in paranormal phenomena has declined during the past century. (I realize that this is contrary to what the surveys that I cited earlier suggest.) Beliefs influence expectations, and numerous experiments in psychology have shown that expectations influence perceptions (Allport & Kramer, 1946; Dixon, 1981). This must also be true of extrasensory perceptions. A disbeliever in apparitions is less likely to see one than is a believer. Some disbelievers may see apparitions despite their skepticism, but the overall effect of an increased skepticism would be to reduce the number of persons sensitive to apparitions and other paranormal experiences also. In addition, disbelief may cause dismissal of a paranormal experience that does occur through quick interpretation of it as "just a hallucination" or "only a coincidence." From the consequent reduction, both of the perception of paranormal experiences and of their recognition as being paranormal when they do occur, fewer of them would be reported.

Indications of interference with paranormal phenomena may be exceedingly difficult to detect. To illustrate this point, I shall mention an observation from our study of the features of persons who claimed to remember experiences when they were recovering from being near death. Greyson and I (1980) found that such persons were much more likely to say that they had had what I call the advanced phenomena of these experiences, such as meeting deceased persons or "beings of light," when their near-fatal crisis occurred at home or outdoors than when it occurred in a hospital or other public place. I want to emphasize that I completely overlooked the importance of this finding for several years, until I happened to have occasion to review our data and suddenly realized the possible significance of this correlation. I have long thought that the attempt of some experimenters to simulate in their laboratories a home-like atmosphere by putting in deeply upholstered chairs and some well-known prints of Picasso's paintings was downright silly. To reach this mock living room, the subjects of such experimenters would usually have had to traverse half a mile of hospital or other institutional corridors which would effectively tell them that they were far from home. The results of our comparison between the experiences of persons having near-fatal crises in their homes and in their hospitals confirmed me in my bias against the use of laboratories to study paranormal phenomena, except for a few restricted purposes.

I shall next consider the possibility that spreading materialism has had an inhibiting effect on paranormal phenomena through paranormal causes. Critics tell us that allegations of their having an adverse effect on the phenomena are mere evasions of the painful truth that they have improved vigilance and tightened controls, so that the alleged phenomena do not occur in the presence of the controls they recommend. This may be true in some instances, and I am far from saying that we can learn nothing from critics. However, we for our part have obtained abundant evidence of the effect of the participants' beliefs on the delicate balance for or against paranormal effects in experimental situations (White, 1976). An atmosphere of completely unqualified belief appears to facilitate and may indeed be essential for the occurrence of paranormal physical phenomena (Batcheldor, 1966; Owen & Sparrow, 1976), and I think this may be equally true of paranormal mental phenomena. If belief facilitates them, disbelief can block them, as Schmeidler's (1943a, 1943b) experiments showed many years ago.

A person adversely affecting an experiment in extrasensory perception does not need to be physically present with the percipient. Schmeidler (1961a, 1961b) showed that the scores of percipients at card-guessing tended to be high or low according to whether an agent was wishing the percipient to succeed or to fail. Some experiments even suggest that unfavorable influences may not reach the level of an overt wish that a percipient would fail; much more subtle negative qualities may come into play (West & Fisk, 1953). Several experiments, principally of the late nineteenth century, have demonstrated a capacity for certain subjects to be put to sleep by suggestion directed at them from a long distance (Adams, 1849–1850; Janet, 1886a, 1886b; Richet, 1886; Vasiliev, 1976). There are even cases on record whose authenticity we have no reason to doubt of persons having died suddenly after they were wished to death at a distance, the victims being unaware of the fatal wishing aimed at them (David-Neel, 1961; Rose, 1965). These observations warrant us in thinking that disbelief can inhibit the occurrence of the phenomena whose authentic existence it denies.

I have made a diagnosis and, as a medical man should, I have also indicated what physicians call etiology, that is, causes. However, I am reminded now of Hilaire Belloc's slighting reference to physicians who,

> . . . answered, as they took their Fees,
> There is no cure for this disease.

Therefore, I should propose some remedies. We cannot—I say with some regret—return to all conditions as they were in the West a century ago. However, our studies may benefit from a new cycle of belief in paranormal phenomena. Perhaps the current wave of gullibility toward alleged paranormal phenomena that we see among many members of the general public, and which most of us deplore, may, by the processes I have conjectured, once again facilitate the occurrence of the major paranormal phenomena.

Let me, however, suggest three other means of finding major paranormal phenomena today. First, we can go to the countries now called undeveloped. I mean most of Asia and Africa, where social conditions are in many respects similar to those of the West in the nineteenth century or perhaps the eighteenth century. In these regions normal communications still depend largely on conveyance by word of mouth. One's own feet and perhaps the bullock-cart are the main means of movement from one place to another in rural parts. Family ties remain close,[4] everyone believes in the reality of telepathy, and the dead are conceived as having survived and being still sometimes able to intervene in terrestrial affairs. Thus impaired normal communications exist along with both a still strong desire to communicate with other persons one loves and a widespread belief that paranormal communication is possible. In these regions the major paranormal phenomena are said still to occur abundantly.

I have myself no personal experience with any form of paranormal phenomena in Asia and Africa other than that of the children who claim to remember previous lives, but I do have much experience of these cases. I have often asked myself why we find such children so much more easily in those parts of the world than elsewhere. An obvious first answer to this question is that the people of these regions nearly all believe in reincarnation, and this belief somehow facilitates and even promotes the children's narrations about previous lives. This is certainly true, but I think it is insufficient as an explanation of what we are trying to understand. There must be other factors contributing to the occurrence of these and other cases of apparent paranormal phenomena in Asia and Africa. I suggest that one cause is that the peoples of these regions still take as normal what we in the West have come to call paranormal. If I were advising a young scientist entering psychical research today, I would reverse Horace Greeley's[5] advice to young Americans of the mid-nineteenth century and say "Go East, young man."[6]

My second recommendation is a careful search for special subjects who have unusual paranormal capacities and are also willing to cooperate in scientific investigations. In the last few decades several persons with alleged or self-proclaimed gifts have appeared in our arena. Unfortunately, nearly all have tended either to become figures in the world of entertainment and mass media or to welcome and attract a circle (or crowd) of adulating and uncritical followers. The former outcome occurs most often in the West, the latter most often in Asia. With both of them conditions for quiet scientific inquiry become ruined. But we should not despair. Our predecessors had the good fortune to work with Eileen Garrett, Olga Kahl, Gladys Osborne Leonard, Stefan Ossowiecki, Eusapia Palladino, Leonora Piper, and a few others of their quality. Their like will surely be seen again; some may even be among us now, if we would just look for them. There will be no quick results in this endeavor. It may take years of sifting before an investigator finds an outstanding subject and perhaps some further years before investigations with the subject can warrant a publication. Still, the rewards from this effort in gains of knowledge might be immense.

My last suggestion might seem like a rebuke to present members of the Society, but I certainly do not intend it as such. I cannot, however, forbear from telling you that in some respects the domain of the Society for Psychical Research has broken up rather in the manner of the Austro-Hungarian Empire after World War I. If we were to pursue this analogy we might say that regions formerly held under one sovereignty have asserted their independence and gone their own ways. The departure of hypnotism after it received at least a modicum of official recognition from medicine was not regretted in the Society; some members even welcomed it as a sign of progress, because the studies of some of our early members, such as Gurney, had signally contributed to the legitimation of hypnosis. So far so good. Consider, however, the following categories: unusual healings, lucid dreams, multiple personality, mystical or religious experiences, and experiences during near-fatal injuries and illnesses. Each of these topics had the attention of our pioneers, and reports of them appear in the early volumes of our Society or in related publications by early members of the Society. And yet today each of these five categories of research has a separate society devoted to the special study of a particular type of experience.[7] I cannot explain why this happened, but I deplore it. I do not think the secession, as I see it, of these territories that we first colonized is beneficial, either to the small newly-created states or to the mother country. Some of those who have founded these smaller societies seem misguided to me, and they may find themselves more isolated from other scientists than we are.

However, our Society may have been as much at fault as those who have failed to find it an appropriate forum for their interests. The Society for Psychical Research may insidiously have come to identify the field of its endeavors as narrower than it once was or should now again become. Some may even say that the Society has begun to resemble a particular chapter of Alcoholics Anonymous in the United States, which gradually became so exclusive that it eventually denied membership to certain applicants on the grounds that they were drunkards. Some of the recently founded groups with more specialized interests than ours may have taken with them, so to speak, some of the major phenomena of which I lament the decline in our reports.

We must ask ourselves what should be the task of the Society in the remaining decade of this century and in all the decades of the next. It is certainly that of continuing to act as a third force between persons who are too credulous and those who are too skeptical. If we maintain the high standards for which we have been known and esteemed, we may once more attract first-rate scientists and scholars. So long as our Society exists, fanatical skeptics cannot say there are no paranormal phenomena to study. Also, so long as it exists, intelligent persons will have some resources against the claims of the self-deceived and the deceivers who abound around the edges of psychical research.

Our survival cannot, however, rest on an assumed position of magisterial authority. We may not be the best judges—we are almost certainly not—of the place from which the next advances in our field will come. Therefore, in maintaining our standards we must avoid any hardened dogmas that allow only familiar ideas to find expression. An open mind is not necessarily an empty one. Let us try to seek out again the major paranormal phenomena—wherever they may be. Careful investigations of these phenomena brought this Society its early fame; and such investigations can bring it a new fame as well.

NOTES

1. Presidential Address to the Society for Psychical Research, April 1989. Reprinted from the *Proceedings of the Society for Psychical Research, 57,* 149–162 (1990).—Ed.

2. This list may not be exhaustive of all those who confidently claimed the proof, or near-proof, of extrasensory perception. I have not read *all* the Presidential Addresses.

3. The circle of persons interested in psychical research and praising the work of the Society (even though not active in it) may have been larger between 1880 and 1920 than this phrase implies. I think the willingness of so many eminent men to stand in the glaring publicity of the Presidency reflects a broader acceptance of the Society's work by intellectual leaders than we can find among their successors today.

4. This is not just one more datum for dissertations by graduate students in anthropology. There are grounds for believing that the more rapid and more durable recovery from severe mental illnesses in undeveloped countries (compared with West-

ern countries) may be due to the stronger family ties that exist in these countries (Waxler, 1974).

5. This well-known phrase is correctly attributed to John B. L. Soule. Horace Greeley borrowed it and used it, but with due acknowledgment to Soule.

6. During a rehearsal of this Address my colleagues quickly told me that the direction to go East was too narrow. They reminded me that the northwest area of North America is not East, while Africa and South America are South. All these are regions where we may still find major paranormal phenomena.

7. Perhaps I should add to this list of secessions that of the skeptics, who have now formed their own group. The Society for Psychical Research has always had—from Frank Podmore on—one or more members who could be described as "skeptics in residence." However, so far as I know, these members, although they often doubted individual instances, never adopted the stance that paranormal phenomena could not be possible; and none ever advocated stopping the search for more and better evidence of the phenomena.

REFERENCES

Adams, N. (1849–1850). Remarkable mesmeric phenomena. *The Zoist, 7,* 79–80.

Allport, G. W., & Kramer, B. M. (1946). Some roots of prejudice. *Journal of Psychology, 22,* 9–39.

Barrett, W. F., Gurney, E., & Myers, F. W. H. (1882). First report on thought-reading. *Proceedings of the Society for Psychical Research, 1,* 13–34.

Batcheldor, K. J. (1966). Report on a case of table levitation and associated phenomena. *Journal of the Society for Psychical Research, 43,* 339–356.

Berger, H. (1940). *Psyche.* Jena: Verlag von Gustav Fischer.

David-Neel, A. (1961). *Immortalité et Réincarnation.* Paris: Librairie Plon.

Dixon, N. F. (1981). *Preconscious Processing.* New York: John Wiley and Sons.

Dodds, E. R. (1934). Why I do not believe in survival. *Proceedings of the Society for Psychical Research, 42,* 147–172.

Eisenbud, J. (1983). *Parapsychology and the Unconscious.* Berkeley, CA: North Atlantic Books.

Flammarion, C. (1923). Presidential address. *Proceedings of the Society for Psychical Research, 34,* 1–27.

Fox, B. (1988). Electronic smog fouls the ether. *New Scientist, 118,* 34–38.

Gallup, G., Jr. (with W. Proctor) (1982). *Adventures in Immortality.* New York: McGraw-Hill.

Galton, F. (1883). *Inquiries into Human Faculty and its Development.* London: Macmillan.

Greyson, B., & Stevenson, I. (1980). The phenomenology of near-death experiences. *American Journal of Psychiatry, 137,* 1193–1196.

Gurney, E., Myers, F. W. H., & Podmore, F. (1886). *Phantasms of the Living.* (2 Vols.). London: Trübner.

Haraldsson, E. (1985). Representative national surveys of psychic phenomena: Iceland, Great Britain, Sweden, USA and Gallup's International Survey. *Journal of the Society for Psychical Research, 53,* 145–158.

Haraldsson, E. (1988-1989). Survey of claimed encounters with the dead. *Omega, 19,* 103–113.

Janet, P. (1886a). Note sur quelques phénomènes de somnambulisme. *Revue Philosophique de la France et de l'Etranger, 21,* 190–198.

Janet, P. (1886b). Deuxième note sur le sommeil provoqué distance et la suggestion mentale pendant l'état somnambulique. *Revue Philosophique de la France et de l'Etranger, 22,* 212–223.

Kalish, R. A., & Reynolds, D. K. (1973). Phenomenological reality and post-death contact. *Journal for the Scientific Study of Religion, 12,* 209–221.

McClenon, J. (1984). *Deviant Science. The Case of Parapsychology*. Philadelphia: University of Pennsylvania Press.
McDougall, W. (1920). Presidential address. *Proceedings of the Society for Psychical Research, 31*, 105–123.
Murphy, G. (1943). Psychical phenomena and human needs. *Journal of the American Society for Psychical Research, 37*, 163–191.
Owen, L. M., & Sparrow, M. (1976). *Conjuring Up Philip: An Adventure in Psychokinesis*. New York: Harper and Row.
Palmer, J. A (1979). Community mail survey of psychic experiences. *Journal of the American Society for Psychical Research, 73*, 221–251.
Persinger, M. A. (1987). Spontaneous telepathic experiences from *Phantasms of the Living*, and low global geomagnetic activity. *Journal of the American Society for Psychical Research, 81*, 23–36.
Prince, W. F. (1930-1931). Presidential address. *Proceedings of the Society for Psychical Research, 39*, 273–304.
Rhine, L. E. (1982). Presidential address: The way it looks. *Proceedings of the Society for Psychical Research, 56*, 367–398.
Richet, C. (1886). Un fait de somnambulisme à distance. *Revue Philosophique de la France et de l'Etranger, 21*,199–200.
Richet, C. (1922). *Traité de Metapsychique*. Paris: Librairie Félix Alcan. (American edition: *Thirty Years of Psychical Research*, S. De Brath, trans. New York: Macmillan, 1923)
Rose, R. (1965). *Living Magic*. New York: Rand McNally.
Salter, W. H. (1946–1949). Presidential address. *Proceedings of the Society for Psychical Research, 48*, 239–252.
Schmeidler, G. R. (1943a). Predicting good and bad scores in a clairvoyance experiment: A preliminary report. *Journal of the American Society for Psychical Research, 37*, 103–110.
Schmeidler, G. R. (1943b). Predicting good and bad scores in a clairvoyance experiment: A final report. *Journal of the American Society for Psychical Research, 37*, 210–221.
Schmeidler, G. R. (1961a). Evidence for two kinds of telepathy. *International Journal of Parapsychology, 3*, 5–48.
Schmeidler, G. R. (1961b). Are there two kinds of telepathy? *Journal of the American Society for Psychical Research, 55*, 87–97.
Sidgwick, H., & Committee (1894). Report on the Census of Hallucinations. *Proceedings of the Society for Psychical Research, 10*, 25–422.
Smith, H. A. (1910). Presidential Address. *Proceedings of the Society for Psychical Research, 24*, 330–350.
Stevenson, I. (1982). The contribution of apparitions to the evidence for survival. *Journal of the American Society for Psychical Research, 76*, 341–358.
Stevenson, I. (1987). Changing fashions in the study of spontaneous cases. *Journal of the American Society for Psychical Research, 81*, 1–10.
Stevenson, I. (1988). Was the attempt to identify parapsychology as a separate field of science misguided? *Journal of the American Society for Psychical Research, 82*, 309–317.
Tart, C. T. (1984). Acknowledging and dealing with the fear of psi. *Journal of the American Society for Psychical Research, 78*, 133–143.
Vasiliev, L. L. (1976). *Experiments in Distant Influence*. New York: E. P. Dutton.
Waxler, N. E. (1974). Culture and mental illness. A social labeling perspective. *Journal of Nervous and Mental Disease, 159*, 379–395.
West, D. J. (1948). A mass-observation questionnaire on hallucinations. *Journal of the Society for Psychical Research, 34*, 187–196.
West, D.J., & Fisk, G. W. (1953). A dual ESP experiment with clock cards. *Journal of the Society for Psychical Research, 37*,185–197.
White, R. A. (1976). The influence of persons other than the experimenter on the subject's scores in psi experiments. *Journal of the American Society for Psychical Research, 70*, 133–166.

White, R. A. (1985). The spontaneous, the imaginal, and psi: Foundations for a depth psychology. In R. A. White & J. Solfvin (eds.), *Research in Parapsychology 1984* (pp. 166–190). Metuchen, NJ: Scarecrow Press.

4

Research on the Question of Survival After Death: Reviews and Representative Case Reports

EWK

In part 2, I discussed Ian's dissatisfaction with prevailing scientific views of human personality as the product solely of the physical body and with the conflation of mind and body in medicine, psychiatry, and psychology that has resulted. In this part, I turn more specifically to examples of the numerous kinds of phenomena that especially convinced him of the need for a greatly expanded view of the nature of human personality.

As we saw in part 3, Ian argued for the importance of studying spontaneous experiences in psychical research. To those who dismiss such cases as mere "anecdotes" and the study of them as "unscientific," Ian called attention to "the revolution accomplished within our generation in the study of animal behavior by modern ethologists. Scorned thirty years ago as mere 'bird watchers', they have shaken the dogmas of men who were content to study animals only in laboratories. Those of us who study spontaneous cases are the ethologists of parapsychology" (Stevenson, 1971, p. 123).

Ian was the premier modern "ethologist of parapsychology." He did more than perhaps anyone else in the 20th century to identify, investigate, and report what he called "major paranormal phenomena." Although in the course of his long career he investigated nearly every kind of such phenomena, he concentrated on those especially relevant to the question whether human personality survives the death of the body. As he and others have pointed out, the phenomena of psychical research in general, suggesting as they do that consciousness can operate beyond the confines of ordinary sensorimotor processes, could be said to support the survival of consciousness beyond the death of the physical body. Yet some phenomena are more directly relevant to this issue than others. Ian explained:

> Any evidence for extrasensory perception is also, in principle, evidence for the survival of human personality after death. This is because extrasensory perception, as the phrase suggests, does not occur through any known sensory organ or brain process. It indicates, on the contrary, a direct communication between two living minds or of information about a physical object to a living mind. If this kind of communication occurs, it is reasonable to suppose that whatever aspect of a living mind mediates it may survive the death of the body with which it is associated. However, evidence of extrasensory perception is only *indirect* evidence pointing toward the possibility of survival after death; and when we discuss the question of survival after death we usually mean to consider *direct* evidence that a particular personality has survived it. (Stevenson, 1982, p. 116)

Over the course of 45 years, Ian investigated and published reports of hundreds of survival-related cases, including apparitions of deceased persons, out-of-body experiences (especially those occurring during serious illnesses or accidents), information given by trance mediums about deceased persons unknown to them, xenoglossy (speaking a language not learned normally), and, most prolifically, cases of the reincarnation type, that is, cases of young children who exhibit apparent memories and physical and behavioral characteristics of a deceased person. In addition, he published numerous papers summarizing and analyzing similar cases investigated and reported by others.[1]

In 1977 Ian published an important paper outlining the history of scientific research on the question of survival after death.[2] He divided the history into three periods, each distinguished by different empirical and theoretical approaches. The first period began in 1882, when a group of distinguished British scientists and scholars founded the Society for Psychical Research, and continued until the 1930s. During this period, research was concentrated in two major areas: the investigation and analysis of large numbers of spontaneous experiences such as apparitions and out-of-body and near-death experiences, and the experimental study of trance mediums.

The investigators gave great attention to addressing the criticisms leveled at such phenomena. In investigating spontaneous experiences, for example, they pioneered the study and evaluation of eyewitness testimony (Gurney, Myers, & Podmore, 1886, chapter 4); and in the research on mediums, they took particular pains to rule out possible fraud and to address the concern that grieving or credulous persons might give undue weight to general or vague statements by mediums. Ironically, however, the most serious objection to accepting survival as the best explanation came from other research that the early psychical researchers themselves had undertaken. They had conducted numerous successful experiments, especially with hypnosis, of telepathy and clairvoyance (what we now call ESP, or psi), and it began to seem possible that the capacity for ESP in living people, and not the activity of a deceased person, might well account for phenomena such as mediumship, apparitions, or out-of-body experiences. This alternative interpretation gave rise to what has become known as the survival/superpsi (or super-ESP) debate.

The second period of research, therefore, began around the 1930s and lasted until about 1960. For many people, the survival-superpsi debate had reached an impasse, and so researchers turned their attention to the seemingly more tractable problem of experimental studies of ESP and psychokinesis. Survival research was almost completed neglected, but as Ian outlined in his 1977 paper, a few people continued to make isolated, but useful, contributions. For example, in the 1950s the sociologist Hornell Hart (1956) analyzed large numbers of apparitional and out-of-body experiences, not only older ones, but some more recent ones that had continued to be reported. In particular, he found "a significant resemblance between the characteristics of apparitions having a living agent and those having *prima facie* a deceased one," a resemblance that led him to suggest that "these latter might be generated (not necessarily volitionally) by persons who had survived physical death" (p. 158).

In this second phase, researchers—most notably the Duke psychologist J. B. Rhine—had advocated dropping survival research until limits to ESP in living persons could be delineated and thus, in essence, a line between ESP in a living person and communication from a deceased person could be established. Scientists such as Ian, however, increasingly questioned the assumption that any such limits even existed, let alone could be established. In the third phase of survival research, therefore, beginning about 1960, scientists returned to the survival question. By 1977, when Ian published his review paper (and continuing to the present), numerous studies in a wide variety of areas had been conducted by Ian himself and others, including experimental studies of out-of-body experiences, investigations and surveys of near-death experiences and death-bed visions, mediumship, and studies of cases of the reincarnation type. As Ian pointed out in his paper, much of the research of this third period was directed toward evaluation of survival versus superpsi explanations. For example, mediumship research, although nowhere near as extensive as that of the first period, focused on what Ian called "drop-in" cases (these will be described and discussed in a later section). Additionally, Ian called particular attention to cases involving unusual skills, such as the rare cases known as "xenoglossy", in which a person (either under hypnosis or in some other altered state) speaks a language he or she did not learn normally. Ian argued that cognitive information, such as names or knowledge of events, is transferrable by ESP; skills, however, are not transferrable by ordinary cognitive processes, and therefore presumably not by extraordinary cognitive processes (ESP) either.

Ian concluded his 1977 paper by summarizing the importance of survival research, and the reasons he himself devoted so much of his career to it. Not only is the question important in and of itself—"the most important that [one] can ask about himself" (p. 168)—but the relevant phenomena strongly suggest the need for "a fresh examination of many old ideas about the nature of human personality. Once considered about as well defined as an orange by its skin or a tree by its bark, human personalities now appear to be much more extensible and penetrable that they were thought to be" (p. 166). He lamented the lack of attention and resources given by scientists to such an important question, and added that if "results in this field of inquiry have been small and remain indecisive, that is because the laborers have been few" (p. 168). Ever optimistic, Ian believed that progress will come, however, once more of us "understand the theoretical issues involved in studying the question of survival after death" and recognize that "despite formidable difficulties, the question is amenable to empirical investigation" (p. 168).

I will begin this part with a brief discussion by Ian of the state of the evidence for survival.[3] The remainder of part 4 will consist of sections that include case reports, reviews, and general comments by Ian about nine specific types of phenomena that he investigated. Before beginning, however, I wish to emphasize two general points. First, in this part we are dealing with empirical phenomena alone and are leaving aside all theoretical objections to the possibility of survival after death. Part 2 addressed Ian's dissatisfaction with prevailing views of mind as wholly dependent on the body and his suggestion that a more satisfactory view might entail a kind of "vehicle," or substance, which he called a "psychophore," that is different in kind from the ordinary physical body. In this part, I ask readers to do only what Ian asked his readers to do: to examine phenomena from the perspective that survival after death is a possibility that may, or may not, be upheld by further observations and more in-depth evaluation of them.

Second, I repeat a point made in the introduction to part 2: that the depth of our understanding is directly related to the breadth of our view. What this means in the present context is that phenomena relevant to the question of survival after death must be evaluated *not* piecemeal but as a whole. As Ian pointed out many times, the strength of the evidence for survival lies in the convergence of many cases, and particularly many *types* of cases, all pointing in the same direction. A single experience may be dismissed as a mistaken observation or a coincidence; many similar experiences call out for a more adequate explanation. Similarly, we will never arrive at an adequate understanding of one type of experience without recognizing how it fits into a larger pattern involving other types of experiences.

Modern society is deeply divided over the question of survival after death. Many people, on the basis of religious faith or personal experience or both, believe in survival or at least take the idea seriously. Many others, on the basis of what current scientific orthodoxy tells us, dismiss the idea outright or at least consider it highly unlikely. Perhaps the most important lesson to be taken away from this part is that there is a large body of empirical observations relevant to the question of survival, and that no one should come down firmly on either side of the issue without considering that evidence seriously. As Ian himself put it, "the only improper stances are denial that there is any evidence worth looking at or assertion that what we have will suffice" (Stevenson, 1982, p. 120).

NOTES

1. As I mentioned earlier, the appendix contains a list of Ian's publications arranged by topic. For other reviews of the evidence for survival, see Braude (2003) and Gauld (1982).

2. I had intended to include this paper in this volume, but unfortunately the publisher would not permit it to be republished in its entirety. I will briefly summarize the paper here, particularly so that readers may get a sense of where Ian's own work fits into the history of survival research; but I encourage all readers to study the paper itself. We have limited numbers of hard-copy reprints available at our offices at the University of Virginia.

3. Although this paper dates to more than 40 years ago, and his 1977 review is more than 35 years old, I think it fair to say that the state of the evidence has changed quantitatively since then, in that we now have more cases of all types and more analyses of the data, but that it has not changed qualitatively, in that the types of evidence and the arguments for and against various interpretations of them have not changed.

REFERENCES

Braude, S. (2003). *Immortal Remains: The Evidence for Life after Death.* Rowman & Littlefield: Lanham, MD.

Gauld, A. (1982). *Mediumship and Survival: A Century of Investigations.* London: Heineman.

Hart, H., & collaborators (1956). Six theories about apparitions. *Proceedings of the Society for Psychical Research, 50,* 153–239.

Stevenson, I. (1971). The substantiality of spontaneous cases (Presidential Address). In W. G. Roll, R. L. Morris, & J. D. Morris (eds.), *Proceedings of the Parapsychological Association 5, 1968* (pp. 91–128). Durham, NC: Parapsychological Association.

Stevenson, I. (1977). Research into the evidence of man's survival after death. *Journal of Nervous and Mental Diseas, 165,* 152–170.

Stevenson, I. (1982). Survival after death: Evidence and issues. In Grattan-Guinness, I. (ed.), *Psychical Research: A Guide to Its History, Principles & Practices* (pp. 109–122). Wellingborough, England: The Aquarian Press.

FOURTEEN

Sources of Evidence Supporting a Belief in Survival

1969[1]

I believe myself that the available evidence does not compel belief in survival, but it does, I think, permit a rational belief in it based on evidence instead of grounded on faith alone. No one need feel any embarrassment about justifying his belief in survival by the available evidence from psychical research. Nor need he feel any embarrassment either from the fact that much of the evidence, especially that from apparitions and from mediumistic communications, is old evidence; evidence that was once strong does not become weaker with the passing of time in the minds of discriminating persons who are well aware that not all periods in history are equally suited to the bringing forth of certain types of evidence.

Above all, the available evidence of both older and more recent types certainly justifies a much more serious endeavor to obtain additional quantities and kinds of evidence bearing on the survival question. The diversity of evidence from many different types of cases suggests also the possibility of our finding completely new types of evidence in some hitherto neglected quarter. Let me say further that I do not agree with those parapsychologists who advise us to postpone studying the question of survival after death until we have learned the limits, if any, of extrasensory perception in the living. According to this view, only some manifestation beyond the limits of extrasensory perception, whenever these are established, would provide valid evidence for survival. Parapsychologists who admonish us thus are presumably talking about limits of distance and scope for extrasensory perception. There may indeed be no limits to these, but there may very well exist other limits to the powers and use of extrasensory perception in living persons. I am thinking, for example, of the impossibility perhaps of acquiring skills by extrasensory perception, or of the improbability that a marked capacity for extrasensory perception would be focused and limited in such a selective way as apparently occurs in some mediumistic communications and in some reincarnation cases. To improve the evidence for survival, perhaps we need a better understanding of human capacities rather than final knowledge of the limits of extrasensory perception. I therefore strongly favor renewed efforts at the present time to investigate directly the question of survival after death. I can even imagine that direct approaches to survival evidence might clarify certain obscurities connected with paranormal processes among the living.

NOTE

1. Excerpts from "Some Implications of Parapsychological Research on Survival after Death," *Proceedings of the American Society for Psychical Research, 28*, 18–35, 1969. Published with permission of the American Society for Psychical Research, Inc. (ASPR), 5 West 73rd Street, New York, New York 10023, Webpage: aspr.com, e-mail: aspr.com.—Ed.

4a

Apparitions

EWK

One of the most important contributions that psychical researchers have made over the past century and more is to show that hallucinations are most emphatically *not* limited to those who are mentally or physically ill. Throughout history people have reported seeing, hearing, or sensing the presence of deceased persons, particularly at or near the time of death (see, e.g., Crowe, 1848/1986). During the early decades after the founding of the Society for Psychical Research, its leaders learned about thousands of such cases, not only from people who reported them spontaneously but also through two large-scale surveys. Hundreds of these were investigated and reported, and the overwhelming conclusion was that such experiences occur, far more often than had previously been suspected, to healthy, awake, and sane people (see, e.g., Bennett, 1939; Flammarion, 1922–1923; Gurney, Myers, & Podmore, 1886; Sidgwick, E., 1922; Sidgwick, H., et al., 1894).

Knowing full well that, even among sane, healthy people, such experiences can be generated by sorrow, expectation, suggestion, or fear, the early investigators emphasized those cases that were what they called "veridical"—that is, experiences that are not simply subjective but objective in the sense that they correspond to real events not known normally to the percipient, a correspondence that can be verified by others. Of particular importance were what came to be called "crisis" cases—cases in which a person saw (or otherwise became aware of) an identifiable person who had died (or had some other serious crisis) close to the time of the experience, even though the percipient had no normal way of knowing or inferring that this event had occurred. Other important kinds of cases included those in which a person known to the percipient to be dead conveyed some unknown information (e.g., Gurney & Myers, 1889; Myers, 1889, 1890), or cases of "hauntings," that is, cases in which several people, independently and on different occasions, have seen a particular deceased person in a particular place (e.g., Mackenzie, 1983).

Such cases are clearly highly relevant to the question of survival, since they imply to many people that the dying or deceased person has somehow made his or her presence known to survivors. Other people, however, have argued that veridical cases suggest, not the survival of a deceased person, but the ability of living persons to learn about the death or other information by some process such as telepathy or clairvoyance. The emphasis began to shift, therefore, to cases more difficult to explain by telepathy or clairvoyance, especially collective cases, those not-infrequent ones in which more than one person simultaneously experiences the same apparition (e.g., Hart & Hart, 1933; Myers, 1886). Still other kinds of cases suggested the actual projection of some aspect of a person to a distant location. These include "reciprocal" cases, in which one person has an out-of-body experience and seems to be at a distant location, while a person at that location simultaneously sees him or her; and "bystander" cases, in which the dying or deceased person appears, not to the loved one to whom he or she would presumably have wished to appear, but to another person, sometimes even a stranger, who was present with that loved one (for references to collective, reciprocal, and bystander cases, see Stevenson, 1982). Numerous people have analyzed and discussed these two major ways of interpreting veridical hallucinations, but so far with no clear consensus in sight (in addition to the sources already cited, see, e.g., Gauld, 1982; Hart et al., 1956; Tyrrell, 1942/1953).

For most of the 20th century, few carefully investigated cases of veridical apparitions were reported. A few people, however, have continued to recognize the importance of such cases (e.g., Green & McCreery, 1975; Haraldsson, 2009, 2012; Mackenzie, 1971). Among these is Ian, who investigated and reported several such cases, including two in the 1960s (Stevenson, 1964, 1965). In the remainder of this section I include his reports of three apparition cases that he investigated, one the more common, non-veridical type, the other two of the veridical, "crisis" type.

REFERENCES

Bennett, E. (1939). *Apparitions and Haunted Houses: A Survey of Evidence*. London: Faber & Faber.

Crowe, C. (1986). *The Night-Side of Nature*. Wellingborough, England: Aquarian Press. (Original work published 1848)

Flammarion, C. (1922–1923). *Death and Its Mystery* (3 Vols.). New York: Century.

Gauld, A. (1982). *Mediumship and Survival*. London: Heinemann.

Green, C., & McCreery, C. (1975). *Apparitions*. London: Hamish Hamilton.

Gurney, E., & Myers, F. W. H. (1889). On apparitions occurring soon after death. *Proceedings of the Society for Psychical Research, 5*, 403–485.

Gurney, E., Myers, F. W. H., & Podmore, F. (1886). *Phantasms of the Living* (2 Vols.). London: Trübner. (Available at www.esalenctr.org/display/phantasms/index.html)

Haraldsson, E. (2009). Alleged encounters with the dead: Importance of violent death in 350 new cases. *Journal of Parapsychology, 73*, 91–118.

Haraldsson, E. (2012). *The Departed among the Living: An Investigative Study of Afterlife Encounters*. Guildford, UK: White Crow Books.
Hart, H., & collaborators. (1956). Six theories about apparitions. *Proceedings of the Society for Psychical Research, 50*, 153–239.
Hart, H., & Hart, E. B. (1933). Visions and apparitions collectively and reciprocally perceived. *Proceedings of the Society for Psychical Research, 41*, 205–249.
Mackenzie, A. (1971). *Apparitions and Ghosts*. London: Arthur Barker.
Mackenzie, A. (1983). *Hauntings and Apparitions*. London: Paladin.
Myers, F. W. H. (1886). Note on a suggested mode of psychical interaction. In E. Gurney, F. W. H. Myers, & F. Podmore, *Phantasms of the Living* (Vol. 2, pp. 277–316). London: Trübner.
Myers, F. W. H. (1889). On recognised apparitions occurring more than a year after death. *Proceedings of the Society for Psychical Research, 6*, 13–65.
Myers, F. W. H. (1890). Appendix to "A defence of phantasms of the dead." *Proceedings of the Society for Psychical Research, 6*, 341–357.
Sidgwick, E. (1922). Phantasms of the living. *Proceedings of the Society for Psychical Research, 33*, 23–429. (Reprinted in 1962, *Phantasms of the Living*. New Hyde Park, NY: University Books.)
Sidgwick, H., & Committee (1894). Report on the Census of Hallucinations. *Proceedings of the Society for Psychical Research, 10*, 25–422.
Stevenson, I. (1964). The blue orchid of Table Mountain. *Journal of the Society for Psychical Research, 42*, 401–409.
Stevenson, I. (1965). The case of the "teddy bear" suit. *Journal of the Society for Psychical Research, 43*, 92–93.
Stevenson, I. (1982). The contribution of apparitions to the evidence for survival. *Journal of the American Society for Psychical Research, 76*, 341–358.
Tyrrell, G. N. M. (1953). *Apparitions*. New York: Pantheon Books. (Original work published 1942)

FIFTEEN

Modern Apparitional Experiences

1995[1]

N.E. CASE

N.E., the percipient of this case, is a woman resident of Charlottesville, Virginia, who was born in 1921. She had an apparitional experience following her mother's death in 1971, when N.E. was about 50 years old. She described the experience to me during a meeting in 1984, and then furnished a more detailed account during another meeting with me in 1993. N.E. said that she has had numerous other apparently paranormal experiences.

N.E. was strongly attached to her mother. She did not believe that she was her mother's favorite child among eight siblings; but she did believe that she was the only one of them to have "psychic" abilities. About one month before her mother died, N.E. asked her mother to try, after her death, to give her (N.E.) a signal of her survival of death. Her mother agreed.

When her mother died, N.E. was grief-stricken. The funeral took place two days after the death. N.E. returned home from the funeral in a desolate state and went to bed. Her husband was also in bed. She did not sleep, but kept thinking about her mother. She became aware of a light, which was so bright that she thought it might be coming from a neighbor's automobile. Then the light came into N.E.'s room. It seemed to be yellow-green. N.E. was at first frightened and pulled the bed covers over her head. She then seemed to receive the word "Mother," and uncovered her head. Then she saw her mother, but not in full length; only the upper part of the body and the face were visible. N.E.'s mother seemed to be laughing at N.E. At first N.E. was so awestruck that she could not talk.

The apparitional figure seemed to move across the room. N.E. was then able to ask it whether she (her mother) was in heaven. The figure bowed, as if to say "yes," but did not speak. N.E. then asked: "Is Daddy with you?" The figure again bowed. By this time it had moved near the window, and then it disappeared.

N.E.'s husband was awakened by the sound of her voice and asked her with whom she was speaking; but she did not reply.

N.E.'s younger sister furnished me with a statement (in 1984) from which I quote the following:

> This is to certify that my sister, N.E., told me [that] two nights after our mother died she was in bed and a great light with different colors appeared in her room and a vision of our mother floated toward the bed. N.E. asked mother if she was in heaven and she smiled and nodded her head. N.E. also told our brother G., and possibly other members of our family, about this.

The statement was also signed by N.E.'s brother G.

N.E. told me that at the time of her vision of her mother she had not been thinking about her mother's pact to communicate with N.E. after her death.

Comment. This apparitional experience is typical of those occurring during bereavement. Although the percipient denied that she was consciously expecting a communication from her mother, the expectation was at least latent in her mind and might have stimulated the experience. For N.E., however, the vision was satisfying evidence that her mother had survived death and rejoined her husband in a heavenly realm. The appearing figure communicated no information outside the knowledge or expectations of the percipient.

R.N. CASE

R.N., the percipient in this case, is a resident of Cardiff, Wales, who was born in 1945. She has had a number of apparently paranormal experiences, including at least two apparitional ones.

The experience of this report occurred on July 20, 1989, in R.N.'s office in Cardiff. I learned about it in 1992 from Mr. Jeffrey Iverson, also a resident of Wales, who put me in touch with R.N. (Mr. Iverson, a television producer, had recently made a documentary film in which my research had figured, and he was aware of my interest in apparitions.) She wrote out for me an account of the experience dated June 3, 1993. Subsequently, on June 7-8, 1993, I met her in Cardiff and discussed details of the experience with her. R.N. took me to the office where she had had her experience. I examined the area and sketched the office, locating the place where R.N. had stood when she saw the apparition and where the apparition had seemed to be. I obtained some additional information later through correspondence.

The person figuring in R.N.'s experience was T.I., who had formerly been employed by the company for which R.N. worked. He had quarreled with his associates (not with R.N.) and quit the company abruptly. R.N. had known T.I. well when they were employed together, but did not keep in touch with him after he left their company. At the time of her experience she had not seen him for what she described as "yonks," meaning a time of indefinite length, not precisely remembered. R.N.'s husband (in a later conversation with me) estimated that a month had elapsed between T.I.'s leaving the company (where he also worked and had known T.I.) and R.N.'s apparitional experience.

The experience occurred on the afternoon of July 20, 1989, at around 3:00 p.m. R.N. remembered that she had had that afternoon an appointment with a fellow-employee whom she was advising. (She showed me the entry in her appointment book for this meeting.) R.N. and her visitor were seated in her office, but several telephone calls interrupted their conversation. When these occurred, R.N. had to get up from her chair and walk over to her desk in order to answer the telephone. The outer wall of the office behind her desk was a full sheet of glass (from floor to ceiling), and this gave a clear view of a flat walkway between two stairs that led from a parking lot to an entrance for the building. As R.N. answered the telephone on one occasion, she noticed T.I. walking past. He was wearing a navy blue shirt, a navy blue sailing sweater, and navy trousers. She remembered his "sailor's gait." (T.I. had sailed a great deal and had developed this kind of gait.) R.N. thought that T.I. seemed to be in a hurry. T.I. ordinarily had a ruddy complexion, but on this occasion—to quote now from R.N.'s account—"he was very red and he looked very troubled. He appeared perfectly solid, and I did not attract his attention through the window. I thought no more about this, it was nothing unusual." The distance between R.N. and the appearing figure of T.I. was about 10–12 feet.

On the following day, July 21, a secretary of the company told R.N. that T.I. had died. R.N. commented that his death must have been sudden, perhaps from a traffic accident, because she had seen him just the day before. The secretary replied that this could not be so, because T.I. had died in the hospital. I was able to obtain a copy of T.I.'s death certificate, which confirmed that he had died in the hospital on July 20, 1989. Mr. Iverson further learned from T.I.'s widow that T.I. had been unconscious for almost the entire day before he died and that he had died late in the evening, perhaps around 11:00 p.m.

I obtained a copy of the "clinical notes" of T.I.'s admission to the hospital. They were lamentably sketchy. The notes for July 20 stated that he was unconscious that day before he died, on the same day. They did not record the time of death.

Comment. According to the ascertained facts, R.N. saw T.I. in clothes that seemed natural for him at a time when he was not dead, but dying and unconscious in a hospital 4 miles away. There he would have been dressed in hospital clothing. For investigators of paranormal phenomena there is nothing especially unusual about a person appearing as an apparitional figure while still alive. In their classic study of apparitions, Gurney, Myers, and Podmore (1886) considered an experience to be coincident with death if it occurred within twelve hours before or after the death. It is also common in such experiences for the percipient to perceive the appearing figure in clothes familiar to the percipient, but different from those in which the appearing person was then dressed.

Some readers may suppose that a stranger unknown to R.N. passed the window of her office as she was at her telephone and that she misidentified this person with T.I. The short distance between R.N. and the appearing figure make this unlikely. Even if R.N. had misidentified a stranger as T.I., however, this would leave unanswered the question of why she mistook the stranger for T.I. instead of for someone else. Because T.I. had left the company, R.N. had no reason to expect that she would see him back at the company where he had worked.

Could R.N. have overheard the secretary talking earlier about T.I.'s illness without registering this consciously and yet having this information influence a misidentification of someone else for T.I.? I cannot exclude this possibility, but it seems unlikely. The apparent sight of T.I. would surely have brought into R.N.'s consciousness an awareness that T.I. was ill and unlikely to be walking around. On the other hand, the hypothesis of misidentification receives some support from R.N.'s noting that the appearing figure looked even ruddier than T.I. usually did.

It occurred to me that perhaps as T.I. was dying he had thought about the company with which he had worked and from which he had parted disagreeably not long before he became ill. He might have—I speculated—even considered meeting his former colleagues and making peace with them. If so, he might have mentally projected himself, as it were, back to the company's building, and this might have stimulated R.N.'s perception of him. I was unable to obtain any confirmation of this conjecture. Mr. Iverson learned from T.I.'s widow that T.I. had not discussed the company with her before he lapsed into unconsciousness. . . .

E.W. CASE

E.W., the percipient of this case, was born in 1907. She has lived all her life in Scotland, much of it in Skye. She had had numerous apparently paranormal experiences and was reputed among persons who knew her and knew about her to have what Scottish Highlanders refer to as "second sight." This phrase refers to a somewhat specialized type of paranormal perception, particularly of persons who are near to death or have died (Cohn, 1994). E.W. contributed a chapter to a book about seership (Davidson, 1989) in which she described some of her experiences, including the one I am here including. I am able to furnish some details that E.W. did not mention in her account.

The case came to my attention through reading the book in which E.W. had given a brief description of her experience. I wrote to E.W. and after some correspondence went to Vatten, Skye, where E.W. was then living, on September 3, 1992. I tape-recorded a long interview with her. In essentials, E.W.'s account of her experience to me did not differ from the one she had published, but it was more detailed.

Subsequently, I went to Dunfermline where I met and interviewed Betty McKay, the widow of the person (Ronald McKay) who had figured in E.W.'s apparitional experience. The experience had occurred in Dunfermline, and in 1992 I saw the place where it had occurred and formed some impression of the distance between E.W. and the appearing figure that she saw. Later, I believed that I had not adequately examined the site of E.W.'s experience. Therefore, when I was in Scotland again in August 1994, I returned to Dunfermline and, accompanied by Betty McKay, examined the site closely. I made a sketch of the relevant roads and buildings.

I also obtained a copy of Ronald McKay's death certificate. I learned about a further detail in subsequent correspondence with E.W.

The experience occurred early on the morning of May 29, 1975. E.W. went to the outside door of her house (which faces the main road) in order to bring inside the delivered bottles of milk that had been left on her doorstep. She later thought she had done this between 10:00 and 10:30 a.m. She looked across the road and saw her neighbor Ronald McKay walking out of the driveway of his house and then along the road or drive as if going toward the nearby factory of which he was the manager. E.W. and her husband had known that the McKays had been away on vacation and believed that they were still away. When E.W. went back inside her house, she said casually to her husband: "I see the McKays are back." Her husband asked her when they had come back. E.W. replied: "I don't know, but I saw Ron go down the drive." About half an hour or perhaps an hour later, a senior employee of Ronald McKay's factory came to the house and spoke with E.W.'s husband. He then asked her when she had seen Ron McKay, and she repeated what she had said earlier. Her husband then said that the factory employee had information that Ronald McKay had died that morning while on vacation in England about 150 miles away from Dunfermline.

The temporal coincidence between E.W.'s apparitional experience and Ronald McKay's death must have been close. The interval could not have been more than 3-4 hours. Ron McKay's widow, Betty McKay, told me that he had died at 7:00 in the morning. She and her husband had not yet dressed for breakfast. Ronald McKay had awakened with a headache, had taken a mild analgesic tablet, and gone back to sleep. A little later, when his wife tried to arouse him, she could not do so and realized that he had died. The death certificate attributed his death to "severe coronary sclerosis."

E.W. saw Ronald McKay wearing a nylon shirt tucked into flannel trousers. Betty McKay told me that this was his customary clothing for work. As mentioned, at the time of his death Ronald McKay had not got up and dressed. He was in fact naked; he always slept naked and was in that state when he died.

I estimate that E.W. had the figure of Ronald McKay in view for at least 10 seconds, because she watched him come out of the driveway behind his house and walk along the road toward his factory. The garage of this house and the driveway to it were at the back of the house as was a door of the house. Part of the driveway near the road was visible from where E.W. stood. She would have seen Ronald McKay's face as he came out of the driveway, but when he turned to walk toward the factory his back would have been toward E.W. The distance between E.W. and the appearing figure would have varied during the period of her observation. When they were closest they might have been about 50 feet apart. The figure was lifelike, and E.W. did not think she had seen a dead person until she learned about Ronald McKay's death an hour or so after her experience.

Comment. Given the facts that the appearing figure came out of Ronald McKay's driveway and that E.W. watched him for, I have estimated, 10 seconds, misidentification seems an unlikely interpretation of the case. Moreover, at the time of E.W.'s experiences there were no other houses in the immediate area except those of E.W. and her husband and the McKays. Betty McKay was quite certain that no other human being would have been walking out of the driveway at the back of their house at the time E.W. had her experience.

In this case, as in the R.N. Case, the percipient saw the appearing figure wearing clothes that the percipient was accustomed to seeing him wear, but that the appearing person was not wearing at the time.

NOTE

1. Excerpts from "Six Modern Apparitional Experiences," *Journal of Scientific Exploration*, *9*, 351–366, 1995. Three of these cases are reprinted here; two others are reprinted in the following section on "Deathbed Visions."

The percipients and informants for these cases, with one exception, have been identified by pseudonymous initials. The exception is the E.W. Case, which has been published in a shorter account with real names.—Ed.

REFERENCES

Cohn, S. A. (1994). A survey on Scottish second sight. *Journal of the Society for Psychical Research, 59*, 385–400.

Davidson, H. E. (ed.). (1989). *The Seer in Celtic and Other Traditions*. Edinburgh: John Donald.

Gurney, E., Myers, F. W. H., & Podmore, R. (1886). *Phantasms of the Living* (2 vols.). London: Trübner.

4b

Death-Bed Visions

EWK

Another kind of apparition involves those experienced by people who themselves are dying. Many hospice workers say that it is extremely common for people close to death to see, hear, or talk with already deceased family members or friends. Some even say that, when such "death-bed visions" begin, they know that death is imminent, usually within hours or days at most. Unfortunately, so far there has been little systematic research on the phenomenon to learn how often, to whom, and under what conditions death-bed visions occur.[1] As a result, many people—families of the dying as well as medical personnel and other onlookers—assume that such experiences are purely subjective hallucinations resulting from drugs, delirium, or the expectation of dying.

Such explanations, however, are clearly not adequate. For example, Osis and Haraldsson (1977/2006) found that drugs and delirium seem to *inhibit*, and not cause, death-bed visions, an observation in line with the view that Ian had long taken on such experiences. He suggested that altered states of consciousness may loosen the normal "filtering" activity of the brain and thereby facilitate access to different levels of reality; I refer readers back to part 2 and the excerpts from Ian's 1957 paper "Comments on the Psychological Effects of Mescaline and Allied Drugs" describing the "loosening" effect that psychedelic drugs seem to have and the expansion of perception or consciousness that often results. Similarly, he believed that the altered state of consciousness accompanying the dying process may bring with it awareness of things not ordinarily perceived; it may, for example, "sometimes give the dying heightened powers of extrasensory perception" (Stevenson, 1959, p. 22). In general, "as death approaches . . . the mind is more detached from the brain than it normally is . . . [and] becomes freer of the usual restrictions that its association with a physical body imposes on it" (Stevenson, 1981, p. 138).

The dismissal of death-bed experiences as subjective hallucinations also fails to take into account experiences that are *not* entirely subjective, but veridical—for example, experiences in which the dying person sees someone whom he or she did not know was dead (for a list of references to such cases, see Kelly et al., 2007, p. 410). In addition, there are cases in which a bystander has seen the death-bed vision, either instead of or in addition to the dying person. In the remainder of this section are two cases of this "bystander" type that Ian investigated.

NOTE

1. Some such research is beginning (see, e.g., Fenwick, Lovelace, & Brayne [2010]).

REFERENCES

Fenwick, P., Lovelace, H., & Brayne, S. (2010). Comfort for the dying: Five year retrospective and one year prospective studies of end of life experience. *Archives of Gerontology and Geriatrics, 51*, 173–179.

Kelly, E. F., Kelly, E. W., Crabtree, A., Gauld, A., Grosso, M., & Greyson, B. (2007). *Irreducible Mind: Toward a Psychology for the 21st Century*. Lanham, MD: Rowman & Littlefield.

Osis, K., & Haraldsson, E. (2006). *At the Hour of Death* (3rd ed.). New York: Hastings House. (Original work published 1977)

Stevenson, I. (1959). The uncomfortable facts about extrasensory perception. *Harper's Magazine, 219*, 19–25.

Stevenson, I. (1981). Can we describe the mind? (Presidential Address). In W.G. Roll & J. Beloff (Eds.), *Research in Parapsychology 1980* (pp. 130–142). Metuchen, NJ: Scarecrow Press.

SIXTEEN

Modern Apparitional Experiences

1995[1]

D.I. CASE

D.I., the percipient of this case was born in 1951. The experience she reported occurred in Groton, Connecticut. She later moved to a small town in North Carolina. Her experience occurred when she was 14 years old. She described it afterward to members of her family, but they told her not to talk about it and forget it. She could not forget it, but she seems to have discussed it with almost no one else until she communicated it to our Division in a letter dated July 17, 1991. I corresponded with D.I. about details of the experience and on February 13, 1993, went to the town in North Carolina where D.I. then lived and tape-recorded a long interview with her. D.I. showed me copies of the death certificates of her maternal grandparents.

By the time I came to investigate this case (in the 1990s) two persons who might, at least to some extent, have corroborated D.I.'s account of the experience—her mother and stepfather—had died. From what she said, however, it is doubtful whether they would have made willing informants.

D.I. was a girl just under 14 years of age at the time of her experience, which occurred on January 4, 1965. Her maternal grandfather was living with her, her mother, stepfather, and two brothers. He was dying of leukemia and in such an enfeebled condition that it had been decided to admit him to a hospital. The day before his transfer to the hospital he had been heard calling for D.I.'s father (not her stepfather, who was a member of the current family). Later, D.I.'s mother thought that her father was calling for her first husband (whom she had divorced) because he wished to become reconciled with him before he (her father) died. Such a wish on the part of a dying person for reconciliation with persons from whom the dying person has been alienated occurs not uncommonly (Callanan & Kelley, 1994).

On the day of this planned transfer to the hospital, D.I. had a throat infection and stayed home with her grandfather. Her siblings, mother, and stepfather were all out of the house, at school or work. Her stepfather was due to return home in time to be there when the ambulance came to take D.I.'s grandfather to the hospital. The apparitional experience occurred in the late morning of that day not long before D.I.'s stepfather was due to return to the home. I quote now from D.I.'s first letter about the experience:

> Granddaddy called to me to give him a drink of water. I failed in my attempts to lift him enough to wet his lips. The disease had reduced his once tall, strong stature to [that of] a frail, weak invalid. I called mom at work to ask for help, but she told me it would have to wait until dad [D.I.'s stepfather] returned from work at noon.
>
> Shortly thereafter I heard granddaddy calling out to his wife, Hazel. Grandmom had died nine years prior [on October 13, 1956], so I thought he must be losing his mind. I ran down the hall to make another attempt to help him. I was amazed to find him sitting up, smiling with his arms reaching out. The room was filled with a warm, bright light. He spoke to grandmom, who was standing at the foot of his bed. Neither of them acknowledged my presence. She was there but a brief moment, and when granddaddy laid back down, his soul escaped with her. He died with a smile on his face.

During my interview with D.I., I asked her about details of her vision of her grandmother. One question concerned her assurance that the figure she saw (and her grandfather seemed to see) was really that of her grandmother. Her grandfather's calling out the name "Hazel" was part of the evidence, but apart from that D.I. had known her maternal grandmother well; D.I. had been five years old when her grandmother had died.

D.I. furnished some further details about the clothing that her grandmother seemed to be wearing, or rather not wearing:

> I remember that question in the first letter [of I. S.] and I have given that a lot of thought and I don't, I honestly don't recall clothes. I just recall that it ... a very bright white light and that her face is there and I see her hands. I can see an image of arms but I don't see clothing. She is either in all white or the white light is so bright I can't see the clothing.
>
> S.: But you saw her face?
> D.I.: Her face, right.
> S.: And her arms?
> D.I.: I can tell that the arms are out reaching but the light is so bright and I am not focusing so much on detail. I don't really recall.

I also asked for more details about how D.I.'s grandfather had called for "Hazel" and how the light had appeared. She replied as follows:

> I heard him calling me. But when he starts calling my grandmother's name I am at the other end of the hallway . . . I don't remember exactly what I was doing but I heard him call, "Hazel." But it was in a very nice voice. It wasn't the command he had given me. And I was trying to figure out why is he calling her. He was calling my father last night and he knows my father doesn't live here and now he is calling my grandmother. . . . I can still visualize it. If this was the room and his bed was here the light came out of that corner there of the ceiling and it came, shone right down at the very foot of his bed. And she was not on the floor. . . . I didn't see her feet. But she was above the floor. And if a conversation was held between them it was not to my ears. You could see very beautiful, peaceful expressions on their faces. That is the most vivid part of it for me. That they both were just so at peace at seeing each other. And he raised up. By the time I get to the room he didn't even acknowledge that I had come to the room. He raises up and he raised his arms up to reach her and he just laid back. And when he laid back down he had a smile on his face and his eyes were open. . . . When I am looking at him, then I look back and she was gone. And I got hysterical because I knew without even knowing how. I didn't know how to check for vital signs or anything. I just knew that he was dead. That he had passed.

Comment. Given that 26 years elapsed between this experience and its first recording in written form some doubts may be expressed about the accuracy of D.I.'s memory. I will discuss the question of the accuracy of memories in these cases later.[2]

If we assume the accuracy in essential details of D.I.'s report, the case fits in the category of what Osis and Haraldsson (1977/2006) described as "takeaway cases." By this term they referred to the phenomenological appearance that the perceived figure has come to receive the dying person into the life after death.

If we assume that D.I.'s grandfather perceived his late wife, Hazel, at the time he was calling out her name—and he certainly acted as if he perceived her—the case is also one of a collective apparitional experience. These are defined as experiences shared by two or more persons present at the time and in a position to perceive the appearing figure; definitions vary slightly according to the detailed requirements for "being present." Among all apparitional experiences collective ones occur in about a third of cases (Sidgwick et al., 1894) or perhaps in as many as 56% (Hart & collaborators, 1956).

B.I. CASE

B.I., the percipient of this case, was born in 1921. He is a physician who practiced as a pediatrician and has lived most of his life in a large city in North Carolina. His apparitional experience occurred on June 30, 1955. He first described it to my colleague Dr. Emily W. Cook [Kelly] (E.W.C.) in July 1983, and she made a written record of it on August 12, 1983. In 1992 I wrote to him and asked him to write an account of the experience, which he sent in a letter dated November 5, 1992. On December 12, 1994, I went to B.I.'s home in North Carolina and had a long interview with him. He mentioned at this time some additional details about his experience.

The experience occurred at the time B.I.'s mother-in-law, F.C., died. His father-in-law, G.C., had died 7 years earlier, in 1948. I quote now from B.I.'s letter of November 5, 1992:

> F.C. had had several minor cerebral vascular accidents in the year before she died, but the one 3-4 days before her death was a devastating one. She never regained consciousness. Her children and her physician agreed to keep her comfortable at home and to avoid any life-extending procedures.
>
> I was standing by her bed and no one else was in the room. She had an agonal inspiration, and at that moment I had a very clear picture of G.C. [her late husband] standing across from me with his arms outstretched, and he said: "Flora, I've been waiting for you."
>
> I did not really have to look to see that my mother-in-law had died, but the physician in me pushed me to verify that.

At our meeting in December 1994, B.I. told me that the figure of his father in-law was quite opaque, as he would have seen him in life. B.I. saw the figure only from the waist up, but he believed that the furniture in the room might have prevented him from seeing more of the figure if it had been visible.

E.W.C. remembered from her conversations with B.I. about his experience that the appearing figure of B.I.'s father-in-law had addressed his dying wife as "Flossie," her nickname in the family. When asked about this discrepancy, B.I. checked with three other members of the family (with whom he had discussed his experience) and found that their memories of the name agreed with that of E.W.C. B.I. said that he deferred to their memories of what he had told them earlier.

On the question of his acquaintance with his father-in-law, B.I. said that he and his wife married in 1950, two years after his father-in-law died. He thought that he might have met his father-in-law once or twice some years before his death. He was, however, familiar with his appearance from photographs in the family.

As a pediatrician B.I. had often treated children who had died. He had sometimes prayed for their sufferings to end. Sometimes, after a child had died, he had a kind of inner "flash of seeing" the child running around and playing after being released by death. B.I. attributed these images to "my own hopes that they were at last free to do so [run and play] and my own somewhat vivid imagination." He was sure, however, that he had no expectation of seeing his father-in-law at the moment his mother-in-law died. He wrote: "I was surprised but comforted by what I saw."

Comment. As with the preceding case, a long interval—in this one 28 years—lapsed between the experience and the first written account of it. Again, we confront the question of the accuracy of the percipient's memory over such a long interval.

Investigators of apparitions classify this case as one of the "bystander type." The phenomenal aspects of the experience, assuming survival after death, suggest that G.C. (B.I.'s deceased father-in-law) had come to receive his wife as she died. He (G.C.) had no special interest in B.I., whom he may have met once or twice. Yet B.I. perceived him, whereas his dying mother-in-law showed no evidence of having done so. (She was in a coma.) This is why the appearing person is described as appearing to a bystander rather than to the person with whom he or she presumably would have wished to communicate. Gurney and Myers (1889) and Haraldsson (1987) reported other bystander cases.

NOTES

1. Excerpts from "Six Modern Apparitional Experiences," *Journal of Scientific Exploration, 9*, 351–366, 1995. Two of these cases are reprinted here; three others are reprinted in the previous section on "Apparitions."—Ed.

2. I have omitted this discussion here, but Ian began it thus: "The folk myth about memories of such cases over a period of time is that they become embellished over the years. The evidence points away from this as a generalization" (p. 363).—Ed.

REFERENCES

Callanan, M., & Kelley, P. (1994). *Final Gifts: Understanding the Special Awareness, Needs, and Communications of the Dying*. New York: Poseidon Press.

Gurney, E., & Myers, F. W. H. (1889). On apparitions occurring soon after death. *Proceedings of the Society for Psychical Research, 5*, 403–485.

Haraldsson, E. (1987). The Iyengar-Kirti case: An apparitional case of the bystander type. *Journal of the Society for Psychical Research, 54*, 64–67.

Hart, H., & collaborators (1956). Six theories about apparitions. *Proceedings of the Society for Psychical Research, 50*, 153–239.

Osis, K., & Haraldsson, E. (2006). *At the Hour of Death* (3rd ed.). New York: Hastings House. (Original work published 1977)

Sidgwick, H., et al. (1894). Report on the census of hallucinations. *Proceedings of the Society for Psychical Research, 10*, 25–422.

4c

Out-of-Body and Near-Death Experiences

EWK

Many people today have heard about near-death experiences—experiences that occur at a time when a person is seriously ill or threatened with death in an accident, but recovers. Frequently the person will say that he or she seemed to be out of the physical body and watching events going on, say, at the scene of the accident or in the hospital room. People also describe feelings of great joy and peace and seeing deceased loved ones, or a bright light, or a place of great beauty. In the past nearly four decades such experiences have become the subject of talk shows, best-selling personal accounts, and scholarly research. Although many people who have such experiences become convinced of survival and lose their fear of death, until recently most researchers neglected the question of whether they do in fact provide evidence for survival, preferring instead to address less controversial questions such as the after-effects of the experience.

Ian long ago recognized that, although many of these experiences, like many apparitions and death-bed visions, are entirely subjective, there are features that provide more objective evidence relevant to the issue of survival after death (Stevenson, 1977, p. 161). In some instances in which the person seems to be detached from the physical body, he or she reports seeing actual, verifiable events going on at a distance. Such veridical out-of-body experiences, while not common, are more common than most people realize, and Ian himself investigated some (Cook [Kelly], Greyson, & Stevenson, 1998; Kelly, Greyson, & Stevenson, 1999–2000; see also Hart & Hart, 1933).

An even more important consideration is that in many near-death experiences, as the brain and body are shutting down, the person's mental processes remain clear or even become more vivid. Such observations are in opposition to what the physicalist model of mind/brain relations predicts: that the mind, totally dependent on the brain, shuts down in lockstep with the brain One analysis of cases that Ian and his colleagues investigated showed that the closer to death a person actually was at the time of the near-death experience, the more likely he or she was to experience such enhanced mentation (Owens, Cook [Kelly], & Stevenson, 1990). Particularly important in this regard are cases occurring during cardiac arrest or under general anesthesia, conditions in which the brain processes currently considered essential for consciousness are abolished (Kelly et al., 2007, pp. 415–421). Like experiences associated with psychedelic drugs, dying, and other altered states of consciousness, near-death experiences suggest that, as the brain's normal filtering mechanisms break down, the mind is in some sense liberated.

For many years beginning in the 1950s, Ian investigated reports of out-of-body experiences, particularly those occurring in connection with illnesses and accidents. In the remainder of this section are some general comments that he made about such experiences, followed by a report of one of the many cases that he investigated.

REFERENCES

Cook [Kelly], E. W., Greyson, B., & Stevenson, I. (1998). Do any near-death experiences provide evidence for the survival of human personality after death? Relevant features and illustrative case reports. *Journal of Scientific Exploration, 12*, 377–406.

Hart, H., & Hart, E. B. (1933). Visions and apparitions collectively and reciprocally perceived. *Proceedings of the Society for Psychical Research, 41*, 205–249.

Kelly, E. F., Kelly, E. W., Crabtree, A., Gauld, A., Grosso, M., & Greyson, B. (2007). *Irreducible Mind: Toward a Psychology for the 21st Century*. Lanham, MD: Rowman & Littlefield.

Kelly, E. W., Greyson, B., & Stevenson, I. (1999-2000). Can experiences near death furnish evidence of life after death? *Omega: The Journal of Death and Dying, 40*, 513–519.

Owens, J. E., Cook [Kelly], E. W., & Stevenson, I. (1990). Features of "near-death experience" in relation to whether or not patients were near death. *The Lancet, 336*, 1175–1177.

Stevenson, I. (1977). Research into the evidence of man's survival after death. *Journal of Nervous & Mental Disease, 165*, 152–170.

SEVENTEEN

Cardiac Arrest Remembered

1971[1]

The interesting letter of Drs. MacMillan and Brown (*Canadian Medical Association Journal, 104,* 889, 1971) on a patient's memories of events during a cardiac arrest prompts me to offer a few comments on similar cases I have studied.

The authors have apparently not encountered such experiences in other patients. A large number of similar cases, however, have been reported, although very few have reached the literature of clinical medicine. Most such reports have been published in the journals of psychical research.

It is true that few are from patients who have had cardiac arrest;[2] most have had sudden loss of consciousness, as on sustaining a severe head injury, receiving light anesthesia[3] (for dental work or at obstetric delivery) or being on the verge of drowning. The descriptions of the experience have certain features in common, viz. the sensation of viewing one's body from a point external to it, the unusual clarity of one's mental processes, the feeling of peace and tranquillity and even of ecstasy, and the sensation of floating and moving rapidly from one location to another.

The paucity of these cases among patients with cardiac arrest may derive from the fact that until recently most such patients died and could not relate their experience. We should also consider the possibility that different physical factors accompanying the abrupt alterations in consciousness may play some part in bringing on the experience.

Large scale surveys of these cases are called for so that recurrent patterns can be analyzed. A survey by Osis (1961) elicited much useful data in this general area but did not devote attention to the feeling of being outside one's physical body and looking down on it.

I have studied nearly 50 cases of this nature and, with my colleagues, am engaged in analyzing them. We shall welcome any information from others. The incidence of these experiences is much higher than most physicians realize. Many subjects have great reluctance to say anything about them to physicians for fear of being derided, being thought hallucinated or psychotic. When physicians themselves are better informed of this situation they will be better able to inquire into these experiences and more likely to hear about them from their patients.

NOTES

1. Letter to the Editor, *Canadian Medical Association Journal, 105,* 689, 1971.—Ed.
2. Now, nearly 40 years later, with improved methods of resuscitation, a great many experiences occurring under cardiac arrest have been reported (for some references to reports of these cases, see Kelly et al., 2007, p. 372).—Ed.
3. Since this letter was published, many cases occurring while the patient was deeply anesthetized have also been published (Kelly et al., 2007, p. 416).—Ed.

REFERENCE

Osis, K. (1961). *Deathbed Observations by Physicians and Nurses* (Parapsychological Monograph No. 3). NY: Parapsychology Foundation.

EIGHTEEN

Comments on "The Reality of Death Experiences: A Personal Perspective"

1980[1]

[Dr. Rodin] speaks to us as a medical man who has himself come close to death and survived. Moreover, he has altered his initial evaluation of his experience. Although he at first believed that he had had a preview of death (and liked it), he later became convinced that what he remembered were mere fragments of a toxic psychosis. Dr. Rodin has not explained how he came to change his first evaluation of his experience, but his use of the expression "toxic psychosis" gives us a clue to his reasons and, at the same time, shows us that these reasons may not be sound. . . .

The dying process usually involves a diminution of the oxygen supply to the brain and a corresponding increase in carbon dioxide reaching it. Cerebral anoxia can certainly induce confusion that may be described as a "toxic psychosis." Mental obfuscation is the core of a psychosis. But is that what most persons who have near death experiences describe? Not at all. They remember themselves as having enjoyed unusual mental clarity at the time of nearly dying. Seldom, if ever, they tell us, have they felt more alive, alert, and mentally clear than they did during the near death experience. And this heightened lucidity and sense of aliveness occurred at a time when, to observers watching the patient's body, he seemed either dead or about to become so. I do not object to describing these persons as "toxic," but I do protest against describing them as "psychotic" when what they remember afterwards is far from what patients with the conditions we usually call psychoses remember later about their experiences. One of the patients whose near death experience I studied had had (during his late childhood) a severe illness with a high fever and delirium. (When I interviewed him he was a physician, and so he knew what we mean by the term "delirium.") Then, as his physical condition worsened (so he was told later), his mental state suddenly changed. He saw himself looking down on his physical body from a position above it; but, more importantly, a condition of mental pellucidity abruptly replaced the mental confusion from which he had been suffering. Surely experiences of this type tell us that we still have only a crude understanding of the relationship between the condition of the brain and our conscious experiences.

NOTE

1. These are excerpts from a paper in the *Journal of Nervous and Mental Disease* (*168*, 271–272, 1980) in which Dr. Stevenson comments on a paper published by a neurologist, Dr. Ernst Rodin (*Journal of Nervous and Mental Disease, 168*, 259–263, 1980), describing an experience that he himself had during surgery.—Ed.

NINETEEN

The Case of Linda McKnight

1998[1]

This case was first drawn to our attention early in 1961 by a psychiatric resident of the University of Virginia Hospital. Mrs. McKnight had been a schoolteacher of the resident's wife, and she had once told her class about her experience; it had remained clear in the memory of the student who later became the psychiatric resident's wife. Mrs. McKnight was 34 years old at the time of the experience, which occurred in 1930. In 1961 it seemed worth investigating, if that were possible. I.S. asked the resident to write to Mrs. McKnight requesting her to send us a written account of her experience. She replied in a letter dated January 20, 1961, from which we quote the following:

And now for my story:

As it would seem to an observer.

The day after a gall-bladder operation, I was supposed to be "doing as well as could be expected," when a friend of mine—[a] former nurse—was allowed to bring me some flowers. She gave one look [at me], rushed out to inquire where my nurse was and said I looked as if I were sinking fast. Then she phoned my husband at his office to tell him to come to the hospital immediately. (This trip with police escorting the taxi took about 23 minutes.) Fortunately, my surgeon was in the hospital and he, the resident, and I think an intern came down immediately. He administered heart stimulants by hypodermic, etc., but when my husband came in, the Doctor said: "It's too late, Sir. And this shouldn't have happened because she was making a good recovery." Then he told the nurses to hold the body so it wouldn't slip and had the men lift the mattress to an upright position. He said they were to drop the mattress on signal. When he gave the signal, the jar of the fall started the heart beating again—and the patient lives.

Now as it occurred to me.

When my friend came in she seemed to move as before a slow motion picture camera laying the bouquet of flowers on the table with much deliberation, turning very, very slowly and moving toward the door. I was aware of a sensation of deep cold, an inner cold, and things grew dark, then black—"blacker than midnight in a cypress swamp" as James Meldon Johnson describes the world before God created day and night. After this coldness and blackness came oblivion. Suddenly it was as if someone had turned on a flood light and I glowed in its warmth. My first thought was "no pain—wonderful—I'm free—I can go where I please!" I went to the window to see what was outside. In the street four stories down a boy was teasing a much smaller girl, trying to take away her skates. I thought I should intervene but before I had really left the room my husband came in. He said: "Linda, why do you leave us?" and I turned back. I remember thinking it odd he was bowed over a figure on the bed instead of looking at me. Then I "heard" the conversation [between the doctor and the husband and between the doctor and the nurses] and saw them raise this body and mattress. Suddenly as if someone snapped a rubber band I was jerked into the room, into cold, into blackness, into oblivion. Then there I was in bed with the pain again and people standing around.

My first reaction was I had dreamed this fantastic thing. I said to my husband: "Did you think I had left you?" He began to cry. When the surgeon came I said: "So you thought you'd lost me, didn't you?" and he said gruffly: "We never lose patients. Who's been talking to you?" By this time, because of their reactions, I felt I must prove this experience. I knew the children wouldn't still be playing on the walk. I tried to recall other details. I remembered seeing a Christmas tree on the balcony below (this was February) and a whole area of sheets flapping in the wind. I asked my nurse what was out the window and she said she didn't know but she'd look. Fortunately I spoke in time. "Don't tell me," I said, "Let me tell you. There's a Christmas tree on the balcony below." She had to open the window and lean out to see this. She confirmed the drying area [of the sheets] behind to the left.

Then I knew I had died and had come back again.

I.S. entered into correspondence with Mrs. McKnight about details and obtained the following additional information.

Mrs. McKnight was sure that she had told the nurse about the sheets drying below the window before the nurse looked out the window. She wrote: "I know I did [this] because I was trying to recall details which I had seen which would prove the reality of an experience."

In reply to a question about whether Mrs. McKnight might have seen the area below her hospital window as she was brought into the hospital, she replied: "I entered the hospital at 3.00 a.m. in agony of a gall-bladder attack. I'd never been there before. I was taken to my room, where I was put to bed against the inner wall. Soon afterward I went to sleep under sedation. The only time I left the bed was to be wheeled to the operating room." I.S., not fully satisfied, pressed for more details about the location of the yard where the sheets had been drying in relation to the hospital entrance. Mrs. McKnight replied: "If a drying yard had been beside its [the hospital's] front door, I wouldn't have seen it the night I entered the hospital about 2.00 a.m. in the throes of a violent gall-bladder attack. I'm sure however when I looked out of the window it [the drying area] was on some side street. I don't remember which direction the room faced."

Mrs. McKnight could not remember the name of the hospital where she had had her experience. She did remember the names of the two principal doctors concerned in her operation and experience; but they had both died before 1961. More than 20 years later we began a systematic search for medical records associated with NDEs. We wrote to Mrs. McKnight again. In reply, her daughter wrote to say that Mrs. McKnight had died on March 28, 1984 at the age of 88. Her daughter remembered hearing her mother describe her experience of nearly dying. She thought her mother had had her operation in a hospital in New York City, which she named. We applied to this hospital for the medical records (for which Mrs. McKnight's daughter, as her next of kin, had signed a release to us), but the records could not be found.

Mrs. McKnight, faced with some skepticism on the part of her surgeon, as described above, wanted to discuss her experience with someone else and had asked to see her minister. He was still alive in 1961, and she gave us his name and address. The Rev. Colin Weston replied cordially to our letter. He said that he remembered listening to Mrs. McKnight recount her experience the day after it happened. Unfortunately, he could remember no details clearly. He wrote: "It seems to me she spoke of being outside a window while her body was inside the house. More than this I cannot say, though, I remember, she was very earnest about the experience."

NOTE

1. Excerpts from Cook [Kelly], E. W., Greyson, B., & Stevenson, I. (1998). Do Any Near-Death Experiences Provide Evidence for the Survival of Human Personality after Death? Relevant Features and Illustrative Case Reports. *Journal of Scientific Exploration, 12*, 377–406. The name is a pseudonym.—Ed.

4d

Mediumship

EWK

Certainly one of the most important bodies of evidence for survival after death is that deriving from research with persons who, usually while in a trance or other altered state of consciousness, seem to be communicating with deceased people. Such persons have been known throughout history and across cultures, and they achieved widespread and highly publicized notice—and notoriety—in the 19th century with the spread of Spiritualism. Serious research with such persons—often called "mediums"[1]—began in the late 19th century and continued in earnest through the first decades of the 20th century. Mediumistic phenomena were quickly recognized by the early psychical researchers as especially important because, unlike most other phenomena relevant to the survival issue, they could be produced deliberately and under controlled conditions. Mediums could be, and were, kept under surveillance; the bereaved persons (called "sitters") could be brought to them anonymously; and the information conveyed by the medium—and, ostensibly, by the deceased persons—could be evaluated objectively.

Under these conditions a vast amount of material was collected, analyzed, and reported.[2] It quickly became apparent that the best mediums were getting accurate information about deceased persons in some "supernormal" way, that is, not by means of ordinary sensory processes. The question was, In exactly *what* way? As we saw in the case of apparitions, there are two main theories. Some investigators adhere to the idea that the phenomenon is what it seems to be—communications from a surviving deceased person. Others favor the idea that the medium obtains the information through telepathy with living persons or clairvoyance of physically remote records, objects, and events, that is, "super-ESP" or "super-psi." Over the years, the investigation of mediums increasingly came to be shaped by attempts to discriminate between these two possibilities, but it eventually became clear that the impasse was not going to be resolved easily, or perhaps *ever*. As a result, by the mid-20th century most psychical researchers and parapsychologists had abandoned the study of mediumship.

Just as he kept alive the study of spontaneous cases when most investigators had abandoned them for experimental studies, and kept alive the question of survival when most investigators had abandoned it too, so did Ian, along with a few like-minded colleagues, keep alive the study of mediumship. His primary contribution here was to call attention to a kind of case not readily explainable by super-psi, involving what in 1970 he named "drop-in" communicators (Stevenson, 1970). In these cases, instead of deceased persons known to the medium or to the sitters, a complete stranger appears and gives enough information to allow subsequent verification of his or her identity.

Whereas one of the strengths of mediumship research is that it allows for conditions to be controlled by the investigator, "drop-in" cases are by definition unexpected and uncontrolled and, as such, easy to fake. Ian clearly recognized this and not only exposed instances when such faking likely occurred (Stevenson & Beloff, 1980) but also provided guidelines for evaluating whether normal explanations can account adequately for a case (Stevenson, 1983).

On the other hand, these guidelines also emphasized situations in which normal explanations are *not* adequate—when, for example, the information can only be verified with multiple sources, in unpublished documents, or by the private memories of survivors. Such cases are important because the motive seems far stronger on the part of the deceased person, who often seems to want to communicate some unfinished business, than on the part of the medium or the sitters, who have no knowledge of, or reason to want to hear from, this particular person. Survival, in short, seems a more likely explanation than super-psi.[3]

Several such cases have been published (e.g., Gauld, 1971, 1982). In 1970 (p. 53) Ian mentioned that he had collected about 60 published reports of drop-in cases and was preparing a monograph on them. Unfortunately, by the time of his death he had not done this.[4] He did, however, investigate and publish five drop-in cases (Haraldsson & Stevenson, 1975a, 1975b; Ravaldini, Biondi, & Stevenson, 1990; Stevenson, 1970, 1973). One of these is, in my view, especially important because a written record of what the medium said was made before the deceased person was identified. The report of this case follows.

NOTES

1. "Medium" is a rather question-begging term, suggesting as it does that the person serves as a conduit between the living and the deceased. As a result, some people have preferred the word "automatist," which emphasizes the subliminal or "automatic" processes (such as automatic writing or trance speaking) by which the phenomena are often produced (Myers, 1890, p. 669).

2. For an excellent review, see Gauld (1982).

3. The survival/super-psi impasse is another area where we desperately need a tertium quid approach (which I mentioned in the General Introduction and will discuss more fully in the Conclusion) that can push us beyond the impasse. I agree with those who find the supposed dichotomy between living-agent and deceased-agent hypotheses to be less than clear-cut, since psi must be operating in either case. And, as Michael Sudduth (2009) has so well demonstrated, arguments that undercut living-agent psi are a double-edged sword and work equally well to undercut deceased-agent psi.

4. I am currently working on the material that he left and plan to publish it.

REFERENCES

Gauld, A. (1971). A series of "drop in" communicators. *Proceedings of the Society for Psychical Research, 55,* 273–340.

Gauld, A. (1982). *Mediumship and Survival.* London: Heinemann.

Haraldsson, E., & Stevenson, I. (1975a). A communicator of the "drop in" type in Iceland: The case of Runolfur Runolfsson. *Journal of the American Society for Psychical Research, 69,* 33–59.

Haraldsson, E., & Stevenson, I. (1975b). A communicator of the "drop in" type in Iceland: The case of Gudni Magnusson. *Journal of the American Society for Psychical Research, 69,* 245–261.

Myers, F. W. H. (1890). Review of A. Aksakof's *Animismus and Spiritismus. Proceedings of the Society for Psychical Research, 6,* 665–674.

Ravaldini, S., Biondi, M., & Stevenson, I. (1990). The case of Giuseppe Riccardi: An unusual drop-in communicator in Italy. *Journal of the Society for Psychical Research, 56,* 257–265.

Stevenson, I. (1970). A communicator unknown to medium and sitters: The case of Robert Passanah. *Journal of the American Society for Psychical Research, 64,* 53–65.

Stevenson, I. (1973). A communicator of the "drop in" type in France: The case of Robert Marie. *Journal of the American Society for Psychical Research, 67,* 47–76.

Stevenson, I. (1983). Cryptomnesia and parapsychology. *Journal of the Society for Psychical Research, 52,* 1–30.

Stevenson, I., & Beloff, J. (1980). An analysis of some suspect drop-in communications. *Journal of the Society for Psychical Research, 50,* 427–447.

Sudduth, M. (2009). Super-psi and the survivalist interpretation of mediumship. *Journal of Scientific Exploration, 23,* 167–193.

TWENTY

A Communicator of the "Drop In" Type in Iceland: The Case of Gudni Magnusson

1975[1]

INTRODUCTION

In a previous article (Haraldsson & Stevenson, 1975) we reported the case of a "drop in" communicator who manifested through the Icelandic medium, Hafsteinn Björnsson. We have also published a report of a successful experiment carried out in the United States with Hafsteinn (Haraldsson & Stevenson, 1974). Since we gave in these papers considerable information about the medium we shall not repeat here what we have earlier written about him.

The case of Runolfur Runolfsson developed differently from that of the usual "drop in" communicator who comes, says what he has to say, and then leaves to be heard from again rarely or never. The communicator Runolfur Runolfsson (nicknamed "Runki") continued to manifest through the mediumship of Hafsteinn, and, as we described in our earlier report, he eventually became, and still remains, the medium's principal control. The case we are now presenting conforms to the more common type of "drop in" communication in that after the communicator established his identity he did not appear again.

CASE REPORT

As in our study of the case of Runolfur Runolfsson, we derived our first information for the report of this case from a book by Elinborg Larusdottir (1946). We have added to this information the results of further inquiries made by ourselves. We present first a summary derived from a translation by one of us (E.H.) of Elinborg Larusdottir's report.[2]

The Communication and Initial Investigations

A sitting with Hafsteinn Bjornsson was held on January 25, 1941, at the home of Gudrun Jonsdottir in Reykjavik. Also attending this sitting were Hansina Hansdottir and Hjalmar Gudjonsson. The latter, a resident of Strandhofn in Vopnafjordur,[3] was visiting in Reykjavik, and it was he who asked that the sitting be held and paid the medium's fee.[4]

Two days after the sitting (January 27, 1941) Gudrun Jonsdottir visited a friend, Asmundur Gestsson, and mentioned the sitting of January 25 to him. Gudrun Jonsdottir complained that the sitting had, in her opinion, been rather a failure since they had had an intruding communicator who seemed particularly to address himself to Hjalmar Gudjonsson. But the latter could not place this communicator and indeed was somewhat annoyed because the stranger seemed to prevent him from receiving messages from deceased persons he had known and hoped to hear from.

Gudrun Jonsdottir told Asmundur Gestsson about some of the details given by the communicator about himself. The latter had mentioned, for example, that he had close ties with a place called Eskifjordur and said that he had died there. This gave Asmundur Gestsson the idea that he could write for verification of these details to a cousin, Gudrun Gudmundsdottir, who was the wife of a physician, Einar Astrads, practicing in Eskifjordur.

On February 26, 1941, Asmundur Gestsson wrote to Gudrun Gudmundsdottir about the "drop in" communicator. He asked in his letter (quoted below) if her husband, who was the only physician in Eskifjordur, had ever had a patient by the name of Gudmundur or Gudni Magnusson (the communicator's name given by Finna, the medium's control) and if so, whether he had been injured by an automobile or in an automobile accident, dying from the injuries. Gudrun Gudmundsdottir replied in a letter (also quoted below) dated March 14. It verified the information contained in Asmundur Gestsson's letter and gave details of how a young man named Gudni Magnusson had died following internal injuries which developed after a long walk made necessary when a truck he was driving ran out of gasoline.

At this point Asmundur Gestsson realized the potential importance of the case and he therefore asked Gudrun Jonsdottir to write to Hjalmar Gudjonsson requesting him to send a written report to her of all the details he remembered of what Gudni had said during the sitting of January 25, 1941. (Unfortunately, no notes had been taken during this sitting.) Gudrun Jonsdottir herself also wrote out a statement about the sitting. We shall give next E.H.'s translation of their reports.

Hjalmar Gudjonsson furnished the following statement, which was dated March 30, 1941:

> The first thing that Finna [Hafsteinn's control at this seance[5]] said to me was that a young man was with me and that he was of average height, blond, and with thin hair at the top of his head. He was between 20 and 30 years of age and was called Gudni Magnusson. She [Finna] could easily see him. She said that he had known some of my relatives, and also that he and his death were connected with Eskifjordur and Reydarfjordur. He had been a car or truck driver.[6] She saw clearly how he had died. He had been repairing his car, had crawled under it, stretched himself, and then had ruptured something inside his body. Then he had been brought by boat between fjords to medical care, but died on the way. That is all I remember.
>
> (Signed) *Hjalmar J. Gudjonsson*

The following statement, dated June 6, 1941, was received from Gudrun Jonsdottir:

> I am writing the following to clarify further what came through at a seance with Hafsteinn Björnsson that was held on January 25, 1941, for Hjalmar J. Gudjonsson. . . . The meeting began in the usual manner. Then Finna, the medium's control, started to tell what she saw [in connection] with Hjalmar.
>
> Hjalmar had never been at a seance before and did not believe this [what Finna told him] since he did not recognize in any way at all the man Finna described to him. I had the impression that he did not want to hear anything further from this unknown man, so I asked Finna about him myself. Finna said: "This man has living parents and I see connected with him a countryside or 'herad'. " I asked: "Can you describe the circumstances in which he died?" Finna then said: "He was alone in a car on his way over a mountain pass and then the car broke down. I see clearly how he crawled under the car and then something inside him tore. He died from that." I asked: "Did he die immediately?" Finna said: "No, he managed to get to his home, and then I see he was carried by boat. He was brought to a doctor. I see the boat between fjords and that he died on the way in the boat." I asked: "Can you tell me between what fjords he was to be brought [for medical care]?" Finna said: "I cannot get that, but Eskifjordur is what he has most on his mind." I asked: "How long do you think it is since he died?" Finna said: "I cannot see that clearly. I believe it to be some months, about four or five, but it could be more or less. This man seems to have become well oriented [in the after-life], but he does not feel secure." I asked: "What do you think he wants from Hjalmar? Something specific?" Finna said: "He just came to him since they are both from the same

> part of the country and he is also trying to get strength from him. You should think well of him. That gives him strength." We talked some more about the young man, but I do not remember any of that so clearly that I feel justified in including it in a written statement.
>
> (Signed) *Gudrun Jonsdottir*

The third sitter at the seance, Hansina Hansdottir, signed Gudrun Jonsdottir's statement with a short sentence saying it was accurate according to her recollection.

Readers of the above two statements, which were written independently, will notice that Gudrun Jonsdottir's statement contains many more details than that of Hjalmar Gudjonsson. Two factors may explain this. First, Gudrun Jonsdottir was an experienced sitter whereas Hjalmar Gudjonsson had never attended a seance before. And secondly, when he lost interest in the communicator, Gudrun Jonsdottir took up the conversation with him. It is thus not surprising that she remembered more details of what the communicator said during the sitting.

As already mentioned, the letter Asmundur Gestsson received from his cousin, Gudrun Gudmundsdottir, in Eskifjordur contained details of the circumstances of Gudni's death, and we now give E.H.'s translation of this letter, which was dated March 14, 1941:

> You are probably surprised by my immediate answer to your letter. You know I am always a lazy writer. Because of what you wrote in your letter regarding an accident, I was asked [by Gudni's parents] to write you immediately and ask for all further information, including where you obtained this little information [shown in Asmundur Gestsson's letter, to his cousin], and if you can say anything more about it. This is the case as we know it:
>
> There is a married couple here [in Eskifjordur] by the name of Anna Jorgensen and Magnus Arngrimsson. The husband has worked for a long time at road building both in Mulasyslu and Thingeyjarsyslu, and in recent years his wife has always lived with him wherever he happens to be working. . . . One of their sons . . . who was about 20-21 years of age [he was actually 24 at the time of his death, see below], was a truck driver and had been for the past two or three years. He had often worked with his father in road building. Last fall this young man, whose name was Gudni Magnusson, was very busy with his truck driving and he left in the morning to go to Vidifjordur, a rather long and strenuous journey. Then later in the day he went to Reydarfjordur. After reaching there he left for home. His truck was not running well and the trip took longer than usual. He was alone. When he was crossing the mountain pass between Reydarfjordur and Eskifjordur, the truck ran out of gasoline. So he left the truck and went down to Eskifjordur to obtain some gasoline in a can. That meant a walk of four miles each way and when he returned home he was exhausted. During the night he experienced extremely severe pain in the stomach. Einar

[Astrads, the writer's husband and the physician of the area] was sent for and went to him, but could not diagnose his condition at first.

The next day Einar had to go to Reydarfjordur and stayed there the whole day. In the evening he received a telephone call at Reydarfjordur asking him to come quickly [back to Eskifjordur] because Gudni's condition had become very critical. Einar was also asked to bring with him the army doctor stationed at Reydarfjordur if that would make it easier to help Gudni. The [two] physicians arrived at nine o'clock in the evening and they saw immediately that the young man was in a very critical condition and probably suffering from some internal rupture or intestinal obstruction. They could do nothing with the patient where he was. They therefore decided to send the young man at once to the hospital at Seydisfjordur. They could not use an airplane because, being October, it was already dark. They therefore took Gudni in a motorboat, but he died on the way between Nordfjordur and Seydisfjordur. This is what we here know about this incident. When I read your letter, I naturally thought of this young man because his name was Gudni Magnusson, and although this was not an automobile accident, the young man was working with a truck and working strenuously. So I decided to let the boy's parents see that part of your letter that dealt with this incident. They found it extremely interesting and asked me by all means to write at once and obtain all further information possible. I hope you will write again and tell me all the details.

(Signed) *Gudrun Gudmundsdottir*

In June, 1941, Asmundur Gestsson visited Eskifjordur, where he stayed with his cousin, Gudrun Gudmundsdottir, and her husband, Dr. Einar Astrads. He wanted to meet Gudni's parents, but they were away for the summer. He left them a letter in which he enclosed copies of the two statements from the sitters which we have quoted above, and also asked their permission for the use of their names in a publication of the case. This Gudni's parents readily gave in a letter of reply.

During his stay in Eskifjordur, Asmundur Gestsson was able to verify some other details in the communication from a woman who knew Gudni and his family well. She told him that Gudni's hair was blond and also that, something rather unusual for such a young man, it was beginning to become thin at the top.

The medium's control, Finna, had mentioned a connection between the young man and "herad." This word in Icelandic refers to any large area of land, but it is also a proper name for a particular section of eastern Iceland known as Fljotsdalsherad or, in a shortened form, as Herad. It was therefore relevant to the communicator.

Asmundur Gestsson did not verify that Gudni or his family had actually known relatives of the sitter Hjalmar Gudjonsson, to whom the communicator seemed particularly attracted. The most that can be said about this point is that since both came from the same (eastern) part of Iceland (which is a thinly populated country) it is possible that the two families did have some acquaintance. It is certain, however, that Hjalmar Gudjonsson had no conscious recollection of ever having met Gudni Magnusson or having heard of his death.

Later Investigations by Ourselves

When E.H. returned from the United States to Iceland in the autumn of 1971 and again in the spring of 1972, he continued the investigation of the case with whatever informants and documents were still available.

Asmundur Gestsson had died in the late 1940s, and Einar Astrads, the physician of Eskifjordur, had also died many years earlier. His wife, Gudrun Gudmundsdottir, was near death when E.H. reached Iceland and died not long thereafter, so she was not interviewed. However, E.H. met her daughter, Inga Einarsdottir, who found and gave E.H. two pertinent letters from Asmundur Gestsson to her mother. In her report of the case (summarized above), Elinborg Larusdottir (1946) did not reproduce these letters. However, we shall do so because the first (which we have already mentioned above) provides an additional summary of the communication written soon after the sitting at which it occurred and before any details had been verified. And the second letter contains some additional details of interest.

Asmundur Gestsson's first letter to Gudrun Gudmundsdottir is dated February 26, 1941, that is, about one month after the sitting:

> For specific reasons I want you kindly to look into and let me know if you have any knowledge of whether a certain man by the name of Gudmundur Magnusson has had an accident by being caught under a car some time ago in Eskifjordur or Reydarfjordur and died from it. Most likely the car had fallen upon him, and the man was under the car repairing it when this happened and he then was injured internally. I do not know with any certainty how long ago; perhaps it was eight to ten months or a year or more. The man probably came from Herad, but this is not certain. I expect that in such a case Einar [Dr. Astrads, Gudrun Gudmundsdottir's husband] would have been called and he could therefore give some information. The man's name might as well be Gudni as Gudmundur. I am not personally involved in this, except that I have been asked to inquire into this . . . but as you see the information is not very clear and it is not certain if the accident happened in Einar's area.
>
> (Signed) *Asm. Gestsson*

As mentioned above, Gudrun Gudmundsdottir replied to this letter on March 14, 1941, and we have already quoted this reply as translated by E.H. from Elinborg Larusdottir's book (E.H. was not able to obtain the original). Asmundur Gestsson wrote his cousin again on April 18, 1941, and we quote the following translated excerpts from his letter:

I must send you a few lines with this ship mainly to thank you for your good letter which I received. . . . I still cannot give you more information, or rather I do not want to at present because this case does not involve myself personally, though I think this so important that I must do something about it. The story that led up to it [the writing of his first letter] is as follows: Last winter there came to me a woman whom I know to be a reliable person [this refers to Gudrun Jonsdottir, in whose home the seance was held]. She is related to my deceased wife. She had a reason to visit me. Then we happened to talk about the fact that she had recently attended a seance with a reliable medium. I asked her if anything interesting had happened. Nothing much as far as she herself was concerned, she said. But a man [Hjalmar Gudjonsson] was with her [at the sitting]. He lives . . . in Vopnafjordur and was a guest in town. This woman says that what happened to him might be a remarkable proof. . . . He who came through, Gudni Magnusson, wanted urgently to give information about himself to the man from Vopnafjordur, who I understand knew little or nothing about the "guest." He [the communicator] stressed that his death had occurred in connection with a car in Eskifjordur, and more that I will not mention now, though I want to state that the information you gave me in your letter [of March 14, 1941] fitted surprisingly well with his story. As the woman [Gudrun Jonsdottir] was telling me [about the seance], I understood from her that it would be impossible to get the necessary information [for verifying the communication] as none of those present knew the "guest" at all. Then it crossed my mind that the man had said he had ties with Eskifjordur, and if his story made any sense, then the physician at Eskifjordur would know about his death. I promised the woman to write to you and make inquiries. We did not expect much from this, but thought it worth while to try. Nor was this a matter of personal interest to the woman or to myself as neither of us knew the "guest," and not even the man from Vopnafjordur [Hjalmar Gudjonsson]. . . .

I will not write more now, only that the woman above [Gudrun Jonsdottir] wrote to Vopnafjordur and asked the man there [Hjalmar Gudjonsson] to whom the "guest" came to give as detailed a report [about the seance] as he could. Now she is waiting for an answer. [This was the statement dated March 30, 1941, which we have cited above. But it had not been received in Reykjavik at the time of the writing of this letter, probably because of the slowness of the mail by sea.]

I would like to hear from you again and learn something about the dead man's parents, especially of their interest in psychic matters, for if this is their deceased son, as it seems, he certainly wants to prove to them that he lives. . . .

(Signed) *Asm. Gestsson*

E.H. met Hjalmar Gudjonsson, who was (in 1971–1972) living in Reykjavik. He said that in 1941 he was living in the eastern part of Iceland and had only been on a short visit to Reykjavik at the time of the sitting there, which he remembered well. He was a relative of Gudrun Jonsdottir. He told E.H. that he had read the account of the sitting in Elinborg

Larusdottir's book (1946) and found it accurate. He added that he had been much impressed by the sitting.[7] At the time it took place he had never been to Eskifjordur, and since then only once. He had never known any relatives of Gudni Magnusson, nor had any of his own relatives, so far as he could ascertain, known Gudni. E.H. asked Hjalmar Gudjonsson if he had received any information—for example, in Gudrun Jonsdottir's letter asking for his statement—about the verifications before he wrote his account on March 30, 1941. He replied that he had not. As indicated above, he had already returned to Vopnafjordur before he was asked for his statement, so he was out of touch with the other sitters except by sea mail.

E.H. also interviewed Gudni's brother and sister, Otto Magnusson (born in 1910) and Rosa Magnusdottir (born in 1918). They both confirmed the accuracy of the report in Elinborg Larusdottir's book. Otto Magnusson provided additional verifications of the communicator's description of himself. He was particularly impressed by the detail of thinning hair at the top of Gudni's head, something unusual for a young man of his age at the time he died. He also verified some of circumstances of Gudni's death, as did Rosa Magnusdottir.

Gudni's family did have one relative in Reykjavik at the time of Gudni's death. This was Kafsteinn Jorundsson, his maternal uncle, who died shortly before E.H.'s arrival in Iceland in the spring of 1972. Kafsteinn Jorundsson would naturally have been notified of Gudni's death soon after it occurred. However, Otto Magnusson was not aware of any connection between his uncle and Hafsteinn Björnsson, nor between Hafsteinn and any other member of Gudni's family. According to Otto Magnusson, his uncle was rather "anti-spiritualist" and probably would not have moved in the same circles as Hafsteinn or ever attended any sittings with him.

The Cause of Gudni Magnusson's Death

E.H. obtained a copy of Gudni's death certificate. (Such records, incidentally, are not accessible to the general public, and E.H. obtained access to it only through special exertions. We do not think that it could have been seen by Hafsteinn.) The officially recorded causes of Gudni's death were "intestinal perforation" and "peritonitis." Otto Magnusson told E.H. that as a child Gudni had developed some kind of intestinal trouble which required surgery, and that during the operation "some of the intestines were cut away and sewed together again." Evidently some exertion during Gudni's truck journey led to a tearing of his intestines at a place of weakness residual from the operation of his childhood. This would then have led rapidly to peritonitis from which he died in a comparatively short time,[8] as indicated in Gudrun Gudmundsdottir's letter cited above.

There was no autopsy, but the known facts of his illness make the official attribution of the causes of death almost certainly correct.

The death certificate did not mention the place of Gudni's death, but gave the date as September 28, 1940. His birth certificate gave his date of birth as September 14, 1916.

Gudni's Obituary Notice

Although Inga Einarsdottir had said she was sure that no account of Gudni's death had appeared in any Reykjavik newspaper (in 1940–1941 no newspapers were published in eastern Iceland), we felt that we should check on this ourselves. The only paper at all likely to have printed an obituary of Gudni was *Morgunbladid,* so during a visit to Iceland of I. S. in September, 1972, we checked its files for the autumn of 1940. (At a later date E.H. searched the three other newspapers published in Reykjavik during 1940–1941, but found no mention of Gudni.) Since Gudni was an obscure person who had lived and died in eastern Iceland, we were somewhat surprised to find an obituary notice about him in the November 7, 1940, issue of *Morgunbladid.* It included a photograph of him and about a third of a column of printed matter. The photograph showed a young man one would judge to be in his twenties. It also indicated that he was blond, but although there was a little recession of hair at the upper left of the forehead, no one would have conjectured from seeing this photograph that the man was becoming bald, with thinning of hair at the top of his head.

The text of the obituary notice gave the date of Gudni's birth (September 14, 1916) and of his death (September 28, 1940), so that his age at death could easily be calculated. The names of his parents were also given. The article, however, contained nothing about the circumstances of Gudni's death nor its cause. It mentioned that he had been buried in Eskifjordur (from which it could be inferred that he had lived there), but did not include the names of the other two places (Reydarfjordur and Herad) that were mentioned in the communication. The short article consisted mainly of an eulogy of the deceased, with some reminiscences about his interests and ambitions.

We concluded that this obituary could not have furnished all the verified information in the communication. But we thought that the author of the article, E. Bjarnason, might have known more about Gudni than he had included in it and had perhaps communicated this information in some manner to Hafsteinn. Fortunately, E. Bjarnason (born in 1895) was still living, and E.H. was able to interview him. He had lived in Eskifjordur until 1949, when he moved to Reykjavik. Although he was much older than Gudni, they had been good friends and shared various activities. E. Bjarnason was a personal friend of the editor (in 1940) of *Morgunbladid,* and it was because of this friendship that the newspaper published the obituary of Gudni. Otherwise it would probably not have taken any notice of the death of a young resident of eastern Iceland.

E. Bjarnason told E.H. that he had never met Hafsteinn, nor did he know any relatives or friends of Gudni living in Reykjavik apart from Kafsteinn Jorundsson, Gudni's uncle mentioned above. . . .

DISCUSSION

This case has the unfortunate weakness that no record of the communication was made until at least a month after it was received. And the sitters did not write out their accounts of the seance until approximately two and four months after it was held.

We consider the letter of February 26, 1941, from Asmundur Gestsson to his cousin Gudrun Gudmundsdottir an important document in the case because it provides a written record of some of the communications made before any were verified. It thus compensates, at least partially, for the defect we have just mentioned, the failure to make notes during the sitting. The statement written on March 31, 1941, by Hjalmar Gudjonsson was, according to him, also written before he had any knowledge of the verifications even though Asmunder Gestsson had by then received the first verifications from Gudrun Gudmundsdottir in her letter of March 14. Gudrun Jonsdottir's statement was not written until June 6, several months after Asmundur Gestsson had verified the main facts of the communication, and thus we cannot be sure Gudrun Jonsdottir's memory of the communicator's statements was uncontaminated by her knowledge of the verifications. But Asmundur Gestsson's letter of February 26, although it does not contain all the details the sitters recalled (especially some of those mentioned by Gudrun Jonsdottir), includes essential items such as the communicator's name, his connection with Eskifjordur and Reydarfjordur, and the cause of his death. Readers will have noted that at the time this letter was written the sitters evidently thought that the communicator had died as a result of an internal injury that was somehow related to the breakdown of a truck. Asmundur Gestsson's letter definitely mentioned the detail of some internal injury.

We do not think that anyone will question our conclusion that the verified details of the communication correspond closely with ascertained facts or justified conjectures about the life and death of a single person, Gudni Magnusson of Eskifjordur. The communicator came from a part of Iceland which the medium had never even visited. The sitters, even including the one person present (Hjalmar Gudjonsson) who was from eastern Ireland, had no connection whatever with Gudni or his family.

The newspaper obituary could not have furnished the medium with all the correctly communicated details, nor could the writer of the obituary, who then lived in eastern Iceland which the medium had never visited. The communicator had an uncle in Reykjavik, but as far as we can learn, he had no connections with the medium. Thus despite extensive inquiries we have not been able to find any channel for normal communication to the medium of the correct information he had about Gudni Magnusson and expressed at the seance under consideration. We conclude, therefore, that despite its obvious weaknesses, the case justifies an interpretation that includes some paranormal process.

The main purpose of this report has been the presentation of another case of a "drop in" communicator that we believe to be authentic. The significance of "drop in" communicators for the question of the survival of human personality after death is a large topic of great theoretical and practical significance. One of us has offered some discussion of this matter in connection with a case of this type reported earlier (Stevenson, 1970), and we do not think it necessary to dilate further on the theme here.

NOTES

1. Excerpts from the *Journal of the American Society for Psychical Research, 69,* 245–261, 1975 (E. Haraldsson, co-author). Published with permission of the American Society for Psychical Research, Inc. (ASPR), 5 West 73rd Street, New York, New York 10023, Webpage: aspr.com, e-mail: aspr.com—Ed.
2. Elinborg Larusdottir made it clear in her book that the case was first investigated by Asmundur Gestsson.
3. We think it will assist readers if we make a few comments here on geographical factors in this case. All places mentioned (except Reykjavik) are in eastern Iceland. During the years concerned in this case, 1940–1941, the roads in eastern Iceland were poor and movement was largely by boat. Boats were also the main means of transportation between the eastern part of Iceland and Reykjavik in the western section of the country.
4. In one of our earlier reports (Haraldsson & Stevenson, 1975) we stated that Hafsteinn is not a professional medium. This is true in the sense that he is a full-time employee of the state radio company in Iceland. But he does accept fees for his sittings.
5. In Hafsteinn's mediumship, communicators sometimes give their messages directly to the sitters without a control acting as an intermediary. This was the case in the communications from Runolfur Runolfsson (Haraldsson & Stevenson, 1975). At other times, however, Hafsteinn's control relays the statements of the communicators to the sitters. The communication from Gudni occurred in this way, with Finna playing a role very similar to that generally played by Feda in Mrs. Osborne Leonard's sittings (Thomas, 1947). In Mrs. Leonard's mediumship some communicators also at times dispensed with Feda and communicated without her participation (Thomas, 1950).
6. In everyday use of their language Icelanders do not distinguish, as do English-speaking persons, between "car" and "truck." The communications refer to a car and so do some of the verifying statements. In fact, Gudni drove a truck and his illness occurred shortly after he returned home from a trip in this truck.
7. Contrary to the impression conveyed by Elinborg Larusdottir's book, Hjalmar Gudjonsson thought that at this sitting he had received a communication from an uncle who had drowned; he told E.H. that he was much impressed by the details this communicator gave concerning the drowning.

8. In the days before antibiotics, death from peritonitis could ensue within 48 hours, and could be hastened if internal hemorrhage occurred. Gudni died about 36 hours after returning home in his truck.

REFERENCES

Haraldsson, E., & Stevenson, I. (1974). An experiment with the Icelandic medium Hafsteinn Björnsson. *Journal of the American Society for Psychical Research, 68,* 192–201.

Haraldsson, E., & Stevenson, I. (1975). A communicator of the "drop in" type in Iceland: The case of Runolfur Runolfsson. *Journal of the American Society for Psychical Research, 69,* 33–59.

Larusdottir, E. (1946). *Midillinn Hafsteinn Bjornsson* [*The Medium Hafsteinn Bjornsson*]. Iceland: Nordri.

Stevenson, I. (1970). A communicator unknown to medium and sitters: The case of Robert Passanah. *Journal of the American Society for Psychical Research, 64,* 53–65.

Thomas, C. D. (1947). A new hypothesis concerning trance communications. *Proceedings of the Society for Psychical Research, 48,* 121–163.

Thomas, C. D. (1950). Personal control in trance sittings. In W. H. Salter, *Trance Mediumship* (pp. 35–40). London: Society for Psychical Research.

4e

Cases of the Reincarnation Type

EWK

We come next to the class of cases that was not only the one studied most extensively by Ian but also virtually discovered by him. As I mentioned in the General Introduction, in 1960 he published a two-part paper in which he described cases, unearthed in his wide reading, of what he came to call "cases of the reincarnation type," or CORT. Over the next 45 years he learned about and investigated about 2500 such cases from all parts of the world, West and East. Most of them involved very young children between the ages of about two and eight who seemed to have memories related to another person's life, such as his or her name, mode of death, family members, occupation, interests, and the like. Many of them showed behavior consistent with that person's life, such as a fear of water when that person had drowned or a strong desire to return to the previous parents, spouse, or children. Many of them also had unusual physical characteristics, such as a prominent birthmark or birth defect, often corresponding to the deceased person's mode of death. In 9 books and more than 60 papers, Ian published detailed reports of over 300 such cases, as well as the methods that he used to investigate them, analyses of features of large groups of them, and evaluations of possible explanations. (A listing of these books and papers may be found in the appendix.)

Ian's ultimate decision to focus primarily on these cases resulted in large part because they, more than any other phenomenon, bear on the two major issues that preoccupied him: the origins of individual differences—physical, mental, and behavioral—and the relationship between mind and brain. With regard to the evidence such cases may provide for survival after death, Ian himself had the following to say:

> Along this line we may in the end obtain more convincing evidence of human survival of physical death than from other kinds of evidence. In mediumistic communications we have the problem of proving that someone clearly dead still lives. In evaluating apparent memories of

> former incarnations, the problem consists in judging whether someone clearly living once died. This may prove the easier task and, if pursued with sufficient zeal and success, may contribute decisively to the question of survival. (Stevenson, 1960, p. 117)

The remainder of this section consists, first, of excerpts from a paper that gives a general overview of research on the question of reincarnation. This is followed by a report of a fairly typical case. The final part of this section is one report from a paper that described three cases of a kind that are especially important: those in which a written record of what the child said was made before the two families had any contact with each other. The importance of such records in *any* kind of spontaneous psi experience has been emphasized since the earliest days of psychical research, but they are unfortunately not easy to come by, primarily because most people are either too caught up in an experience, especially when it happens suddenly, to make a written record, or do not realize the importance of such records as objective corroboration of the experience. Nevertheless, such cases do exist (e.g., that of Gudni Magnusson in the previous section), including 33 CORT cases (see Keil & Tucker, 2005, for a list of references to these cases)[1].

NOTE

1. For an analysis of the number and accuracy of statements made by the subjects in cases with written records as compared with cases without them, see Schouten and Stevenson (1998).

REFERENCES

Keil, H. H. J., & Tucker, J. B. (2005). Children who claim to remember previous lives: Cases with written records made before the previous personality was identified. *Journal of Scientific Exploration, 19,* 91–101.

Schouten, S. A., & Stevenson, I. (1998). Does the socio-psychological hypothesis explain cases of the reincarnation type? *Journal of Nervous & Mental Disease, 186,* 504–506.

Stevenson, I. (1960). The evidence for survival from claimed memories of former incarnations. Part II. Analysis of the data and suggestions for further investigations. *Journal of the American Society for Psychical Research, 54,* 95–117.

TWENTY-ONE

Reincarnation: Field Studies and Theoretical Issues

1977[1]

INTRODUCTION

The word *reincarnation* refers to the concept that human beings (and perhaps subhuman animals) consist of two separable components, a physical body and a psychical entity or soul. At the death of the physical body the soul persists and, after a variable interval, becomes associated with a new physical body. As will be seen later, this is merely a short working definition which does not take account of the varying ideas held by different peoples about the nature and details of reincarnation. Although this chapter will be mainly concerned with describing and analyzing the evidence for reincarnation, the evaluation of such evidence requires some understanding of the beliefs held about it throughout the world. This makes appropriate a summary account of some of these beliefs.

THE EXTENT OF THE BELIEF IN REINCARNATION

Many different peoples have believed in reincarnation, and many believe in it today. Among Westerners the belief is most commonly associated with the Hindus and Buddhists of Southeast Asia, but this is probably due to the availability in the West of writings about Hindus and Buddhists and by them, and of translations of the scriptures which expound their beliefs. Western readers are usually less familiar with the fact that many other peoples of the world have also believed in reincarnation and do so at present. The scope of this chapter precludes a survey of all the peoples of past times who have believed in reincarnation. (Interested readers may consult Head and Cranston [1967] as a valuable introduction to the vast literature of this topic.) Students of this subject, however, need to understand how widespread have been the reports of the belief in reincarnation published by authors writing even within the present century. The belief has been reported among such groups as the following: some Islamic sects of western Asia such as the Alevis (Stevenson, 1970) and Druses (Stevenson, 1966/1974); numerous natives in North America, especially of the northwest areas, including Alaska (de Laguna, 1972; Slobodin, 1970; Stevenson, 1966, 1966/1974); many tribes of East and West Africa (Besterman, 1968; Deschamps, 1970; Noon, 1942; Parrinder, 1954, 1956; Thomas, 1968; Uchendu, 1964; Zahan, 1965); the Trobriand Islanders of the South Pacific (Malinowski, 1916); the northern tribes of Central Australia (Spencer & Gillen, 1904); and the Ainu of northern Japan (Munro, 1963). The foregoing list is not intended to be exhaustive, but should suffice to show that even in modern times many peoples outside Southeast Asia have believed in reincarnation and still do. The belief is in fact so widespread outside the culture of Europe and its derivatives in the Americas as to suggest the idea that all peoples not influenced by European ideas hold it. This, however, would be incorrect. Recent inquiries have shown that the Alevis of Anatolia do not believe in reincarnation (Bayer, 1970–1971), although they may once have done so, as other Alevis of south central Turkey still do. Similarly, the Ismailis, an Islamic sect of the Shiite branch, no longer believe in reincarnation (Makarem, 1972, 1973) although their ancestors once did. And Van de Castle (1973) found no evidence of the belief in reincarnation among the Cunas of Panama.

Many Europeans and Americans (of South and North America), apart from the native groups mentioned above, also believe in reincarnation. A Gallup poll taken in 1968 in eight countries of western Europe showed that an average of 18 percent of persons in these countries believed in reincarnation. A similar poll carried out in the United States and Canada showed that 20 percent of the Americans and 26 percent of the Canadians questioned believed in reincarnation (Gallup International, 1969).

A consideration of the occurrence of a belief in reincarnation in widely separated cultures raises the question: How does (or did) the belief arise in these different cultures? In some instances we know or can surmise that the belief spread by normal means of communication. For example, there has been some communication between India and western Asia since protohistoric times and it is not improbable that the belief in reincarnation in India had some influence on its occurrence in western Asia. (There are also, however, important differences in the particular ideas about reincarnation found in Southeast Asia and in western Asia.) But such normal communication could not possibly account for the occurrence of the belief in reincarnation in northwestern Canada and West Africa, both of which have been effectively isolated (at least with regard to cultural influences) from Southeast Asia since man began to develop different cultures thousands of years ago. We are therefore on quite safe ground in supposing that the belief in reincarnation arose independently in different places and at different times.

It is possible to reach the idea of reincarnation through philosophical argument. The quickest route by this method is to assume the existence of a soul and its immortality and then to ask whether a soul that has no terminus to its existence can have had a beginning. Schopenhauer used this argument when he wrote: "Whoever believes that man's birth is his beginning must also believe that his death is his end" (Schopenhauer, 1908, vol. 2, p. 558; my translation). And from the concept of the prenatal existence of the soul it is a short step to the idea that the soul had incarnated in other physical bodies before the birth of its present one.

Although other philosophers besides Schopenhauer have believed in reincarnation on purely rational grounds (McTaggart, 1915; Plato, 1910), it is unlikely that the belief arose in such a complicated way among groups of food gatherers and primitive cultivators. It seems more probable that they came to it through the examination of experiences that fell within their purview. These would be described by persons who claimed that they could actually remember having lived before. Such persons would presumably communicate their experiences at least within their own village and often, perhaps, to groups outside it. To the extent that observation in modern times has been possible, persons having such experiences have been found in every culture where the belief in reincarnation is strong and also in some where it is not.

We know, however, that some peoples in the past believed in reincarnation without our having received from them accounts of anything like the experiences of apparent memories and evidence that can be found today. In India, for example, the belief in reincarnation can be traced as far back as the later Vedas; but although early scriptures and myths of India contain scattered allusions to persons having memories of previous lives, we do not have any account of a fully developed case, such as this chapter will be mainly concerned with, until the eighteenth century A.D. Similarly, we know that some of the ancient Greeks believed in reincarnation, and Greek philosophers such as Plato (1910) argued the merits of the concept in detail, but without citing supportive case material of which, as in ancient India, there exist some fragmentary accounts. E. R. Dodds (1971) explained this by supposing that, if there had been any acceptable case material in ancient Greece, philosophers like Plato would have considered it irrelevant and almost undignified to descend from the heights of rational argument to the lower levels of empirical inquiry. A third example derives from the history of the Cathars, a heretical sect which flourished in southern France during the twelfth and thirteenth centuries (Madaule, 1961; Nelli, 1972). Reincarnation formed an important tenet of their creed, but from them also we have received almost nothing comparable to modern case material. The explanation of this instance may lie in the systematic destruction by the Inquisition of the writings of the Cathars, with the result that most of what we know about them today derives not from their own documents, but from those of their persecutors and exterminators.

Notwithstanding the above examples from earlier times, it seems likely that empirical evidence from personal experiences has either established the belief in reincarnation or strengthened it where it already existed. Such evidence has probably contributed more than other factors to sustaining the belief, especially in the face of strongly held opposing systems such as those of Christians, orthodox (Sunni) Moslems, and most present-day scientists. A later section of this chapter will return to the topic of the relationship between the belief in reincarnation and the occurrence of cases, but it may be helpful to say here that the relationship is almost certainly circular: The cases sustain the belief, although they are not necessary for it, and the belief fosters the cases by creating an ambiance favorable to their development and reporting.

THE TYPES OF EVIDENCE SUGGESTING REINCARNATION

Of the several different types of evidence adduced in support of a belief in reincarnation the weakest by far consists of statements made by one person, usually a sensitive, medium, or yogi, concerning the supposed previous life or lives of another person. In no department of parapsychology, if it may be called such, is the volume of utterance so disproportionately large in comparison with the weakness of presented evidence. In nearly all instances of this type the statements of the person claiming to "read" another person's previous lives consist of completely unverifiable assertions about the previous life allegedly perceived. Some persons have exploited claims to "read" other persons' past lives in sordid commercialism with regard to which one does not know whether to deplore more the cupidity of the profiteers or the gullibility of the deceived. The simple and not too expensive device of having several such "sensitives" make statements about the same person seems rarely to be adopted, although it would quickly unmask the pretensions of most of the practitioners in this field.[2] This topic cannot be dismissed, however, without acknowledging that very rarely several sensitives have made the same (or very similar) statements about a presumed previous life of one person and that also very rarely mediums have made statements concerning the previous life of a person that were concordant with spontaneous memories the person himself had had. In these instances the most we can say by way of interpretation, assuming no normal leak of information, is that they provide evidence of extrasensory perception on the part of the medium or sensitive making the statements. They are not necessarily evidence of reincarnation, although harmonious with that interpretation.

On a slightly higher level of evidential merit are experiments with hypnosis and regression to presumed previous lives. But here again, interest and enthusiasm on the part of the general public has far outrun respectable data. The nature of the hypnotic state, and even its existence as an authentically different form of consciousness, have been much debated for more than a century. It can be agreed, however, that suggestions accepted by a subject may induce in him a condition in which he is more suggestible than usual, and that in this latter state he may be induced to experience images that, like the content of many dreams, ordinarily remain unconscious. Recall of childhood memories sometimes becomes greatly increased, with the recovery of surprising details previously forgotten but verified as correct (Reiff & Scheerer, 1959). Given this fact, it is possible to suppose that subjects could also easily be "taken further back" until they would remember real previous lives. But several difficulties interpose themselves before such a simple explanation. As already mentioned, the subject under hypnosis is in a condition of increased suggestibility, and he usually feels a strong inclination to conform to the wishes of the hypnotist. Therefore, when the hypnotist instructs the subject to "go back to a previous life," he will attempt to do so to the best of his ability; it matters little how explicit the instructions are because the subject responds almost as obediently to implied suggestions as to specific ones. Secondly, the hypnotic state (which was compared above to dreaming sleep) facilitates the mobilization of memories of all kinds that ordinarily remain dormant. These may include forgotten memories of books read, films seen, or radio and television programs heard. Some of these latent memories may furnish the materials for the construction of plausible, and even impressive, "previous lives" that are nevertheless completely imaginary. In some instances the "previous lives" may contain a mixture of fact and fiction as historical novels do. But even when they do include verifiable information the task of the investigator has only begun, because he must then show that the subject could not possibly have acquired the correct information by normal means of communication. This is formidably difficult and not made easier by the fact that in a number of instances the content of a hypnotically induced "previous life" has been traced to a book or other normal source of information to which the subject had been exposed. The subject is usually completely unaware of such exposure, a fact that leads to calling such instances "cryptomnesia"[3] instead of examples of fraud. But this possibility also increases the difficulty in interpreting hypnotically induced "previous lives" and makes the need for caution particularly great. The fact that some of the "previous personalities" emerging during experiments with hypnosis show an impressive range of apparently appropriate emotions and much consistency over months or years has no bearing on the provenance of the details included in the "previous personalities" and merely shows, as dreams do, the dramatizing powers of levels of the mind that ordinarily remain unconscious.

When all the above has been admitted, however, there still remains a small number of cases of hypnotic regression in which something valuable has emerged. Two cases of responsive xenoglossy were developed during experiments with hypnosis (Stevenson, 1974a, 1976). And in the case of Bridey Murphy (Bernstein, 1956) the hypnotized subject mentioned recondite details about life in Ireland of which it seems extremely unlikely that she could have had normal knowledge (Ducasse, 1960). This case has not been improved upon in the many books since written for the general public that have reported experiments with hypnotic regression. Most of these contain absurd anachronisms and other solecisms. Nevertheless, the few substantial results from the use of hypnosis in such experiments justify a more extensive exploration of the technique with better controls. The possibility of developing additional authentic cases of responsive xenoglossy would alone warrant this effort. (These, however, may be better interpreted as evidence of discarnate survival than of reincarnation.) But as of now, by far the best evidence of reincarnation comes from the spontaneous cases of claimed memories of previous lives.

SPONTANEOUS CASES OF THE REINCARNATION TYPE

Kinds of Spontaneous Cases of the Reincarnation Type

Memories of apparent previous lives may occur to persons under a variety of conditions. They have been reported in the form of vivid (and recurring) dreams, during intoxication with certain drugs such as lysergic acid diethylamide (LSD), and during meditation. When the apparent memories occur during adulthood the same question arises as with experiments using hypnosis: Could the subject have acquired the content of his apparent memories—whether verifiable or not—from some source to which he had been normally exposed? The difficulties of answering this question in the majority of adult subjects, not with certainty, but just with reasonable probability, have made cases which begin when the subjects are young children seem much more promising. With them, one can in most instances achieve satisfactory assurance concerning whether the apparent memories could have come from normally acquired information. This is simply because the parents of a child of 2 or 3 (the age at which most children with spontaneous memories of previous lives begin to talk about them) usually know who has been in contact with the child, and they can give this information to an investigator. The possibility of greater control over normal sources of information has been responsible for the fact that most scientific investigations bearing on the evidence of reincarnation have started with cases having young children as subjects. This being so, most of the remainder of this chapter will be devoted to data derived from the investigation of such cases.

Features of Typical Cases of the Reincarnation Type

As already mentioned, the typical case of this type starts when a child between the ages of 2 and 4, but occasionally older, begins to narrate details of a previous life that he claims to have lived before his birth. The child often begins talking about this previous life as soon as he gains any ability to speak, and sometimes before his capacity for verbal expression matches his need to communicate so that he mispronounces words that are later better understood or uses gestures to supplement what he cannot yet say clearly with words. The subjects of these cases vary greatly both in the quantity of their utterances and in the richness of the memories of the previous lives talked about. Some children make only three or four different statements about a previous life, but others may be credited with 60 or 70 separate items pertaining to different details in the life remembered. It is conjecturable that in all cases the subject remembers more than he tells because his telling depends very much both on his own related emotions that lead him to confide in others about his memories, or to conceal them, and on the willingness of other persons to listen to him. (Even in Asia busy parents often do not make suitable audiences for the talk of small children.) In most cases the volume and clarity of the child's statements increase until at the age of between 5 and 6 he usually starts to forget the memories; or, if he does not forget them, he begins to talk about them less. Spontaneous remarks about the previous life have usually ceased by the time the child has reached the age of 8 and often before.

Unexpected behavior of various kinds nearly always accompanies the statements the child makes about the previous life he claims to remember, or occurs contemporaneously with them. This behavior is unusual for a child of the subject's family, but concordant with what he says concerning the previous life, and in most instances it is found to correspond with what other informants say concerning the behavior of the deceased person about whom the subject has been talking, if such a person is traced. (It has become conventional to refer to this person as the "previous personality" of the case; this phrase can be used without commitment to any interpretation of the case, and also without regard to whether a particular person has in fact been identified as corresponding to the subject's statements.) This unusual behavior may take the form of phobias, such as for guns or bladed weapons, or of philias, such as special interests and appetites for particular foods, motor vehicles, books, and other objects, as well as attachments to certain persons. The child often also shows "adult" attitudes and behaves with gravity, wisdom, and sometimes patronizing condescension toward other children. The latter conduct apparently derives, in instances with unusually vivid memories, from the conviction on the part of the subject that he is still an adult, not a child. Very often the child asks, or even clamors, to be taken to the place where he says he lived before, and shows marked concern over the people "he" left there. The unusual behavior on the part of the subject that relates to the previous life usually diminishes at about the time he stops talking about the previous life, but residues of it may persist for many years and long after the child has forgotten the imaged memories he once had of the previous life.

Nearly always, upon the insistence of the child or to satisfy their own curiosity, his parents take him to the place where he says he lived, and they try to find the family he is talking about. In most Asian cases this is not too difficult because the child usually gives enough details concerning proper names so that a corresponding person can be found without much effort. In some cases this person may already be known if the child refers to a previous life as a deceased member of his own family. In other instances, the subject gives so little detail that no one corresponding to his statements can be traced.

In many cases the subject has some birthmark or congenital deformity that corresponds in location and appearance to a wound (usually fatal) on the body of the related previous personality. The child may point to the birthmark as the place where "he" (in the previous life) was (for example) stabbed or shot. Or the birthmark may be noticed at the subject's birth and judged by his parents to indicate the identity of the "incoming" personality before the child himself has made any statements about a previous life. This occurs frequently in cases among the Tlingits of Alaska (Stevenson, 1966, 1966/1974). In some cases the subject suffers from an internal disease that corresponds with one from which the related previous personality suffered but of which other members of his family have been free.

In addition to the features of typical cases mentioned above, several others occur in some cases, particularly in those of certain regions. In some cultures a person before he dies makes a prediction about his next incarnation. This may take the form of selecting the parents he has chosen for his next incarnation, indicating a certain mark on his body the appearance of which on his next body will identify him, or expressing some wish about the conditions and circumstances he will experience in that next life, such as not having flat feet or a stutter. In a small number of cases expressed wishes of these kinds appear to have been fulfilled according to the evidence of the case as later developed. Their chief present significance undoubtedly lies, however, in the fact that the expression of such wishes nearly always alerts other people, such as the intended next parents, concerning the possibility that this person will reincarnate in a particular family. And expectations thus aroused can influence the parents in their observation and reporting of the indicated child's statements and behavior; furthermore, the parents and other adults may encourage such statements and behavior in the child in a manner that does not occur when they have no acquaintance whatever with the person of whom the child is speaking. Thus cases with the feature of a pre-mortem prediction have the strength that a particular development was foretold, but also the weakness that self-fulfillment may have entered into the realization of the prediction.

The expression "announcing dreams" has been coined to indicate dreams experienced during a pregnancy, usually by the expectant mother but sometimes by a relative or friend, in which a deceased personality indicates to the dreamer his intention to reincarnate as the baby of the pregnant woman. In a dream of this type the "communicator" may seem to state his intention verbally and explicitly or may indicate it only symbolically, as when the deceased personality (in the dream) appears at the front door of the dreamer's house with his suitcase as if he were arriving for a long visit. In a few instances the dreamer does not recognize the deceased person who seems to be coming to announce his rebirth. More often, however, he is recognized, and in these cases, as with the pre-mortem predictions mentioned above, the stage may be arranged for the parents to influence statements and behavior of their child that correspond to what is known or inferable about the identified deceased person.

The cases occur in all social strata of the cultures in which they are found, from the richest to the poorest. Not infrequently the two families concerned belong to widely different social classes, the subject being born in a poor family and remembering a previous life in a wealthy one, or vice versa. In the majority of cases, however, the subject remembers a previous life in his own culture and in a place within 15 miles of that where his family lives. However, numerous cases have occurred in which the two families concerned are much more widely separated. There is also an appreciable number of "international" cases in which the subject remembers a previous life as a person of another country (and culture); for reasons not well understood "international" cases tend to be weak in verifiable details or totally lacking in them.

The interval between death and presumed rebirth varies considerably. For Turkish (Alevi) cases the average interval is 9 months, for Sri Lanka (Sinhalese) cases it is 21 months, for Indian cases it is 45 months, and for Tlingit cases it is 48 months. The reasons for these differences are not yet understood.

The period of childhood when the memories are strongest is often fraught with conflict for the subject and his family. Any such turbulence usually passes away, however, as the child grows older and forgets, or stops talking about, the memories of the previous life. With rare exceptions the subjects of these cases develop normally during the years after the age of 10. (For further remarks on the later development of the subjects, see Stevenson, 1966/1974, 1975.) . . .

Brief History of the Investigation of Cases of the Reincarnation Type

As already mentioned, some ancient writings of India and Greece contain allusions to persons who claimed to remember that they had lived before. Almost nothing, however, that corresponds to the typical fully developed modern case of this type was reported earlier than the late nineteenth century. Between then and 1940 sporadic reports of such cases began to appear, sometimes in single reports, sometimes in small groups of reports (Gupta, Sharma, & Mathur, 1936; Hall, 1898; Hearn, 1897; Osborn, 1937/1974; Sahay, 1927; Sunderlal, 1924). In 1924 Delanne published a remarkable compilation of reports of cases which he had garnered from previously printed sources and his own correspondents. Although his collection reproduced some newspaper reports characterized by journalistic brevity and inattention to detail, it also included a small number of cases that had evidently received rather careful observation and documentation.

By 1960 it was possible to show that the quality of at least some reports of cases suggestive of reincarnation justified a systematic investigation of any additional cases that could be located (Stevenson, 1960). No one then seems to have realized how numerous such cases are in many different parts of the world. In the following year (1961) I began field investigations in India and Ceylon (now Sri Lanka) and gradually extended them to many other parts of the world. The first results of these endeavors were published in 1966 (Stevenson, 1966, 1966/1974) with further articles and books following in subsequent years (Stevenson, 1970, 1975, 1977, 1980, 1983a; Stevenson & Story, 1970; Story & Stevenson, 1967).

Most of the case reports published between the 1890s and 1960 were included in books written for the general public or from the point of view of Spiritualists. They thus fell outside the literature and the growing tradition of psychical research which developed into modern parapsychology. It should be noted, however, that three reports of Indian cases published in the 1920s, two by Sahay (c. 1927) and one by Sunderlal (1924), included the important feature of a written record made before any attempt at verifying the subject's statements was begun. The advances in the investigation of these cases since 1960 include, first, the more systematic collection of data from a large number of cases; second, the more careful recording of data obtained from firsthand informants; third, the analysis of each case with regard to interpretations alternative to reincarnation; and fourth, the increased attention given to observations of the physical and behavioral resemblances between subjects and related previous personalities of the cases. Some of these topics will next be considered in more detail.

The Distribution of Cases of the Reincarnation Type

As already mentioned, cases of the reincarnation type are reported (and found) much more frequently in those areas of the world where the belief in reincarnation is held by the majority of the population. Yet cases have also been reported and investigated in cultures having a majority of persons uninformed about reincarnation, uninterested in it, or actually opposed to the belief in it. In recent years more cases have been found in such groups, which include the Christians of Lebanon and Sri Lanka, the Sunni Moslems of India, and the Christians of Europe, the United States, and Canada. It cannot be said as yet whether this has resulted from a softening of former opposition to the idea of reincarnation (and the related fear of seeming to endorse it by presenting a case), to better methods of finding cases, or to a combination of these and other factors.

The incidence of reported cases of the reincarnation type provides a quite inadequate guide to the real incidence of cases of this type. . . . Present methods of case-finding are haphazard and therefore far from satisfactory. But they are particularly deficient with regard to improving our understanding of the real incidence of the cases. This will require systematic surveys made with proper sampling methods in a variety of cultures. Considering the inadequacy of the methods of case-finding and the paucity of persons actively engaged in locating and studying cases, it is perhaps surprising that the University of Virginia's collection of cases now numbers nearly 1,600. It should be emphasized, however, that these 1,600 cases are of uneven quality with regard to the richness of detail they have, the thoroughness of the investigations they have received, and the judgments of authenticity based on such investigations. About two-fifths of the cases have received extensive investigation by myself. Another (approximately) two-fifths have been investigated less thoroughly—either by myself or by one of my assistants who has worked as an interpreter with me in the study of other cases. One-fifth of the cases I have accepted into the series on the basis of published reports that seemed to justify credence or because I obtained reports about them from persons in whom I had confidence even though they were not working directly with me. All of the 1,600 cases have been provisionally accepted as authentic so that they have been included in a computerized analysis of the data of the entire collection to which I shall refer later. At least several hundred other cases have been notified to me, but set aside as insufficiently authentic and not meriting inclusion in the group to be studied further. Some of these latter cases could be dismissed on initial examination, others only after they had been given some investigation.

Probably more cases of the type than have come to my attention have occurred and are still occurring in many parts of the world. At the same time readers should not conclude from the rather large number of cases known about or conjectured, especially in Asia, that many persons remember previous lives. Cases of this type are rather rare even in Southeast Asia where, in comparison to the incidence of cases in the West, they occur relatively frequently. Thus in India it is unusual to find more than one case in a family or more than one in a village although some families do have several cases. It is more common to find two or several cases in the same family among the Druses of Lebanon and the natives of northwest North America.

Methods of Investigation

The methods of investigation used for these cases, described in more detail elsewhere (Stevenson, 1966/1974, 1975), derive from those developed by the early investigators of spontaneous cases in psychical research (Gurney, Myers, & Podmore, 1886; Myers, 1903). With due acknowledgment of the greatness of these pioneers I have made some efforts to improve upon their methods and also to modify them as required for the special features and circumstances of cases of the reincarnation type.

As with other types of spontaneous cases in parapsychology, the investigator of cases of the reincarnation type can rarely study the case while its main events are still unfolding. In the investigations of recent years it has been possible to reach more cases during this stage, but even when this happens the investigator in most instances has still the task of reconstructing as well as he can events that took place before he came on the scene. For this, reliance is placed mainly on interviews with firsthand informants, preferably several or more of them, and preferably also including a second interview (or more) with at least the main informants. . . . Every effort is also made to corroborate the oral testimony by whatever written documents are at hand or obtainable. These include birth certificates or horoscopes, diaries, notebooks, and school records.

After the investigation has been carried as far as it can be with the subject and his family, at least in its initial stages, the entire procedure of interviewing firsthand informants is repeated with the family of the deceased person about whom the child has been talking. If no such person has been identified and if the subject has given an apparently sufficient number of verifiable details, the investigators themselves try to find a person corresponding to the child's statements. It has happened, however, that in nearly every case in which the child has given sufficient details to permit verification its family has taken it to the previous family before an investigator reached the scene. It has been possible in fewer than 15 cases for the investigator to be the first person to trace the concerned previous family. For examples of these rare, but extremely valuable cases, see Stevenson (1966/1974, 1975, 1977).[4]

Great importance is given to independent verification of the child's statements, the mere assertion by the child's parents that he was correct in a certain item being regarded as quite insufficient confirmation that he was. At the same time, when the two families have already met, care has to be taken that the family of the deceased person concerned does not compliantly, even if unintentionally, furnish false information that erroneously indicates the subject to have been more accurate than he really was. The investigators try to see buildings and objects mentioned by the child and to meet themselves any persons named by him who are still living. In this way they check on the accuracy or incorrectness, as the case may be, of many of the statements the child has made.

The data derived from field investigations are analyzed both with regard to individual cases and with regard to characteristics that recur in many cases. These types of analysis will next be considered separately.

Analyses of the Data of Individual Cases

The material derived from interviews and whatever written documents have become available are analyzed for consistencies and discrepancies among the statements of different informants and among those of one informant at different times. The information thus derived, together with any other evidence bearing on the reliability of the informants, is then taken into account in a consideration of various alternative interpretations of the case. The most important of these are the following.

Fraud

Dishonestly contrived cases have occurred, and at least some of them have been exposed.[5] These have betrayed themselves by radical departures from the features of a typical case. It would be difficult to simulate a case with a young child as the subject. Small children are not easy to coach for the assumption of roles that do not seem natural to them. In a typical case the subject even up to the age of about 5 would still be talking about the previous life he remembered, and he could therefore be questioned about it. Also, in a typical case the child has made at least some remarks to informants other than his parents, such as uncles, aunts, and neighbors. Suspicion would be aroused by any case that depended on the unsupported statements of the subject's parents, although in some cases that seem from all other indices to be authentic, the child has made only a few statements about a previous life and these only to his parents. We have other clues to fraud besides the ones mentioned above, but it does not seem necessary to describe these here.

Apart from the practical difficulties of perpetrating a fraud, few motives exist for anyone to try, at least in Asia. Although in the West books may be written and fortunes made on fictitious and insubstantial cases, such opportunities do not exist in Asia, at any rate for the villagers among whom the majority of genuine cases occur. A few fraudulent cases in Asia have, however, been traced to unscrupulous journalists and "investigators."

Paramnesia

As already mentioned, the two families concerned in these cases have nearly always met before an investigator reaches the scene and begins to make written records of what has happened up to that time. Under these circumstances the families concerned may mingle their memories of what the child said with what they learn or remember about the identified previous personality, and they may then attribute to the child more knowledge about the previous personality than he really had before the two families met. In an extreme development of this kind the informants could elaborate a rather detailed case on the basis of a few statements made by the child. This could, at least in theory, happen without the people concerned being aware of what they are doing and without any intention to deceive.

The hypothesis of paramnesia may apply to a small number of cases, especially those in which the child has given out only a few details about the previous life he claims to remember, or is said to remember. But it seems an unlikely explanation for the many cases that are rich in apparently remembered details. Moreover, in at least some of the latter cases, that is, those richer in details, the informants are educated and thoughtful persons who have given their statements to investigators within a few weeks or months of the main events of the case. To account for such cases on the basis of faulty memory is to attribute to these informants deficiencies of observation and remembering for which there is no other evidence. Finally, the hypothesis of paramnesia cannot apply at all to those cases (unfortunately still very few) in which someone made a written record of what the child said about the previous life before any attempt at verification was made.[6]

Cryptomnesia[7]

In the hypothesis of paramnesia the child is credited with knowing more about the previous personality than he did; in cryptomnesia his knowledge about the previous personality is not in question, but he is thought to have come by it normally. In a small number of mediumistic cases, a medium has communicated information which she had acquired normally, perhaps through reading, although she had completely forgotten her exposure to the material which emerged in the communications.

There is no question here of dishonesty, only that of a simple forgetfulness of what one had read or otherwise seen or heard. In some instances the medium may not even have been aware, at the time, of her exposure to the material later communicated, so that even the process of perception was unconscious.

Although cryptomnesia has been adduced as an explanation for at least some cases of the reincarnation type, no case has been identified yet as a proven example of cryptomnesia. Despite this weakness of the hypothesis—that it lacks examples from empirical studies—it remains an important possibility in certain cases. And it deserves special consideration when the two families concerned in a case have known each other before the case developed. In such instances members of one or the other family may well pass on to the subject more information about the deceased personality he later talks about than he or they afterwards recall. On the other hand, cryptomnesia does not seem a likely explanation for those quite numerous cases in which the two families concerned live in villages or towns separated by 50 or more miles and in which the persons on the two sides of the case assert, with good grounds for believing them, that they never had any acquaintance with each other prior to the development of the case. The very early age—2 or 3 years—at which most subjects begin to speak about the previous lives makes it unlikely that anyone could have had contact with such a child sufficient to communicate the information it seems to remember without the contact being known and remembered by its parents.

Extrasensory Perception and Personation

As explained above, certain cases may be explained by supposing normal channels of communication to the subject of information about the related previous personality. But this interpretation cannot reasonably apply to cases in which the two families concerned live in widely separated communities, in which the child begins to talk about a previous life at a very early age and with abundant detail, and in which the investigators reach the case when memories of events are still reasonably fresh. This has led to the proposal that the subjects are really gifted with extrasensory perception and that, using their paranormal powers, they obtain knowledge about a deceased person with whom they then identify themselves. The main sources for the information paranormally obtained by the subject are presumably the surviving relatives and friends of the deceased person. The previous personality thus constructed is viewed as a pathological secondary personality cast into a reincarnationist form under the influence of the culture surrounding him in which memories of a previous life are acceptable and expected. The hypothesis requires attribution of some degree of paramnesia to the subject himself, though not necessarily to other informants. He, however, comes to believe that information obtained contemporaneously derives from memories and so he falsely sets it in the past instead of in the present of his experiences. Chari (1962a, 1962b) and Murphy (1973) have persuasively argued the merits of this interpretation which they (with variations) favor. It is essential to include in this hypothesis the unusual behavior shown by the subject that corresponds to behavior reported for the related previous personality; a hypothesis of paranormal cognition alone will not suffice.

The hypothesis accounts quite well for the greater frequency of reported cases in cultures favoring the belief in reincarnation; it also accords with the fact that in the majority of cases the families concerned (those of the subject and the related previous personality) live in the same general geographical area. This would make easier paranormal communication to the subject through so-called psychometric objects that had been associated in some way with the deceased person or his family. The hypothesis does not, however, adequately account for the exceptions to the above general principles; that is, for cases that crop up in families and cultures unsympathetic or even hostile to the belief in reincarnation and those, alluded to above, with wide geographical separations between the families concerned. The most serious objection to it comes from the fact that, with rare exceptions, the subjects of these cases show no trace of paranormal powers apart from the memories of the previous lives they claim to remember. If the accurate details in their statements derive from the use of paranormal cognition of an "ordinary" kind, it is surprising, to say the least, that it manifests so powerfully with regard to one particular person and no other, and for a few years of childhood and not thereafter. This argument seems to me strong, but it is not compelling since it has been found that some persons show paranormal abilities in only one particular task or situation (Pratt, 1973).

There are also difficulties for the hypothesis of extrasensory perception and personation in the subject's accurate knowledge of the condition of buildings and objects during the lifetime of the related previous personality and his (usual) ignorance of changes occurring to them after the previous personality's death. Nor is it clear how a theory of "ordinary" paranormal cognition could by itself account for the unusual behavior that almost invariably accompanies the subject's statements about the previous life he remembers. This behavior, as mentioned earlier, often extends over 5 years and sometimes many more. It may include attitudes and sometimes strong emotions and skills which it is not easy to conceive as being transmitted by "ordinary" extrasensory perception.

Other Hypotheses

Several other hypotheses have been put forward to account for these cases. Each may apply to some of the cases, without being applicable to all of them.

Retrocognition is a variant of the hypothesis of extrasensory perception, and as such is liable to the same criticisms. Why, for example, should a child show strong retrocognitive ability in relation to only one particular deceased person and no other?

"Inherited memory" may apply to certain cases in which it is possible for the subject to be a lineal descendant of the previous personality, whether or not such genetic linkage is known to exist. Even in such cases, however, the hypothesis of "inherited memory" would be proposing transmission through genetic linkages of detailed imaged memories, something that is not envisaged in present-day theories of inheritance, although it is not for that reason impossible. The hypothesis of "inherited memory" could not apply to the majority of cases of the reincarnation type in which the subject is born just a few years after the death of the previous personality in a family totally unrelated to the other one concerned. Thus the subject could not possibly be descended from the previous personality or have inherited any qualities from him.

"Possession" of the subject, whether temporary or permanent, by a discarnate personality has been put forward as an explanation for cases of the reincarnation type since at least as far back as the eighteenth century when Swedenborg (1758/1906, p. 155) espoused it. Its gravest weakness is its failure to account for the cessation of the unusual statements and behavior expressed by the subject as he becomes older. As mentioned above, most subjects gradually cease talking spontaneously about the previous lives between the ages of 5 and 8, and their associated unusual behavior also diminishes, if sometime later. This process is much more often gradual than abrupt, and it is difficult to understand why "possessing spirits" would all (or mostly) withdraw themselves in such a fashion and when the subjects were of about the same age.

Reincarnation

In reincarnation research, as in other branches of parapsychology, one reaches paranormal interpretations, and especially those including survival as a part of them, only after trying to eliminate interpretations along normal lines or those that take account of processes for which we already have independent evidence. This means that reincarnation should only be considered the best interpretation of any case after the alternative interpretations mentioned above have been considered and found unsatisfactory, or at least less satisfactory than reincarnation in accounting for all the facts of the case. A later section of this chapter will attempt to summarize the present status of the evidence for reincarnation, but first I will consider the value of the analysis of large numbers of cases.

Analyses for Recurrent Characteristics in Numbers of Cases

Investigators in the early years of psychical research found it helpful to study the recurrent characteristics or patterns discoverable in large numbers of spontaneous cases considered together (Gurney et al., 1886; Sidgwick, Sidgwick, Johnson, Myers, Myers, & Podmore, 1894). The method was further developed by Green (1960), Hart (1956), Rhine (1953, 1954), and Sannwald (1959a, 1959b). In recent years the development of computers has made possible the handling and analysis of large amounts of data from many cases with less effort and time than was hitherto needed. In the application of this method to the data of cases of the reincarnation type two kinds of uniformities have emerged.

Characteristics Recurring in Cases from All Cultures Studied

Certain features have recurred, with some exceptions, in the cases of all cultures so far investigated. Examples of such features are: the usual age (2 to 4 years) when the subjects first start speaking about the previous lives; the usual age (5 to 8 years) when they stop talking about the previous lives; the high frequency of violent death in the related previous personalities (Stevenson, 1966/1974, 1974b, 1980, 1983a); and the prominence of events connected with the death of the previous personality, or just preceding it, among the subjects' memories. These and other recurrent features found in cases of many different parts of the world appear to have two significances.

First, since at least some of the cultures in which these features have been found are effectively isolated from each other with regard to possibilities for mutual influence, and have been so for centuries, the occurrence of similar features in their cases is an indication of the authenticity[8] of the cases. These "universal" features could not be explained as resulting from local cultural influences. They suggest instead some widespread human experience. This conclusion would not by itself tell anything about paranormal interpretations. Obviously other features of human experience have recurred in many (or perhaps all) different cultures which men have developed. The making of myths is certainly one of these, and the widespread occurrence of reincarnation cases could be an example of this mythopoeic tendency.

Second, the understanding of features that can be expected in a case of this type assists in the delineation of a "standard" case in comparison with which new cases can be evaluated. This may aid in such different matters as the earlier detection of fraudulent cases and reassurance to parents of a young subject of a case who are worried about whether he will later develop normally. The concept of a "standard" case is naturally modified from culture to culture by taking account not only of the "universal" features, but also of those that are culture-bound.

Culture-Bound Recurrent Features of the Cases

At least some of the features described as found in all cultures where cases of this type have been investigated vary to some extent from culture to culture. For example, although a high incidence of violent death has been found for the previous personalities in the cases of all cultures so far studied, the actual percentage of violent deaths ranges from a low of 38 percent in Sri Lanka cases to a high of slightly more than 78 percent in the Druse cases of Lebanon and Syria (Stevenson, 1974b, p. 409). Other features of the cases vary so much from one culture to another that we may properly speak of them as culture-bound. An impressive example of such a culture-bound factor in the patterns of the cases is the markedly variable incidence of those in which the subject claims to remember a previous life as a person of the opposite sex. No case of this type has been found among approximately 220 cases of the Alevis of south central Turkey and the Druses of Lebanon and Syria. Nor has any case of the "sex change" type been found in 85 cases occurring among the Tlingits of southeastern Alaska. (De Laguna [1972, p. 779] mentioned cases of the "sex change" type reported to her by two informants of the Yakutat Tlingits farther north.) At the other extreme, Slobodin (1970) has reported in incidence of 50 percent "sex change" cases in 44 cases that he studied among the Kutchin of northwestern Canada. In the University of Virginia collection of cases those of Burma and Thailand (consisting together of about 250 cases) have an incidence of approximately 20 percent of the "sex change" type. In all other cultures (not previously mentioned in this paragraph) the incidence of "sex change" cases is about 5 percent.

"Announcing dreams" and birthmarks also show a marked variation from one culture to another. Although these two features occur to some extent in the cases of all cultures so far studied, they have both been found much more abundantly in the cases among the Burmese, the natives of northwestern North America, and the Alevis of south central Turkey.

The connections between the subject and the family of the previous personality also vary significantly from one culture to another. For example, among the Tlingits of southeastern Alaska the subject and previous personality were related on the side of the subject's mother in 70 percent of the cases. Among the neighboring Eskimos (in a much smaller group of cases) subject and previous personality were related on the mother's side in only 27 percent of the cases. The incidence of such connections between the two families concerned in other cultures is extremely low, and although exact figures are not yet available for these, the incidence can be estimated as probably not higher than 2 percent among cases of Southeast Asia. For further information about apparently culture-bound variations in the characteristics of the cases, see Stevenson (1966, 1970, 1973a, 1974b).

An interesting and probably important concordance occurs between the patterns in the cases of a particular culture and the beliefs held about them in that culture. For example, inquiries among the peoples where no cases of the "sex change" type occur almost always elicit the statement that "sex change" is "impossible." Beliefs concerning this and other features of the cases seem often to be held inflexibly and applied as standards assumed to be true for cases all over the world when the person making such an assertion has obviously had no experience of cases outside his own culture and perhaps of few within it. In interpreting the connections between beliefs and the patterns of the cases one naturally thinks that the local beliefs favor the development of cases congenial to the culture; the development of cases that seem discordant could be discouraged and even suppressed by scolding a subject whose memories seemed to depart from the norm acceptable in a particular culture, that is, the characteristics of that culture's typical case. We should remember, however, that an agreement between beliefs and patterns in the cases is not incompatible with reincarnation, and is indeed what we should expect if reincarnation occurs. It is altogether possible that the belief held by a person before he dies may influence what actually happens to him after he dies and if and when he reincarnates. Such an idea has been taught in Buddhism for centuries (Evans-Wentz, 1957).

THE PRESENT STATE OF THE EVIDENCE FOR REINCARNATION

Although systematic investigations of cases of the reincarnation type have been undertaken for less than 16 years, a considerable body of data has already been collected. Some parapsychologists have been surprised at the quantity of data that has been recorded and published so far, and most appear to agree that the results justify further investigations in this area.

Parapsychologists vary much more in their opinions concerning the interpretation as evidence for the survival of bodily death of the data so far obtained from these cases. Before 1960 few parapsychologists would have been willing to consider reincarnation as a serious interpretation for cases of this type, if they were aware of any. Today probably most parapsychologists would agree that reincarnation is at least entitled to inclusion in any list of possible interpretations of the cases, but not many would believe it the most probable interpretation.

All the cases (and all their reports) have deficiencies, as have most cases and reports of other types of spontaneous paranormal phenomena. The perfect case can be conceived (Stevenson, 1973b), but probably met only in fantasy and not in field work. We cannot reasonably expect to find any single case that will provide conclusive proof of reincarnation, nor is such proof a likely result from the study of all the cases considered together. Instead we may look for an accumulation of evidence, first from a larger number of cases, and second from an improvement in their average quality. The quality of the cases should improve as more scientifically trained persons of the countries where they occur begin to investigate them and reach them at early stages of their development more often than has been possible up to now. Some hopes may be expressed also for the results from the further investigation of cases having birthmarks and deformities. Cases with these features obviously require more than extrasensory perception for their interpretation. If it is argued, as some persons have done, that in such cases the account of a previous life has been made up to account for the birthmark or deformity, the latter themselves still have to be explained. If reincarnation seems a better interpretation of such cases, this suggests that some psychic "force" can influence human fetuses *in utero*, sometimes rather drastically.

OTHER THEORETICAL ISSUES RELATED TO REINCARNATION

Most of the hypotheses and theories with regard to reincarnation may be considered within two main categories: those concerned with alternative interpretations of the empirically derived evidence of reincarnation and those concerned with the processes of reincarnation, if it occurs. Because systematic research in this area is new, emphasis has been given to developing and analyzing evidence that indicates reincarnation as at least a reasonable hypothesis justifying further investigation. Previous sections of this chapter have already considered this category of theoretical issues.

With regard to theories of process, the field of reincarnation research is even less far advanced than other branches of parapsychology. We may, however, briefly consider such theories of process as have been developed, first by the peoples among whom the cases occur most frequently, and second by investigators working in the scientific tradition.

The peoples of regions where cases frequently occur often have some beliefs about the processes of reincarnation. Indeed, in some such areas, such as those of Southeast Asia where Hinduism and Buddhism predominate, there exist a number of scriptures alluding to concepts about reincarnation. What we may call local concepts of reincarnation vary considerably from one culture to another. For example, Hinduism decrees no fixed interval between death and presumed subsequent rebirth. But the Druses of Lebanon and neighboring countries believe that reincarnation occurs instantly at death, the released soul entering immediately into the body of a newly born baby (Stevenson, 1966/1974, 1980). The Jains of India have a somewhat similar belief but hold that the new connection between the recently deceased soul and its new physical body occurs at the moment of the conception of that body (Stevenson, 1975). Beliefs of this kind—and there are many of them—tend to be held dogmatically, and they can hardly be dignified with the name theory since they are promulgated as doctrines and not presented as testable hypotheses. Moreover, to the extent that they are confirmed by observation of cases occurring in the same area, this result may derive from a self-fulfilling prophecy as suggested in an earlier section of this chapter.

The few ventures in theorizing that Western scientists interested in this subject have made push our ideas only a little way ahead of the reasonably established facts. One example is the "law" mentioned above which suggests that what a person believes will happen to him after death will in fact happen to him. (But this idea, as already mentioned, has come to us from Buddhism.) Another tentative generalization derives from the observation mentioned earlier that the family of the subject usually lives within about 15 miles of the previous personality's family. Many exceptions have occurred to this general observation, but it has suggested another provisional "law" according to which, other things being equal, persons tend to be reborn near where they die. The tendency just mentioned and some other often observed features of the cases offer the hope of an eventual understanding of the factors which, if reincarnation occurs, influence a deceased person so that he is reborn in one particular family rather than in another of all those in which he might be reborn.

Some thought has been given, on the assumption that reincarnation occurs, to what it is that reincarnates. But here also concepts do little more than loosely connect observations. The subjects of the cases show three qualities corresponding to similar ones in the related previous personalities: imaged memories, behavioral traits, and physical characteristics, the last two occurring in some cases only. It may be supposed then that, if reincarnation occurs, some intermediate "body" comprised of nonmaterial "substances" acts as a carrier (during the interval between death and rebirth) between the previous personality and the new physical body in which its memories and other qualities will later manifest. Broad (1958) called this intermediate "something" a "psi-component," thus properly emphasizing its paranormal characteristics.

If, as now seems possible, the evidence for reincarnation increases and improves in the years ahead, more advanced theories related to it will be developed and tested. Already some predictions about the occurrence of birthmarks under certain conditions have been found accurate, and it seems likely that more and bolder predictions will be offered in the future. It is not difficult even to imagine in the future a whole demography of reincarnation that would attempt to study characteristics of groups of people from the point of view of the hypothesis of reincarnation.

Although research on cases of the reincarnation type developed to some extent away from traditional topics of inquiry in parapsychology (but not from traditional *methods*), nevertheless some links can already be discerned between the data of cases of the reincarnation type and those elicited in other branches of parapsychology. For example, "announcing dreams" purport to be communications from discarnate personalities. As such they relate closely to other types of apparent discarnate communications such as those conveyed through mediums, in some paranormal dreams not concerned with reincarnation, and in apparitional experiences. Another example of a connection with other areas of parapsychology occurs in the frequent claims by subjects of reincarnation cases in parts of Southeast Asia, especially Burma, Thailand, and Vietnam, that they remember events happening to them after death in the preceding lives and before their presumed rebirths. Such a subject may report having seen "his" previous physical body being buried or cremated and may also claim to remember having been in some kind of "intermediate body" during the "intermission" period between death and rebirth. Experiences of this kind have important affinities with those of living persons who, usually after some serious accident or during a near-fatal illness, seem to leave their physical bodies and later remember that while "out-of-the-body" they seemed to see their physical bodies, lying inert, as from a different position in physical space. Persons having this latter type of experience recover and afterwards narrate what they remember to other persons; the mentioned subjects of reincarnation cases having somewhat similar experiences of being "out-of-the-body" say that they did not recover, but died, were reborn, and preserved memories of these experiences in their new lives.

In conclusion, something may be said about the potential contribution of the investigation of cases of the reincarnation type to branches of knowledge outside parapsychology. The other types of evidence bearing on the question of the survival of human personality after death do not impinge except peripherally on orthodox theories of child development and human personality. This is because the persons having the experiences from which such evidence derives, mediums for example, are (usually) adults and merely acting as temporary conduits or registrars of communications from ostensibly discarnate persons. In this process their own personalities, which are already in adult form anyway, become only transiently altered by the communications which they transmit. On the other hand, the subjects of the best reincarnation cases are young children whose personalities are not fully formed, and they often manifest unusual behavior during several years or more. Such children show a mixture of behavior that might be expected of children in their families and behavior that seems quite surprising. The unexpected behavior, however, may make sense if reincarnation is taken seriously as an explanation of it. Furthermore, there are many other children who, although they have no imaged memories of previous lives, nevertheless manifest strange, unexpected behavior that cannot be adequately accounted for either by heredity or by early environmental influences, but which might derive from patterns of conduct learned in previous lives. For example, in our efforts to understand children who are confused about gender identity it may be helpful to add reincarnation to the presently considered interpretations of this disorder. This suggestion receives support from some of the cases of the "sex change" type mentioned above; some subjects of such cases show behavior characteristic of a person of the opposite sex (Stevenson, 1973c, 1966/1974, 1975).

The study of cases of the reincarnation type thus holds out prospects for enriching our understanding of child development and, beyond that, of biology and medicine. If this occurs, an understanding of reincarnation will not replace present knowledge of heredity and environmental influences, but will supplement it. The greatest contribution from its investigation, however, will certainly derive from whatever additional evidence it adds to that already obtained, or to be obtained by other researches in the future, bearing on the important question of the fate of human personality after physical death. Future investigations of the evidence of reincarnation may confirm the prediction made many years ago by the English philosopher McTaggart (1915) who wrote: "If we succeed in proving immortality, it will be by means of considerations which would also prove pre-existence" (p. 113).

NOTES

1. Excerpts from Part VII, Chapter 2, in B. B. Wolman (ed.), *Handbook of Parapsychology* (pp. 631–663). New York: Van Nostrand Reinhold.—Ed.
2. Ian himself did this: "Eight persons have independently read my own purported previous lives. Not a single one of these readings has agreed with any of the others. . . . [Moreover] several of the readings placed me in different countries during the same periods of time" (1987/2001, p. 272).—Ed.
3. For a review of cases of cryptomnesia, see Stevenson (1983b).—Ed.
4. This number has now grown to 33 (see Keil & Tucker, 2005).—Ed.
5. See Stevenson, Pasricha, and Samararatne (1988).—Ed.
6. For an analysis of the hypothesis of paramnesia that compares cases with written records and cases without them, see Schouten and Stevenson (1998).—Ed.
7. For a general discussion of the phenomenon of cryptomnesia, see Stevenson (1983b).—Ed.
8. Ian (1971, p. 93, note 3) drew the following distinction between "authenticity" and "paranormality" or "evidentiality":

> By "authentic" I mean a high reliability of the witnessing and reporting so that one can justifiably believe the perception and other related events to have happened as reported. By "evidential" I mean authenticity plus a justified interpretation that the case has paranormal features.

For a more detailed discussion of this important distinction, see Stevenson, Palmer, & Stanford, 1977).—Ed.

REFERENCES

Bayer, R. (1970–1971). Personal communications.

Bernstein, M. (1956). *The Search for Bridey Murphy*. Garden City, New York: Doubleday.
Besterman, T. (1968). Belief in rebirth among the natives of Africa (including Madagascar). In T. Besterman, *Collected Papers on the Paranormal* (pp. 22–59). New York: Garrett Publications.
Broad, C. D. (1958). *Personal Identity and Survival* (the Thirteenth Frederic W. H. Myers Memorial Lecture). London: Society for Psychical Research.
Chari, C. T. K. (1962a). Paranormal cognition, survival and reincarnation. *Journal of the American Society for Psychical Research, 56*, 158–183.
Chari, C. T. K. (1962b). Paramnesia and reincarnation. *Proceedings of the Society for Psychical Research, 53*, 264–286.
De Laguna, F. (1972). Under Mount St. Elias: The history and culture of the Yakutat Tlingit. *Smithsonian Contributions to Anthropology, 7*, 776–781.
Delanne, G. (1924). *Documents pour servir à l'étude de la réincarnation*. Paris: Editions de la B.P.S.
Deschamps, H. (1970). *Les Religions de l'Afrique Noire*. Paris: Presses Universitaires de France.
Dodds, E. R. (1971). Personal communication.
Ducasse, C. J. (1960). How the case of *The Search for Bridey Murphy* stands today. *Journal of the American Society for Psychical Research, 54*, 3–22.
Evans-Wentz, W. Y. (Ed.) (1957). *The Tibetan Book of the Dead* (3rd ed.). London: Oxford University Press.
Gallup International (1969). *Report of Polls Concerning the Belief in Reincarnation in West Europe, Canada, and the United States.*
Green, C. (1960). Analysis of spontaneous cases. *Proceedings of the Society for Psychical Research, 53*, 97–161.
Gupta, L. D., Sharma, N. R., & Mathur, T. C. (1936). *An Inquiry into the Case of Shanti Devi*. Delhi: International Aryan League.
Gurney, E., Myers, F. W. H., & Podmore, F. (1886). *Phantasms of the Living* (2 vols.). London: Trübner.
Hall, H. F. (1898). *The Soul of a People*. London: Macmillan.
Hart, H., and collaborators (1956). Six theories about apparitions. *Proceedings of the Society for Psychical Research, 50*, 153–239.
Head, J., & Cranston, J. L. (1967). *Reincarnation in World Thought*. New York: Julian Press.
Keil, H. H. J., & Tucker, J. B. (2005). Children who claim to remember previous lives: Cases with written records made before the previous personality was identified. *Journal of Scientific Exploration, 19*, 91–101.
Madaule, J. (1961). *Le drame albigeois et le destin français*. Paris: Bernard Grasset.
Makarem, S. (1972). *The Doctrine of the Ismailis*. Beirut: The Arab Institute of Research and Publishing.
Makarem, S. (1973). Personal communication.
Malinowski, B. (1916). Baloma: The spirits of the dead in the Trobriand Islands. *Journal of the Royal Anthropological Institute of Great Britain and Ireland, 46*, 353–430.
McTaggart, J. M. E. (1915). *Human Immortality and Pre-Existence*. London: Edward Arnold.
Munro, N. G. (1963). *Ainu: Creed and Cult*. New York: Columbia University Press.
Murphy, G. A (1973). Caringtonian approach to Ian Stevenson's *Twenty Cases Suggestive of Reincarnation*. *Journal of the American Society for Psychical Research, 67*, 117–129.
Myers, F. W. H. (1903). *Human Personality and Its Survival of Bodily Death* (2 vols.). London: Longmans, Green.
Nelli, R. (1972). *Les Cathares*. Paris: Grasset.
Noon, J. A. (1942). A preliminary examination of death concepts of the Ibo. *American Anthropologist, 44*, 638–654.
Osborn, A. (1974). *The Superphysical* (rev. ed.). London: Frederick Muller. (First published in 1937)
Parrinder, E. G. (1954). *African Traditional Religion*. Westport, CT: Greenwood Press.

Parrinder, E. G. (1956). Varieties of belief in reincarnation. *Hibbert Journal, 55,* 260–267.

Plato. (1910). *The Meno* (F. Sydenham, trans.). London: J. M. Dent.

Pratt, J. G. (1973). A decade of research with a selected ESP subject: An overview and reappraisal of the work with Pavel Stepanek. *Proceedings of the American Society for Psychical Research, 30,* 1–78.

Reiff, R., & Scheerer, M. (1959). *Memory and Hypnotic Age Regression.* New York: International Universities Press.

Rhine, L. E. (1953). Subjective forms of spontaneous psi experiences. *Journal of Parapsychology, 17,* 77–114.

Rhine, L. E. (1954). Frequency of types of experience in spontaneous precognition. *Journal of Parapsychology, 18,* 93–123.

Sahay, K. K. N. (c. 1927). *Reincarnation: Verified Cases of Rebirth after Death.* Bareilly: N. L. Gupta.

Sannwald, G. (1959a). Statistische Untersuchungen an Spontanphänomenen. *Zeitschrift für Parapsychologie und Grenzgebiete der Psychologie, 3,* 59–71.

Sannwald, G. (1959b). Zur Psychologie paranormaler Spontanphänomene: Motivation, Thematik and Bezugspersonen "okkulter" Erlebnisse. *Zeitschrift für Parapsychologie und Grenzgebiete der Psychologie, 3,* 149–183.

Schopenhauer, A. (1908). *Die Welt als Wille und Vorstellung* (2 vols.). Leipzig: F. U. Brockhaus.

Schouten, S. A., & Stevenson, I. (1998). Does the socio-psychological hypothesis explain cases of the reincarnation type? *Journal of Nervous & Mental Disease,* 186, 504–506.

Sidgwick, H., Sidgwick, E. M., Johnson, A., Myers, F. W. H., Myers, A. T., & Podmore, F. (1894). Report on the census of hallucinations. *Proceedings of the Society for Psychical Research, 10,* 25–422.

Slobodin, R. (1970). Kutchin concepts of reincarnation. *Western Canadian Journal of Anthropology, 2,* 67–79.

Spencer, B., & Gillen, F. J. (1904). *The Northern Tribes of Central Australia.* London: Macmillan.

Stevenson, I. (1960). The evidence for survival from claimed memories of former incarnations. *Journal of the American Society for Psychical Research, 54,* 51–71, 95–117.

Stevenson, I. (1966). Cultural patterns in cases suggestive of reincarnation among the Tlingit Indians of Southeastern Alaska. *Journal of the American Society for Psychical Research, 60,* 229–243.

Stevenson, I. (1970). Characteristics of cases of the reincarnation type in Turkey and their comparison with cases in two other cultures. *International Journal of Comparative Sociology, 11,* 1–17.

Stevenson, I. (1971). The substantiality of spontaneous cases (1968 Presidential Address). In W. G. Roll, R. L. Morris, & J. D. Morris (eds.), *Proceedings of the Parapsychological Association 5, 1968* (pp. 91–128). Durham, NC: Parapsychological Association.

Stevenson, I. (1973a). Characteristics of cases of the reincarnation type in Ceylon. *Contributions to Asian Studies, 3,* 26–39.

Stevenson, 1. (1973b). The "perfect" reincarnation case. In W. G. Roll, R. L. Morris, & J. D. Morris (eds.), *Research in Parapsychology 1972* (pp. 185–187). Metuchen, NJ: Scarecrow Press.

Stevenson, I. (1973c). Some new cases suggestive of reincarnation. IV. The case of Ampan Petcherat. *Journal of the American Society for Psychical Research, 67,* 361–380.

Stevenson, I. (1974). *Twenty Cases Suggestive of Reincarnation* (2nd rev. ed.). Charlottesville: University Press of Virginia. (First published in 1966)

Stevenson, I. (1974a). *Xenoglossy: A Review and Report of a Case.* Charlottesville: University Press of Virginia. (Also published as *Proceedings of the American Society for Psychical Research, 31,* 1–268, 1974)

Stevenson, I. (1974b). Some questions related to cases of the reincarnation type. *Journal of the American Society for Psychical Research, 68,* 395–416.

Stevenson, I. (1975). *Cases of the Reincarnation Type. Vol. 1. Ten Cases in India.* Charlottesville: University Press of Virginia.

Stevenson, I. (1976). A preliminary report on a new case of responsive xenoglossy: The case of Gretchen. *Journal of the American Society for Psychical Research, 70,* 65–77.

Stevenson, I. (1977). *Cases of the Reincarnation Type. Vol. 2. Ten Cases in Sri Lanka.* Charlottesville: University Press of Virginia

Stevenson, I. (1980). *Cases of the Reincarnation Type. Vol. III. Twelve Cases in Lebanon and Turkey.* Charlottesville: University Press of Virginia.

Stevenson, I. (1983a). *Cases of the Reincarnation Type. Vol. IV. Twelve Cases in Thailand and Burma.* Charlottesville: University Press of Virginia.

Stevenson, I. (1983b). Cryptomnesia and parapsychology. *Journal of the Society for Psychical Research, 52,* 1–30.

Stevenson, I. (2001). *Children Who Remember Previous Lives: A Question of Reincarnation* (rev. ed.). Jefferson, NC: McFarland. (Original work published 1987, Charlottesville: University Press of Virginia)

Stevenson, I., Palmer, J., & Stanford, R. G. (1977). An authenticity rating scale for reports of spontaneous cases. *Journal of the American Society for Psychical Research, 71,* 273–288.

Stevenson, I., Pasricha, S. P., & Samararatne, G. (1988). Deception and self-deception in cases of the reincarnation type: Seven illustrative cases in Asia. *Journal of the American Society for Psychical Research, 82,* 1–31.

Stevenson, I., & Story, F. (1970). A case of the reincarnation type in Ceylon: The case of Disna Samarasinghe. *Journal of Asian and African Studies, 5,* 241–255.

Story, F., & Stevenson, I. (1967). A case of the reincarnation type in Ceylon: The case of Warnasiri Adikari. *Journal of the American Society for Psychical Research, 61,* 130–145.

Sunderlal, R. B. S. (1924). Cas apparents de reminiscences de vies antérieures. *Revue Métapsychique,* No. 4, juillet-août, 302–307.

Swedenborg, E. (1906). *Heaven and its Wonders and Hell.* Boston: New-Church Union. (First published in Latin, London, 1758)

Thomas, L. V. (1968). *Cinq Essais sur la mort Africaine.* Dakar: Université de Dakar.

Uchendu, V. C. (1964). The status implications of Igbo religious beliefs. *The Nigerian Field, 29,* 27–37.

Van de Castle, R. L. (1973). Personal communication.

Zahan, D. (ed.) (1965). *Réincarnation et Vie Mystique en Afrique Noire.* Paris: Presses Universitaires de France.

TWENTY-TWO

Some New Cases Suggestive of Reincarnation: The Case of Ampan Petcherat

1973[1]

INTRODUCTION

This case is not as rich as many others in the number of statements made by the subject about the previous life. Its principal interest lies in the fact that the subject, a girl, claimed to remember details in the life of a boy and, when she was young, showed a number of definitely masculine traits. The incidence of "sex change" as a feature of these cases varies widely from one culture to another. There are no cases of this type among approximately 200 cases from Alevis of Turkey, Druses of Lebanon and Syria, and Tlingits of Alaska. And, at the other extreme, approximately 20 percent of cases in Burma and 17 percent of cases in Thailand show this feature. Among cases from most other countries, e.g., Ceylon, India, Europe, and the United States (apart from Tlingit cases), the incidence of "sex change" is about 5 percent.[2]

SUMMARY OF THE CASE AND ITS INVESTIGATION

Ampan Petcherat was born in Song Klong, Thailand, in March, 1954. She was the daughter of Yod "Ngoi" Petcherat and his wife, Kim Suan. Ampan was Kim Suan's third child. Her parents later separated and Ampan stayed with her mother. In 1966 they were living in the town of Klong[3]

Darn, which is seven kilometers north of Song Klong and about thirty kilometers southeast of Bangkok.

When Ampan was about a year old she began to tell her mother that she had another mother and father at Klong Bang Chag near Klong Bang Plee. She said she had been a boy in the life with those parents. She described a house and objects in it, and also narrated how she had drowned after being bitten by a snake. Ampan would cry in talking about the previous home and ask to be taken to it. She repeated the story of her drowning from time to time. She gave no names of the previous family, only that of the place where she said she had lived.

Ampan's mother had the habit of paddling in a boat over to the area of Klong Bang Chag (about 20 kilometers from Klong Darn) each year at harvest time. From the time when Ampan was very small she took her on these trips. On one of them Ampan recognized the village of Bang Chag (which her mother would have known anyway), but they did not attempt at that time to trace the previous family Ampan talked about. As to why she did not look for the previous family earlier, Kim Suan said that Ampan expressed fear of a ghost which she said was in the village of Bang Chag.

In 1961, when she was seven, Ampan spontaneously recognized a woman on the street of Klong Darn whom she addressed as "my aunt." This woman was later identified as Joy Ruang Gun, a maternal aunt of the child whose life Ampan claimed to be remembering. It seems that on the first occasion of seeing her Ampan merely pointed to her and said to her mother: "That is my aunt." Later Ampan called Joy Ruang Gun "aunt" as they passed on the road and Joy Ruang Gun stopped and asked Ampan how she knew her. Ampan then said: "You are my mother's older sister." She was in fact the older sister of Tong Bai Puang Pei, of Bang Chag, who had lost a son, Chuey, by drowning in 1950.[4] She took Ampan and her mother to Klong Bang Chag to meet the family of this boy. At Klong Bang Chag Ampan made some additional statements about the previous life and some additional recognitions. Later she was taken to Wat Bang Plee Noi, where she recognized Chuey's older brother, Chuan, and one of his cousins. Ampan's statements fitted very closely facts of the life and death of Chuey Puang Pei who was a boy of about four when he drowned at Klong Bang Chag in 1950.

This case came to my attention in 1963 when a correspondent in Bangkok, T. Magness, sent me some preliminary information about it which he had obtained from a newspaper report. I was unable to investigate the case until July, 1966, when I spent several days interviewing members of both families. Francis Story participated with me in this investigation. In March, 1969, I returned to the area and interviewed several of the main informants again as well as two new ones. Ampan and her mother had in the meantime moved south to Sattahib, about 250 kilometers south of Bangkok. In March, 1971, I returned to the area once more and had further interviews with members of the previous family. I have not met with Ampan and her mother since I saw them in 1969.

PERSONS INTERVIEWED DURING THE INVESTIGATION

In Klong Darn I interviewed:

Ampan Petcherat
Kim Suan Petcherat, Ampan's mother
Ladda Lak Yam, Kim Suan Petcherat's cousin

In Song Klong I interviewed:

Yod "Ngoi" Petcherat, Ampan's father ("Ngoi" is a nickname meaning "lame")
Ben Ja Gauchainiem, an acquaintance of Ampan

At Wat Bang Plee Noi I interviewed:

Ven. Phra Chim Dhamma Choti
Ven. Phra Thong Yoi Uttamo

At the village of Bang Chag, on Klong Bang Chag, I interviewed:

Tai Puang Pei, Chuey's father
Tong Bai Puang Pei, Chuey's mother
Tong Puang Pei, Chuey's paternal great-aunt
Klah Puang Pei, Chuey's paternal uncle
Chuan Puang Pei, Chuey's older brother
Joy Ruang Gun, Chuey's maternal aunt (Tong Bai Puang Pei's older sister)
Pad Ruang Kham, Chuey's maternal aunt (older sister of both Tong Bai Puang Pei and Joy Ruang Gun)

Of the above informants I have set aside the testimony of two as being largely worthless. Ampan's father, Yod "Ngoi" Petcherat, said that he did not remember much and in comparison with other informants his testimony showed an unusually large number of discrepancies. He did not, however, discredit the case. Ben Ja Gauchainiem was a young woman of about 20 years of age who in 1969 helped me to trace Ampan and her mother at their new home in Sattahib. She, however, cast doubts on the case and impugned the veracity of Kim Suan Petcherat. But when I questioned her about her knowledge of the case, I found she had not herself ever talked with Ampan about it and (almost certainly) not with Kim Suan Petcherat either. She also reversed her own statements about her knowledge of the case and, in my opinion, disqualified herself as a reliable informant.

The testimony of the remaining informants hung together well. The members of the two families concerned supported each other's accounts of the case in all substantive matters. In 1966 I did not interview the Puang Peis independently of Ampan and her mother, who came along in the boat to Bang Chag to show us the way. But they were not with me in 1969 or 1971 when I visited the village of Bang Chag again and went over many of the details once more. And the Puang Peis were naturally not present when I saw Ampan and her mother again in Sattahib in 1969.

Two of the interpreters who worked with me on the case in 1966 were not adequately qualified and some of the discrepancies in the testimony are due, I believe, to faults of translation. The testimony of this case does include more discrepancies than the average case of the type, but these discrepancies seem to me to be, as usual, about details rather than about the main facts and events reported.

RELEVANT FACTS OF GEOGRAPHY AND POSSIBLE NORMAL MEANS OF COMMUNICATION BETWEEN THE FAMILIES CONCERNED

Song Klong, where Ampan was living with her mother up to the time the two families met in 1961, is 37 kilometers south of Bangkok and about 15 kilometers from Klong Bang Chag and the village of Bang Chag which is off this klong. In those days the only feasible way of traveling between these two places was by boat on the klongs. The main highway south from Bangkok runs through both Klong Darn and Song Klong. Since they are marketing towns, persons from the smaller villages such as Bang Chag are likely to visit them rather often. In 1971 a new highway going south came close to Wat Bang Plee Noi, although I still had to reach Bang Chag by boat along Klong Bang Chag.

Both of the families concerned in the case denied having any previous acquaintance with each other before Ampan was brought to Bang Chag by Chuey's maternal aunt in 1961. I think this claim is additionally supported by the failure of Kim Suan to look up Chuey's family on her annual visits to Klong Bang Chag between 1956 and 1961. I believe it unlikely that she was deterred by Ampan's fear of a ghost and that if she had had any knowledge of a family corresponding to Ampan's statements who had lost a boy by drowning, she would have gone to them to verify Ampan's statements.

THE DEATH OF CHUEY PUANG PEI

Chuey's parents were not present when he drowned so they were not firsthand informants of how this occurred. The two firsthand informants I interviewed were Chuey's paternal uncle, Klah Puang Pei, and his older brother, Chuan Puang Pei. Their accounts of the event, which they were remembering many years later, differed in some respects, but not in the fact that no one really knew how Chuey had come to drown.

Chuan was himself a boy of not more than eight or nine when Chuey drowned. He said that he, Chuan, and a cousin, Sa Ing, had been playing in and around the water, but he thought that Chuey had not been in the water, although he was nearby. According to Chuan, Chuey could not yet swim, but only walked in shallow water. (This disagrees with the statement of Klah Puang Pei, who said that Chuey could swim well.) Evidently Chuan paid no attention to what Chuey was doing until somehow he noticed that he was missing. So far as he remembered, Chuey had been sitting on the bank and they did not think he had gone into the water until he was found to be missing. Chuan then gave the alarm. He told me that he pulled Chuey's body out of the water; Klah Puang Pei said that he and he alone pulled the body out of the water. (I have not considered this a serious discrepancy since it is very likely that Chuan in some way helped his uncle get Chuey's body out of the water.)

Since children often drown in the klongs of Thailand the accident was found regrettable but almost "natural." No one considered the possibility that Chuey had been bitten by a snake and so no one examined his body for evidence of a snake bite. That a snake had bitten Chuey was at no time suspected by his family until Ampan's first visit to them in 1961.

There are poisonous snakes in the klongs of Thailand. But even if Chuey was bitten by a poisonous snake it is unlikely that death would have occurred so quickly from the venom. It is more probable that the small boy was startled and frightened by the bite, if it occurred, and then began to aspirate water and sank. So I believe that Chuey died from drowning even though he may have been bitten by a snake just before drowning. It is also possible that Chuey was bitten by a snake while sitting on the bank and then, after being bitten, rolled or jumped into the water and drowned.[5]

Klah Puang Pei said that Chuan had playfully pulled Chuey's leg before the drowning, but the family did not think this contributed to the drowning in any way. Chuan denied to me, however, that Chuey had been playing in the water. Since "leg-pulling" at the time of the drowning figured in Ampan's memories the point is of some importance, but I cannot decide whether Chuan or his uncle had the more accurate memory of exactly what happened. Since Chuan was a young boy at the time, I am inclined to credit the version of his uncle over his own, but not with firm confidence.

Chuey's paternal great-aunt, Tong Puang Pei, put a spot of red ochre[6] on the upper chest of Chuey's body before it was cremated. Unfortunately, in 1966 she did not remember on which side of the chest she had made the mark. Chuey's body was taken to the nearby wat at Klong Bang Plee and cremated.

In 1966, Chuey's father indicated his age at death as being about four years. In 1969 Chuey's mother said he was between three and four years old. In 1971 she changed her estimate and suggested that he was about five years old. His brother Chuan put Chuey's age at death as between four and six. I think it is safe to conclude that Chuey was about four years old when he died, certainly not much less and probably not much more.

STATEMENTS AND RECOGNITIONS MADE BY AMPAN

In the Tabulation I have listed all the statements and recognitions made by Ampan and approximately in chronological order. Statements 1-19 were made before the two families had met. (The time of occurrence of Item 4 is doubtful; it may not have taken place until Ampan went to Bang Chag.)

The recognition of Item 20 also occurred before the two families had met. Items 21–25 occurred at the time of Ampan's meeting with Joy Ruang Gun in Klong Darn. Items 26–31 occurred at the time of Ampan's first visit to Bang Chag. Items 32–33 occurred at Wat Bang Plee Noi.

I have included a few statements made to me by Ampan herself in 1966 and one from 1969. In 1966 her memories had faded considerably, but she said she still remembered some details. I have not, however, listed her as the sole informant for any item.

Item 4 requires some particular comment. Chuey's older brother, Chuan, was about eight or nine when Chuey drowned in 1950. Many young Thai men, perhaps most, spend several months or a year in a wat at some time or other in their lives. Chuan joined a monastery, Wat Bang Plee Noi (near Klong Bang Chag), when he was about 20 and remained there for approximately eight months. But he only decided to become a monk about a month before he actually entered the monastery, which he did just a few months before Ampan's first visit to Bang Chag in 1961. He was a monk at the wat when Ampan was taken there to see if she could recognize him. At the end of his eight months in the monastery he disrobed, became a farmer, and married. If Ampan had really said that Chuey's brother was a monk she would have been showing apparent extrasensory perception of the present circumstances of the previous family. But I think that Yod "Ngoi" Petcherat may have gotten this item mixed up. Chuey's mother, Tong Bai Puang Pei, told me Ampan said that Chuey had had a brother who was *going to be* a monk. Now it is quite possible that even a boy as young as Chuan was when Chuey died could have expressed the wish or intention of becoming a monk. Many boys in their teens or younger enter the monasteries as samaneras or novices. I have no evidence that Chuan expressed any such intention when Chuey was alive, but if my surmise that he did is correct, then Ampan's otherwise somewhat strange remark that she (in the former life) had a brother "who was going to be a monk" could be placed among Chuey's memories.

Seven of the items in the Tabulation relate to Chuey's death. Ampan had insisted that he was bitten by a snake and thereafter drowned. This has not been verified and, as I have already said, was not even conjectured by Chuey's family until Ampan mentioned it to them more than 10 years later. Discrepancies occurred in the testimony for Item 17. I cannot resolve them completely and I think that some at least are due to faulty translation. Both of Ampan's parents seem to have formed the idea that she was blaming Chuey's brother for the drowning by saying he had pulled Chuey's leg. Klah Puang Pei, Chuey's uncle, stated that there had been some "leg-pulling" in the water and I imagine the usual "horseplay" of boys swimming. Chuan denied to me in 1971 that there had been any "leg-pulling" between himself and Chuey before Chuey drowned, although he said he had been playing around in the water with Sa Ing. In 1966 Ampan seemed to preserve some rather clear memories of the previous life. Her testimony on this item was inconsistent on two days, but I think this was due to poor translation. In her clearest statement she described how Chuey had been playing at pulling legs with his brother before he was bitten by the snake and drowned. Ampan said that Chuey was not with Chuan at the time he drowned. I suppose then that Ampan had given her parents a somewhat similar account of the events earlier and that they had interpreted this incorrectly to imply that she was blaming the drowning on Chuan. But Ampan's parents further said that when Ampan met Chuan (in 1961 at Wat Bang Plee Noi), she had reproached him for drowning Chuey. The Ven. Phra Thong Yoi Uttamo, who was present at the wat when Ampan met Chuan, remembered no such comment. Nor did Chuan, who said that he and Ampan did not discuss the drowning when they met at the wat. Ampan's mother said that her father was not even present at the monastery when Ampan first met Chuan, so his testimony, not very reliable to begin with, was second hand on this point. It is odd, however, that Kim Suan Petcherat, who did seem to be a reliable witness, was the only person who remembered that Ampan had made reproaches about the drowning to Chuan. Possibly Ampan muttered these in a low voice that her mother could hear and the others could not.

In my effort to understand the discrepancies and incorrect items of this case it occurred to me that perhaps Ampan (or other informants) mixed up memories of leg-pulling (if this occurred) before Chuey drowned with those of the pulling of Chuey's body out of the water after the drowning. Ampan described how Chuey's body was taken to Wat Bang Plee Noi for cremation. Since this event obviously occurred after the recovery of the body from the water, she may have had partially distorted memories of the body being "pulled" from the water.

In 1966 Ampan told me that she had remembered the name of the previous personality, Chuey, but had not told anyone the name earlier because "there was no one to tell." This seemed like a strange remark since she had told her mother a number of details about the previous life. But her mother, who was rather a simple person, probably expressed little interest in the matter and certainly did not seem to have encouraged Ampan to tell more details. But neither did she suppress her. Ampan's father was out of the house (and I think out of the household) during much of Ampan's early years.

THE BIRTHMARK ON AMPAN'S CHEST

Ampan had a birthmark on the upper left chest below the left clavicle. In 1966 it consisted of a circular area of darker pigment about a half inch in diameter. It had the appearance thus of a pigmented, flat naevus. This birthmark may correspond in location with the red ochre mark placed on Chuey's body before cremation by his great-aunt, Tong Puang Pei. Unfortunately, since she had forgotten on which side of his chest she had placed the red ochre mark, we cannot be positive about the correspondence. I learned about the birthmark on Ampan's upper left chest before I knew that a member of Chuey's family had put red ochre on his upper chest before the cremation of his body. Since, however, the two families had met by that time, it is possible that they had informed each other about the possible correspondence between the birthmark and the red ochre mark.

Ampan said that Chuey was bitten on the right leg by a snake in the water. No one seems to have examined her legs to see whether she had a birthmark corresponding to a wound of a snake bite on the body of Chuey.

AMPAN'S BEHAVIOR RELATED TO THE PREVIOUS LIFE

Circumstances Stimulating Ampan's Statements about the Previous Life

One of the first occasions when Ampan spoke about how she died in the previous life occurred when she was playing in the water with her brothers. (Since Chuey had only one brother, I believe that here, as often in Asia, the word "brothers" was used loosely to mean cousins or other children of the neighborhood as well as biologically related siblings.) This situation then seems to have reminded her of the circumstances of the death of Chuey who was playing in (or near) the water with his "brothers" just before he drowned.

A visit with her mother in a boat on Klong Bang Chag also stimulated Ampan's memories for she then recognized the area of Bang Chag where Chuey had lived.

The Emotions Shown by Ampan in Talking of the Previous Life

Ampan cried when she expressed her wish to visit the previous family before she had done so. She seems to have had a strong desire to see its members and when at the age of seven she spontaneously recognized Chuey's aunt, Joy Ruang Gun, she embraced her and asked her to take her to her (previous) family. When Ampan first met Chuey's mother, Tong Bai Puang Pei, she also embraced her tightly. Kim Suan Petcherat and Chuan Puang Pei both said that Ampan wept when she met Chuan at Wat Bang Plee Noi. (Kim Suan Petcherat also said that Chuan wept, but he did not mention this to me himself.)

Ampan distinctly rejected Yod "Ngoi" Petcherat as her father during these early years. According to her mother she said: "Nai[7] Yod in not my father. I have another father." The absence of Yod "Ngoi" Petcherat from the home could well have stimulated such rejecting remarks; but Ampan made similar remarks about her mother, saying that Kim Suan was not her mother and that she had another mother.

After the first meeting of the two families, they continued to exchange visits at least up to 1966 when Ampan and her mother were living in Klong Darn. Chuan visited Ampan in Klong Darn and Ampan went to Bang Chag from time to time. She and her mother accompanied us there in 1966.

Masculine Traits in Ampan

Ampan, both according to her mother and from her own statements, had distinctly masculine interests and inclinations when she was a child. In 1966 her mother said that Ampan liked to dress as a boy and wear trousers or pants. And she liked boys' games such as boxing. (Boxing is a distinctly masculine sport in Thailand as it is everywhere else.) Ampan told me she would prefer to be a boy because they have a freer life than girls. At that time, she impressed me as being rather boyish in her dress (she was wearing shorts) and in her gait. She seemed to me to have a boyish way of swinging her arms as she walked.

In March, 1969, when I saw Ampan again, she was 15 years old. She had begun to menstruate just three or four months before this date, which (I was told) was late for Thai girls. Ampan's mother said that (in 1969) Ampan had only "learned to dress" in girls' clothes two years earlier, that is, at the age of 13. By this expression I think she meant to say that Ampan had then begun to dress in girls' clothes voluntarily without being pressured or forced to wear them.

In appearance Ampan seemed in 1969 to have definitely moved to the feminine side since my last meeting with her nearly three years before. She was wearing a long sarong-like skirt and blouse of distinctly feminine type and her figure was filling out into feminine proportions. She was beginning to use makeup. But her mother said that she chose her friends among tomboy girls and had little interest in boys. On the other hand, an American soldier from the nearby base at Sattahib had taken an interest in her and she showed me his photograph.

Ampan said she still liked boxing and still engaged in boxing herself. She also said that she still would prefer to be a boy since she would be freer as a boy than as a girl.

As a gift I offered Ampan a choice between a boy's knife and a bottle of perfume and she chose the latter.

To explore her sexual orientation a little further I asked her to do the extended draw-a-person test (Whitaker, 1961). Her first (free choice) drawing was of a boy; her second (with directions to draw a member of the opposite sex) was of a girl; and her third (free choice) drawing was of a girl. But the figure of this third drawing seemed to me extremely masculine. The hair was short and the person was wearing what seemed to be a shirt with buttons down the center. I thought Ampan had drawn another boy or man until she told me the drawing was supposed to be of a girl.

In summary, Ampan when younger showed more masculine traits than most girls of her age. And at the age of 15 she still showed some definitely masculine traits and preferences, including a wish to be a boy.[8] At the same time she had moved definitely toward the feminine side in her overall sexual orientation.

Other Behavior of Ampan Related to the Previous Life

In view of the fact that Chuey had died of drowning it was of interest to me to learn whether Ampan had manifested any fear of the water. Both Ampan and her mother positively asserted that she had never shown any fear of the water. She enjoyed swimming from a fairly early age.

According to Ampan, she had a dislike for snakes that persisted up to 1966, but afterwards this receded because she said in 1969 that she liked snakes and enjoyed playing with small ones. I do not think that Ampan ever had a marked phobia of snakes because her mother in 1969 could not remember that she had ever been afraid of them.

RELATIVE DELAY IN FADING OF AMPAN'S MEMORIES

In 1966 Ampan spoke quite freely about her memories of the previous life which seemed then still quite fresh. At that time she was 12 years old. Three years later (almost) she said the memories had largely faded, but not entirely. She still recalled and reviewed with me details of the drowning of the previous personality. It seems then that the memories faded in Ampan at a rather later age than is usual in these cases.

After the first meeting of the two families in 1966 they continued to exchange visits at least up to 1966 when Ampan and her mother were living in Klong Darn. Chuan visited Ampan in Klong Darn and Ampan went to Bang Chag from time to time. She and her mother accompanied me there in 1966. After the removal of Ampan and her mother to Sattahib visits between the two families became more difficult, but in 1971 Chuey's mother said they had seen Ampan the previous year at Klong Darn, presumably when members of both families were visiting there. The visits between Ampan and the previous family may have contributed to the persistence of her memories.

Ampan dropped out of school at the end of the third year which would be at the age of about eight years. But she was by no means a recluse and seemed to be leading (apart from inattendance at school) a normal social life for a girl of her age both in 1966 and 1969.

COMMENTS ON THE EVIDENCE OF PARANORMAL PROCESSES IN THE CASE

I cannot exclude in this case the possibility that the two families may have had some slight, casual contact at some time or other prior to the development of the case. The Puang Pei family would certainly have gone into the larger towns of Klong Darn and Song Klong along the highway and it was on one such visit of Chuey Puang Pei's aunt that Ampan recognized her. But this did not happen until Ampan was seven and if the Puang Peis had frequently visited the area of Song Klong (which is not a large town), where Ampan first lived, one might have expected that she would have recognized one or another of them earlier. I feel confident anyway that the two families had no significant contact with each other prior to Ampan's first statements. Each family denied any prior familiarity with the other and I see no reason to doubt their statements on the matter.

Both families are of approximately equal social and economic status. Ampan and her mother had nothing to gain by her attaching herself to some not very well-to-do farmers in a village 15 or so kilometers away.

In this case extrasensory perception (at least between Ampan and other living persons) seems a less plausible interpretation than it may be for some other cases. For one thing, Ampan showed knowledge of conditions of the house and family as they were during the lifetime of Chuey; that is, she remembered a house that had been taken down, a red dog that was no longer there, trees that had been removed, and a brother who was going to become a monk. If she got all this information through extrasensory perception she was reaching into the past. It was a past known to surviving members of the family to be sure, but still it was their past situation rather than their present one.

Table 22.1. Summary of Statements and Recognitions Made by Ampan

Item	*Informants* [1]	*Verification*	*Comments*
1. She[2] had a house at Klong Bang Chag near Klong Bang Plee.	Yod "Ngoi" Petcherat, Ampan's father Kim Suan Petcherat, Ampan's mother	Tai Puang Pei, Chuey's father Tong Bai Puang Pei, Chuey's mother	Both informants said Ampan had mentioned both names. Bang Plee is not so much the name of a klong as of a fairly large area. Klong Bang Plee runs through it and past the temple called Wat Bang Plee Noi.
2. She had another father and mother.	Kim Suan Petcherat	Tai Puang Pei Tong Bai Puang Pei	
3. She had two older brothers.	Kim Suan Petcherat	Tong Bai Puang Pei	Chuey had only one older brother, Chuan, who was about 8-9 years old when Chuey drowned. Ampan may also have been counting Chuey's cousin, Sa Ing, as a "brother." He had an older sister, Mia, who died the same year Chuey drowned. There may have been an error of translation in the statement of Kim Suan.
4. One brother was a monk.	Yod "Ngoi" Petcherat Tong Bai Puang Pei	Incorrect	This item may not have occurred until after the two families had met. Yod "Ngoi" Petcherat may have been a secondhand informant for it. Tong Bai Puang Pei said Ampan told her Chuey had had a brother who was going to be a monk. This is also what Tong Bai Puang Pei said (as a secondhand informant) that Ampan had told Chuey's aunt.
5. She had an uncle.	Kim Suan Petcherat	Klah Puang Pei, Chuey's paternal uncle	

6. She had an aunt.	Kim Suan Petcherat	Tong Bai Puang Pei Joy Ruang Gun, Chuey's maternal aunt	Joy Ruang Gun was the aunt Ampan recognized in Klong Darn.
7. She had one younger sister.	Kim Suan Petcherat	Tong Bai Puang Pei	Chuey had a younger sister called Khao.
8. There was a red dog where she lived.	Kim Suan Petcherat Joy Ruang Gun	Tong Bai Puang Pei	The dog had died by the time Ampan visited Klong Bang Chag. The item is in no sense specific since it seem to me that about a quarter of all dogs in Thailand are reddish or rust brown in color. Joy Ruang Gun said Ampan had mentioned two red dogs at the house and she said this was correct. But her sister, Tong Bai Puang, said there was only one red dog.
9. There were three buffaloes.	Kim Suang Petcherat Joy Ruang Gun	Tong Bai Puang Pei	The Puang Pei family had two adult buffaloes and one baby buffalo during Chuey's lifetime. Joy Ruang Gun said Ampan mentioned only two buffaloes, which she said was correct, perhaps thinking only of the adult ones.
10. Red trousers belonging to her were hanging on the second floor.	Kim Suang Petcherat	Tong Bai Puang Pei	Some red cloth for a sarong, not for trousers, was hanging up in the house when Chuey drowned. But the sarong was Chuey's.
11. She was a boy in the previous life.	Kim Suang Petcherat	Tong Bai Puang Pei	Chuey was a boy of about four when he drowned.
12. The house looked like a stable.	Kim Suang Petcherat	Doubtful	The house, which I visited in 1966 and 1969, was elevated on stilts like most houses along the klongs in Thailand. Animals could sometimes get under the floor of the upper part, but I would not have described this house as resembling a stable.

13. Before she died she had been playing hide-and-seek and swimming.	Kim Suang Petcherat	Unverified	I did not learn at what the children had been playing before going into the water. Chuan and another boy, Sa Ing, had been playing together in the water.
14. She had been bitten by a snake.	Kim Suang Petcherat Ladda Lak Yam, cousin of Ampan's mother Ampan (1966)	Unverified	See text for full discussion of drowning of Chuey. Ampan said the snake bit Chuey on the right leg while he was in the water. (See the following item.)
15. She then fell into the water and drowned.	Kim Suang Petcherat Ampan (1966)	Klah Puang Pei	Ampan herself said in 1966 that Chuey was in the water when bitten by the snake.
16. Her two brothers were there when she drowned.	Kim Suan Petcherat Ampan (1969)	Chuan Puang Pei, Chuey's older brother Tai Puang Pei	Chuan was nearby when Chuey drowned. One other child, a cousin, Sa Ing, who could be loosely called a "brother," was present also. In 1969 Ampan said that, in addition to Chuey's brother, a boy who was his cousin was present. She did not give his name, but referred to him as "pee-nawng" which means in Thai a brother, sister, or cousin. Tai Puang Pei was away from the house when Chuey drowned, and so was a secondhand witness.
17. One of her brothers pulled her ankle and held her under the water.	Kim Suan Petcherat Yod "Ngoi" Petcherat	Unverified	In 1966 Ampan herself gave discrepant testimony on two different days and each of her statements differed from what her mother said she had said earlier. Yod "Ngoi" Petcherat's account of what Ampan had said also differed from that of his wife. He said Ampan had claimed that Chuey's brother had drowned him by putting his foot on his neck. Klah Puang Pei, Chuey's uncle, thought Chuey and Chuan had been playing together in the water and that Chuan had pulled Chuey's leg, although he did not think this had anything to do with Chuey's

			drowning. But Chuan said he had only been playing in the water with the other boy, Sa Ing, before they noticed Chuey was missing.
18. Her elder brother took her out of the water, but she was already dead.	Ladda Lak Yam	Doubtful	Klah Puang Pei said he alone removed body from the water. But Chuan said that he had pulled Chuey's body from the water. Perhaps they helped each other. In 1966, Ampan herself "withdrew" this item and said she did not know who pulled the body from the water. She did not, however, deny that earlier she said that Chuan had done so.
19. Her body was taken to Wat Bang Plee.	Kim Suan Petcherat Ampan (1966)	Tong Bai Puang Pei	Ampan said that Chuey's father took Chuey's body to the wat for cremation.
20. Recognition of Bang Chag	Kim Suan Petcherat		Ampan repeatedly asked her mother to take her to the place of the previous life. So Kim Suan Petcherat took Ampan along when she had occasion to paddle over to Klong Bang Chag. On one of these occasions Ampan recognized Bang Chag, where Chuey had lived. But she and her mother did not approach Chuey's house or family at that time.
21. Recognition of Chuey's aunt, Joy Ruang Gun	Joy Ruang Gun Kim Suan Petcherat		Kim Suan Petcherat was with Ampan when she saw Joy Ruang Gun in Klong Darn and said: "That is my aunt." Ampan seems not to have talked with Joy Ruang Gun on this first occasion of seeing her. However, later she passed her on the street and called her "aunt." Joy Ruang Gun heard her, stopped, and asked Ampan how she knew her. Ampan then said that she (Joy Ruang Gun) was Chuey's mother's older sister. Joy Ruang Gun then asked Ampan: "Who are your parents?" and received the answers of the

			following two items. Kim [illegible] varied what she said (on different occasions) Ampan had called the strange woman they saw in the street. At first she said Ampan had referred to her as "aunt," but in later discussion said Ampan had used a word that means "mother." (This discrepancy may have arisen in a difficulty with translation since Ampan later left no doubt that she had thought of the woman recognized as her previous aunt.) Ampan and her mother said she had recognized Chuey's aunt at Song Klong, but Joy Ruang Gun said she met Ampan first at Klong Darn. Faults of memory may have occurred here or the two occasions mentioned above may have occurred at different towns.
22. Her father was called Tai.	Joy Ruang Gun	Tai Puang Pei	Ampan made this and the remark of the next item as she met Chuey's aunt and tried to establish her previous identity with her.
23. Her mother was called Bai.	Joy Ruang Gun	Tong Bai Puang Pei	
24. There was a bamboo tree in front of the house.	Joy Ruang Gun	Joy Ruang Gun	
25. There were two red jars at the house.	Joy Ruang Gun Tong Bai Puang Pei	Tong Bai Puang Pei	Joy Ruang Gun said Ampan told her, *before* she came to Bang Chag, that there were two red jars at the house, which Joy Ruang Gun and Tong Bai Puang Pei said was correct. Ampan also made a similar remark at Bang Chag, but then mentioned only one red jar. When I visited the Puang Pei home in 1966 they still had a large red jar. If one had been there in 1961 when Ampan visited she might have seen it, although her remark was mentioned to me as an

			indication of her knowledge of objects around the house in Chuey's time. But even if Ampan had not seen a red jar at the house, the item is not at all specific since perhaps half the homes along the klongs keep drinking water in red jars. (The other jars are nearly all a kind of bistre brown.)
26. Recognition of Chuey's mother, Tong Bai Puang Pei	Tong Bai Puang Pei Ladda Lak Yam		This item occurred at Bang Chag. Ampan went to Tong Bai Puang Pei, embraced her tightly, and said: "Mother." Ampan knew she was going to Bang Chag and naturally expected to meet the previous mother and father.
27. Recognition of Chuey's father, Tai Puang Pei	Ladda Lak Yam Tai Puang Pei		When Ampan and her mother arrived at Bang Chag, Chuey's father was not at home, but later arrived with two other men. While they were sitting in the boat before landing, Ampan was asked to say which was the previous father. She correctly pointed to Tai Puang Pei. Attempts were made to mislead her, but she insisted on the identification she had made.
28. There were banana and coconut trees at the house.	Tong Bai Puang Pei	Tong Bai Puang Pei	Ampan made this remark when she went to Bang Chag. These trees were no longer standing at the time of Ampan's visit. Not at all a specific item, but not without some value since the trees were no longer there.
29. There had been two houses where she lived.	Tong Bai Puang Pei	Tong Bai Puang Pei	Ampan made this remark when she went to Bang Chag. One of the houses had been removed by the time of Ampan's visit there.
30. Recognition of site where Chuey was drowned.	Tong Bai Puang Pei Ladda Lak Yam		This recognition is of doubtful value. Ampan pointed to a place in the water near the house. She did not indicate the exact spot where Chuey had drowned. Children would obviously swim

		near the boat dock on the klong and so this is the most likely site for drownings.
31. Recognition of Chuey's sister, Khao	Kim Suan Petcherat	Ampan pointed at Khao and said: "Sister," but did not give Khao's name.
32. Recognition of Chuey's brother, Chuan	Kim Suan Petcherat Ven. Phra Thong Yoi Uttamo, monk of Wat Bang Plee Noi Chuan Puang Pei Ampan (1966)	This recognition occurred at Wat Bang Plee Noi, where Chuan was then living as a monk. Chuan was among a group of other monks variously estimated as 10 and 30 in number. Chuan said that Ampan had picked him out of the group of monks sitting together at the wat. But he wavered on the question of whether she had indicated him spontaneously and said: "You are my brother," or whether someone had asked her to pick out Chuey's brother from the group. Ampan wept when she met Chuan and he also, according to Kim Suan Petcherat, was moved to tears. Ampan's recollection of the scene was that she was asked to say which of the monks was her previous brother and pointed to Chuan correctly. The other two informants indicate the recognition was more spontaneous, but it appears Ampan herself had said Chuey's brother was at the wat and asked to go there. She therefore expected to see him there.
33. Recognition of Sak, Chuey's cousin	Joy Ruang Gun Chuan Puang Pei	Sak was another young monk in the group at Wat Bang Plee Noi. According to Joy Ruang Gun, Ampan indicated him and said: "This phra [monk] is Nang Pad's son." Sak was Nang Pad's son; Nang Pad was the elder sister of both Tong Bai Puang Pei and Joy Ruang Gun. Chuan did not say that Ampan had mentioned Sak's name, but said she spontaneously pointed to two other monks (Sak and Sa Ing) and said they were

			Chuey's cousins, which was correct. It would have been improper for Ampan to have mentioned a monk's own name. "Nang" is an honorific in Thai corresponding to "Mrs."

Notes:

[1] The *Informants* column lists the witnesses of what Ampan said or did relating to the previous life, while the *Verification* column names the persons who vouch for the accuracy of what she said or did with regard to the previous personality.

[2] "She" actually refers to the male previous personality, but to avoid confusion I have used the feminine pronoun in this Tabulation. Also to reduce misunderstanding I have referred in the Comments to Ampan saying that Chuey had done this or that. In fact, although Ampan said she had remembered the name Chuey, she does not seem to have mentioned it to anyone when she was first talking about the previous life. Instead her statements would be phrased with the first person singular as subject, e.g., "I was bitten by a snake."

NOTES

1. Reprinted from the *Journal of the American Society for Psychical Research, 67,* 361–380, 1973. Published with permission of the American Society for Psychical Research, Inc. (ASPR), 5 West 73rd Street, New York, New York 10023, Webpage: aspr.com, e-mail: aspr.com.—Ed.

2. In addition to the present case, other cases in which the subject remembered a previous life as a member of the opposite sex are those of Paulo Lorenz (Stevenson, 1966/1974), Gnanatilleka (Stevenson, 1966/1974), Dolon Champa Mitra (Stevenson, 1975), and Ruby Kusuma Silva (1977).

3. Readers will find this case easier to understand if I explain now that this part of Thailand has numerous connected klongs or canals running through it. The klongs actually have some sluggish current and resemble the bayous of southern Louisiana. Formerly they provided the chief routes of transport in the area and even today, although many roads have been built, are still much used for travel and transport. Towns and villages along the klongs often have the same names as the klongs on which they are located. So do some of the wats, as Buddhist temples are called in Thailand, if they are located on klongs.

4. Dates for birth and death in this case are approximate only.

5. North American readers familiar with the prominent local reactions produced at the site of a bite by a pit viper, e.g., a rattlesnake, may find almost incredible the failure of Chuey's family to notice on his body marks and other signs of a snake bite if one occurred before he drowned. It is important to understand, however, that the hematoxic venoms of the vipers produce much more local reaction at the site of the bite than do the neurotoxic venoms of snakes such as cobras and other members of the Elapidae family. "The bitten part shows little local reaction in the case of neurotoxic venoms but is swollen, discolored, and painful when infiltrated by the hematoxic type" (Mackie, Hunter, & Worth, 1954, p. 620).

Since we do not know that Chuey was bitten by a snake it is perhaps idle to speculate about what species of snake may have bitten him. But an important candidate would be the Monocled Cobra (*Naja naja kaouthia*). It is quite common in the area of Klong Darn and many cases of snake bite occur there each year, although most of them happen when the person bitten is on land. These cobras are good swimmers and can remain under water for considerable time. Cobras usually bite only in self-defense, but may strike if stepped upon inadvertently. They inject a neurotoxic venom.

In the case of Chuey, if he was bitten by a snake, local reaction at the site of the bite would have been further reduced by the fact that he drowned and died immediately after the bite.

6. Such marks are sometimes made on bodies as a tag of identification that will be reproduced on the next body of the reincarnating person. The practice is fairly widespread in Burma (Mi Mi Khaing, 1962) and Assam (Parry, 1932) as well as in Thailand, where I have recently studied two more cases of the type. [Since this paper was published, many more cases of this type have been identified. To date, 74 cases have been identified by Ian and his colleagues, and case reports of 24 of them have been published (Stevenson, 1997, 1:803–879; Tucker & Keil, 2002–2005).—Ed.]

7. "Nai" is an honorific in Thai meaning "Mr." It might be used by a child in referring to its father.

8. Ampan's expressed desire to change sex should be considered in the light of other facts and circumstances. First, she was a 15-year-old girl, not a grown woman when she made the remark. Secondly, Asian women (particularly those of Buddhist countries) express a wish to be men more often than do western women. This difference derives, I think, from the generally inferior social status of women in Asia and, in Buddhist countries, from the lower status accorded women with regard to possibilities for spiritual development. Women can attain enlightenment, but they cannot become monks. And since monks have more opportunities for meditation and other actions that promote spiritual advancement men have an advantage over women in their

ability to take up a monk's life. Many women in other parts of the world also express a wish to be men, but I believe the wish is more often and more strongly expressed by women in Asia than it is by women in Europe and North America.

REFERENCES

Mackie, T. T., Hunter, G. W., & Worth, C. B. (1954). *A Manual of Tropical Medicine* (2nd ed.). Philadelphia: W. B. Saunders.

Mi Mi Khaing. (1962). *Burmese Family*. Bloomington: Indiana University Press.

Parry, N. E. (1932). *The Lakhers*. London: Macmillan.

Stevenson, I. (1974). *Twenty Cases Suggestive of Reincarnation* (2nd ed.). Charlottesville: University Press of Virginia. (First published in 1966)

Stevenson, I. (1975). *Cases of the Reincarnation Type. Vol. 1. Ten Cases in India*. Charlottesville: University Press of Virginia.

Stevenson, I. (1977). *Cases of the Reincarnation Type. Vol. 2. Ten Cases in Sri Lanka*. Charlottesville: University Press of Virginia.

Stevenson, I. (1997). *Reincarnation and Biology: A Contribution to the Etiology of Birthmarks and Birth Defects* (2 vols.). New York: Praeger.

Tucker, J. B., & Keil, H H. J. (2002-2005). Experimental birthmarks: New cases of an Asian practice. *International Journal of Parapsychology, 13*, 1–18.

Whitaker, L. (1961). The use of an extended draw-a-person test to identify homosexual and effeminate men. *Journal of Consulting Psychology, 25*, 482–485.

TWENTY-THREE

Three New Cases of the Reincarnation Type in Sri Lanka with Written Records Made Before Verifications

1988[1]

. . . In the interest of brevity we omit from the case reports that follow many of the details that a complete report of each case would include. For example, we shall only mention the names of informants where doing so would help readers to identify persons referred to more than once. We also omit some details of the subjects' behaviors that related to their statements. Instead, we shall focus attention on the following two features of each case: the key statements made by the subject that were verified as corresponding to events in the life and death of a particular deceased person and the possibilities for the normal communication of information about the previous personality to the subject or the subject's family.

CASE REPORT

The Case of Thusitha Silva

Thusitha Silva was born near Payagala, Sri Lanka, on July 29, 1981. Her parents were Gunadasa Silva and his wife, Gunaseeli. Gunadasa Silva was a tailor. Thusitha was the sixth of the family's seven children.

When Thusitha was about three years old she heard someone mention Kataragama, and she began to say that she was from there. She said that she lived near the river there and that a dumb boy had pushed her into the river. She implied, without clearly stating, that she had then drowned. (Thusitha had a marked phobia of water.) She said her father was a farmer and also had a boutique for selling flowers which was near the Kiri Vehera (Buddhist stupa). She said that her house was near the main Hindu Temple (Devale) at Kataragama. She gave her father's name as Rathu Herath and said that he was bald and wore a sarong. (Thusitha's father wore trousers.) Thusitha did not give a name for herself in the previous life and indeed gave no proper names apart from "Kataragama" and "Rathu Herath." She never explicitly said that she had been a girl in the previous life, but she mentioned frocks and also objected to having her hair cut; so her parents inferred that she was talking about the life of a girl.

Tissa Jayawardane learned of this case in the autumn of 1985 and visited Thusitha and her family for the first time on November 15, 1985. Having recorded the above statements and some others he went to Kataragama. Here we should explain that Payagala is a small town (population in 1981: 6,000) on the western coast of Sri Lanka south of Colombo, and Kataragama, a well-known place of pilgrimage, is in the southeastern area of the island, in the interior (Obeyesekere, 1981; Wirz, 1966). Kataragama is approximately 220 km by road from Payagala. It is also a small town (population in 1987: approximately 17,500) and consists almost entirely of temples and supporting buildings together with residences for the persons who maintain the temples and supply the needs of the pilgrims. A moderately large river, the Manik Ganga, runs through the town.

T.J. went first to the police station in Kataragama, where he inquired for a family having a son who was dumb. He was directed to a double row of flower stalls along the pavement of the main road to the Buddhist stupa, known as the Kiri Vehera. (The vendors at these stalls sell flowers to pilgrims for their use in worship.) Upon inquiring again among the flower vendors he was told to go to a particular flower stall, and at that one he asked whether a young girl of the family had drowned. He was told that a young daughter of the family had drowned in the river some years earlier, and one of her brothers was dumb. According to T.J.'s notes, Thusitha had made 13 verifiable statements and all but three of these were correct for the family with the dumb child who had lost a girl from drowning.

In the second phase of the investigation (in December 1985), G.S.[2] learned about 17 additional statements that Thusitha had made, and he recorded these. The two families still had not met (and, so far as we know, this is still true), so that, as mentioned earlier, we consider our record of these statements uncontaminated by any contact between the two families. Two of these 17 additional statements were unverifiable, but the other 15 were correct for the family of the drowned girl. A few of these statements, such as that one of the houses where the family had lived had had a thatched roof, were of wide applicability. A few others, such as that there were crocodiles in the river, could be regarded as part of information generally known about Kataragama. However, several of the additional statements that G.S. recorded were about unusual or specific details, and we will mention these. Thusitha said that her father, in addition to being a farmer and selling flowers, was also a priest at the temple. She mentioned that the family had had two homes and that one of them had glass in the roof. She referred to the water in the river being low. She spoke of dogs that were tied up and fed meat. She said her previous family had a utensil for sifting rice that was better than the one her family had. She described, with imitative actions, how the pilgrims smash coconuts on the ground at the temple in Kataragama.

Western readers unfamiliar with Sri Lanka may not immediately appreciate the unusualness of the details in several of these statements. For example, there are plenty of dogs in Sri Lanka, but most of them are stray mongrels who live as scavengers; few are kept as pets. Also, most Sinhalese who are Buddhists would abhor hunting, although Christian Sinhalese might not. It happened that the family of the drowned girl had neighbors who hunted, and they fed meat from the animals they killed to a dog chained in their compound. This would be an unusual situation in Sri Lanka. Another unusual detail was that of a glass (skylight) in the roof of the house. Devotees at Hindu temples other than the one at Kataragama may smash coconuts as part of their worship; however, Thusitha had never had occasion to see this ritual.

In the third phase of the investigation, I.S. (accompanied by G.S. and T.J.) went to Thusitha's family and then to Kataragama. Each family was visited twice in this phase, once in November 1986 and again in October 1987. We learned that the girl who had drowned, who was called Nimalkanthi, had been not quite two years old when she died, in about June 1974. Nimalkanthi had gone to the river with her mother, who was washing clothes there. She was playing near her mother with two of her brothers one of whom was the dumb one. Her mother apparently became absorbed in her washing, and then suddenly noticed that Nimalkanthi was missing. The brother who could speak could not say where she had gone. Nimalkanthi's mother raised an alarm, a search was made, and Nimalkanthi's dead body was recovered from the river. It is unlikely that the dumb brother had pushed Nimalkanthi into the water, but all three children had been playing around just before she disappeared. It seems probable that she lost her footing and slid or fell into the water; she could not swim. Thusitha's statement that the dumb brother had pushed her into the river thus remains unverified, and it is probably incorrect. However, the brother may have pushed her playfully just before she drowned accidentally.

Two of Thusitha's verifiable statements were definitely incorrect. She said that her father of the previous life was bald, but Nimalkanthi's father (whom we interviewed) had a good head of hair. She said his name was Rathu Herath, but it was Dharmadasa. There were, however, two bald men in the family—Nimalkanthi's maternal grandfather and a maternal uncle—and Nimalkanthi would have seen them often. And a cousin by marriage, whom Nimalkanthi saw from time to time, was called Herath (not Rathu Herath). Thus one could argue that Thusitha's memories included some confusions of the adult men in her family, but we do not wish to emphasize this explanation.

Another of Thusitha's statements was incorrect for Nimalkanthi's lifetime, but not for the period after her death. She said that she had sisters (but did not say how many). Nimalkanthi had one sister, and about 18 months after her death, her mother gave birth to another daughter.

Concerning the possibilities for previous acquaintance between the families concerned, we are confident that they had none. Nimalkanthi's family had never even heard of Thusitha when we first met them. Nimalkanthi's father had never been to Payagala; he had passed through it only on his way to a larger town called Kalutara, also on the west coast of Sri Lanka. Thusitha's family had never gone to Kataragama in an effort to verify her statements. Gunadasa Silva said he had hoped to do this, but for various reasons—largely the needs of his tailoring business—he had never got around to this.

In the years 1980–81 Gunadasa Silva had gone "very often" to Kataragama. On one visit only, when she was two months pregnant with Thusitha, his wife, Gunaseeli, had gone with him. Gunadasa had bathed in the river in the usual way of pilgrims and had purchased flowers from the flower stalls near the Kiri Vehera. He could not remember the name—if he ever knew it—of the flower vendor from whom he purchased most of the flowers he bought. Thus he had gone to Kataragama after Nimalkanthi's death, but had stopped going there before Thusitha's birth. Thusitha, incidentally, said that she had seen her father at Kataragama, a reference on her part to a presumed discarnate existence between the death of Nimalkanthi and her own birth.[3]

We made inquiries in Kataragama about the frequency of drownings in the river. The police station had records available only for the three years of 1985–87. There had been one drowning in 1985, none in 1986, and one (up to October) in 1987. The coroner of Kataragama had died in 1986 and his records were not available. The coroner of the neighboring town of Tissamaharama, who had been acting coroner at Kataragama for almost a year (since the death of its regular coroner), had no detailed figures of drownings in the river at Kataragama; however, he estimated that one occurred about every two years, mostly among pilgrims. The registrar of births and deaths at Kataragama did not keep records beyond each year, at the end of which the records were sent to the government office (kachcheri) of the next largest administrative area. The records were not classified according to causes of death. The registrar said that there had been no drownings so far in 1987 (contrary to the police records). She estimated that two children drowned in the river each year, a much higher estimate than other sources suggested.

There were 20 stalls of flower vendors on either side of the broad avenue that leads to the Buddhist stupa (Kiri Vehera) in Kataragama. On the day of our inquiries one stall was unattended, but we asked the vendors at all the others whether any member of their family was dumb and whether any member had drowned. One vendor's family had a cousin who was dumb; no other family (apart from Nimalkanthi's) had any dumb member. No family except Nimalkanthi's had lost a member through drowning.

Comment

Despite Thusitha's failure to state correctly any proper names other than that of Kataragama, we have no doubt that we have identified the only family to which her statements could refer. The single detail that her (previous) father had a flower stall near the Kiri Vehera in Kataragama immediately restricted the possibilities to about 20 families. Of these, only one had both a son who was dumb and a daughter who drowned in the river. The various other details Thusitha mentioned are hardly necessary for increasing the correctness of the identification of the family to which Thusitha's statements correspond, although they do provide additional confirmation. . . .

DISCUSSION

. . . During the nearly 30 years that have passed since the systematic investigation of these [CORT] cases began, a variety of interpretations for them have been put forward, both by us and by other persons who have read our reports. The leading interpretations are: fraud, cryptomnesia (source amnesia), unintentional distortion of memories on the part of the informants (paramnesia), extrasensory perception on the part of the subject, possession, and reincarnation. We shall not review the arguments for and against each of these interpretations. Interested readers may study full discussions of them elsewhere (Stevenson, 1966/1974, 1975, 1987). Suffice it to say here that although each of the interpretations that are alternative to reincarnation may be correct for a few cases, all but one break down when applied to most of the cases. The exceptional interpretation, however, is extremely difficult to exclude. We refer to that of paramnesia, which means that, without being aware that they have done so, the informants for the families concerned in a case have so muddled their memories of what the subject said and of what was true about the identified deceased person as to vitiate the case. This possibility has become further elaborated into what we may call the sociopsychological interpretation of the cases. According to it, in a culture having a belief in reincarnation a child who seems to speak about a previous life will be encouraged to say more. What he says then leads his parents somehow to find another family whose members come to believe that the child has been speaking about a deceased member of their family. The two families exchange information about details, and they end by crediting the subject with having had much more knowledge about the identified deceased person than he really had had. Chari (1962, 1987) has been a particularly articulate and long-standing exponent of this interpretation. Brody (1979) gave a succinct as well as a fair exposition of it.

Because we recognize the plausibility of the sociopsychological interpretation, at least for some cases, we attach great importance to the cases of the present group: ones in which someone (ourselves preferably) makes a written record of the subject's statements before they are verified. . . .

NOTES

1. Excerpts reprinted from the *Journal of Scientific Exploration, 2,* 217–238.—Ed.
2. G.S. is Godwin Samararatne, Ian's coinvestigator and coauthor of this paper.—Ed.
3. Most children who claim to remember previous lives say nothing about events after death in the previous life and before their birth. Memories of a discarnate existence are particularly rare in Sri Lanka cases. The case of Disna Samarasinghe (Stevenson, 1977) is exceptional. When the children do make comments about such "intermediate" experiences, they frequently include the child's explanation of how it came to be in its family, instead of in some other family.

REFERENCES

Brody, E. B. (1979). Review of *Cases of the Reincarnation type. Volume II. Ten Cases in Sri Lanka.* By Ian Stevenson. Charlottesville: University Press of Virginia, 1977. *Journal of Nervous and Mental Disease, 167,* 769–774.

Chari, C. T. K. (1962). Paramnesia and reincarnation. *Proceedings of the Society for Psychical Research, 53,* 264–286.

Chari, C. T. K. (1987). Correspondence. *Journal of the Society for Psychical Research, 54,* 226–228.

Stevenson, I. (1974). *Twenty Cases Suggestive of Reincarnation.* Charlottesville: University Press of Virginia (2nd rev. ed.). (First published in *Proceedings of the American Society for Psychical Research, 26,* 1–362, 1966.)

Stevenson, I. (1975). *Cases of the Reincarnation Type. I. Ten Cases in India.* Charlottesville: University Press of Virginia.

Stevenson, I. (1977). *Cases of the Reincarnation Type. II. Ten Cases in Sri Lanka.* Charlottesville: University Press of Virginia.

Stevenson, I. (1987). *Children Who Remember Previous Lives: A Question of Reincarnation.* Charlottesville: University Press of Virginia.

4f

Cases of the Reincarnation Type with Birthmarks and Birth Defects

EWK

I have reserved a separate section for a class of CORT that became increasingly important in Ian's eyes as his research progressed—namely, cases involving children who were born with unusual birthmarks or birth defects corresponding to similar marks or wounds on the deceased person. (Ampan's case in the previous section provides one example.) Although he had noted such cases as early as his first paper on CORT (Stevenson, 1960a, pp. 54, 62) and published examples in his first book on CORT (Stevenson, 1966/1974, the cases of Ravi Shankar, Wijeratne, William George Jr., and Henry Elkin), as the cases accumulated their implications became more evident. First, the correspondence between the birthmarks and wounds could not plausibly be attributed to chance in the vast majority of cases. The marks and defects were often highly unusual ones, many instances involved more than one, and other aspects of the case (such as the child's memories or behavior) also had to be accounted for. Second, many of the cases clearly involved more than potentially faulty memories of the informants, since autopsy reports or hospital records objectively documented the correspondence. The cases also present a serious challenge to the super-psi explanation: even if the child obtained information about the deceased person by ESP—an explanation Ian found unsatisfactory from the beginning (e.g., Stevenson, 1960b, pp. 101–104; 1987/2001, pp. 159–161)—ESP certainly did not cause the mark or defect. The influence of a deceased person, in whatever manner, seems more plausible. As we will see in the next section, there is another possible explanation in some cases, but nonetheless these birthmark/birth defect cases as a whole strain super-psi explanations. Finally, these cases also became increasingly important in Ian's eyes because they promised to shed light on the questions that lay behind his early interests in medicine, psychosomatic medicine, and psychiatry—the influence of mind on body and the sources of individual differences in health and disease. As a result, for many years Ian focused his efforts most intently on studying cases of this type.[1]

In the remainder of this section I have first included two pages from *Reincarnation and Biology*, pages that he said "summarize the question that has preoccupied me for my whole career" (2000, personal communication). This is followed by a paper in which Ian provided a brief review of the birthmark/birth defect cases, preliminary to the three large volumes published four years later that included reports of over 200 of these cases (Stevenson, 1997a, 1997b). Finally, I include a report of one such case.

NOTE

1. The enormous scope of this project initially escaped even Ian. Some years ago I came across a letter from the late 1970s in which Ian had told his correspondent that he was working on a monograph on cases involving birthmarks and birth defects, to be published "sometime next year." The monograph finally came out nearly 20 years later (Stevenson, 1997a, 1997b)—and certainly not because of any indolence on Ian's part. Unfortunately, like so many people who have unusual experiences, I failed to make a note of what I had seen. The letter was re-filed and remains buried somewhere in Ian's vast files of correspondence!

REFERENCES

Stevenson, I. (1960a). The evidence for survival from claimed memories of former incarnations. Part I. Review of the data. *Journal of the American Society for Psychical Research, 54*, 51–71.

Stevenson, I. (1960b). The evidence for survival from claimed memories of former incarnations. Part II. Analysis of the data and suggestions for further investigations. *Journal of the American Society for Psychical Research, 54*, 95–117.

Stevenson, I. (1974) *Twenty Cases Suggestive of Reincarnation* (2nd ed., rev.). Charlottesville: University Press of Virginia. (Original work published 1966)

Stevenson, I. (1997a). *Reincarnation and Biology: A Contribution to the Etiology of Birthmarks and Birth Defects* (2 vols.). New York: Praeger.

Stevenson, I. (1997b). *Where Reincarnation and Biology Intersect*. Westport, CT: Praeger.

Stevenson, I. (2001). *Children Who Remember Previous Lives: A Question of Reincarnation* (rev. ed.). Jefferson, NC: McFarland. (Original work published 1987)

TWENTY-FOUR

Excerpt from *Reincarnation and Biology*

1997[1]

In addition to contributing to the evidence of reincarnation, the cases I describe here suggest a hitherto neglected factor in the etiology of birthmarks, congenital malformations, and some other diseases. Some persons who have heard of a case of this type have suggested that the subject's statements and associated reported behavior are invented to explain a birthmark or congenital malformation the subject may have.[2] I think that this may happen in a few cases, and I have studied several in which I think it did happen. Yet even if we explain the other features of a case by a congenital malformation, we have not necessarily explained the malformation itself. The concept of reincarnation may, however, do just that. If cases of this type are best interpreted as instances of reincarnation, reincarnation helps us to understand the occurrence of some birthmarks and birth defects.

During the last century medical research has increased our knowledge of some of the proximate physical causes of birth defects. A variety of factors, such as genetic abnormalities, certain diseases of pregnant women, and alcohol and certain drugs taken by them, have been shown capable of causing them. But causing them in which persons? Why is one person born with a birth defect when another—his twin brother perhaps—is not?

This is not a question that could interest committed materialists. They can ask about mediating causes and say, for example, that a certain baby was born with congenital heart disease because its mother had German measles in the first trimester of her pregnancy with it. But they cannot—without violating their principles—ask about more ultimate causes, such as why a particular *person*, as opposed to a particular *body*, has a congenital malformation. To materialists there is no person in the body, because there can be no person other than a body. To ask why one person has a congenital malformation and another has not is, for them, like asking why, when several dice are shaken in a cup and thrown out, one of them rolls so that six faces up, but the other five dice do not. It is, they would say, just a matter of chance.

The Western concept of chance can be traced back as far as Empedocles, but it seems to have become widely developed among scientists only during the past 300 years, beginning perhaps with the desire of gamblers and insurers to lessen their losses and increase their gains. In the 18th century Edward Gibbon (1796/1907) wrote contentedly that "I have drawn a high prize in the lottery of life . . . the double fortune of my birth in a free and enlightened country, in an honourable and wealthy family, is the lucky chance of an unit against millions" (p. 217). The concept of chance has become deeply incorporated in modern biology. First, evolution is said to occur almost entirely by natural selection acting on mutations that occur by chance. Second, chance is said to govern the sorting of the gene-carrying chromosomes into the gametes: spermatazoa and ova. Yet much remains unexplained, especially about the uniqueness in body and behavior of each living being when born. Also in the 18th century, Alexander Pope (1733/1966) could write:

> All Nature is but Art, unknown to thee;
> All Chance, Direction, which thou canst not see;

A vindication of the research reported here would not nullify the role of chance in human and other matters; but it would show chance to have less influence in our lives than most scientists now believe it to have. Chance may lie farther back in the chain of causes leading to our present existences than we realize.

Returning to materialism—as a complete doctrine of human personality—those who think it gives an incomplete account of the nature of man can legitimately ask why one person has a congenital malformation while another does not. Moreover, inquirers willing to take reincarnation seriously also find it reasonable to ask a further question: why does a congenitally malformed person have the *particular* malformation he or she has and not some other one?

This work is, therefore, considerably more than a treatise on birthmarks and birth defects. It is also a study of the reasons for some of the differences between individual persons. Geneticists say we are all unique because of the random distribution of genes among the chromosomes of our parents during the formation of the gametes (sperm and ova), the union of which is the conception of an embryo that will become a new person. They would add that a further contribution to individuality comes from environmental influences after conception—uterine and postnatal. I am not denying the importance of genes and recognized environmental influences in contributing to the uniqueness of individuals; but I am presenting evidence that this uniqueness may derive also from another factor: reincarnation. Most scientists today believe that a person only comes into existence at the time his or her body is conceived by the union of the parents' gametes. However, we now have evidence suggesting that at least some persons have had existences before the conception of their bodies and that the events of these existences have influenced the conditions of their lives and contributed to their uniqueness as individuals. This evidence is not as strong as it may become; it certainly does not compel a belief in reincarnation, but it provides a rational (as opposed to a religious) basis for that belief. I believe that the cases of this volume provide additional justification for the belief.

NOTES

1. *Reincarnation and Biology: A Contribution to the Etiology of Birthmarks and Birth Defects* (vol. i, pp. 5–6), Ian Stevenson, M.D. Copyright © 1997 by Ian Stevenson. Reproduced with permission of ABC-CLIO, LLC, Santa Barbara, CA.—Ed.

2. My associate in Burma, U Win Maung, often reminded me that in Hindu-Buddhist cultures one does not require a *specific* explanation for a birth defect, because a *general* one lies at hand—in the doctrine of karma. Thus if a child is born with missing fingers, his parents simply attribute the malformation to some event in one of the subject's previous lives. They usually have little curiosity—and may have none whatever—concerning a particular event that might account for the defect in a more detailed manner. It is thus a matter of indifference to them whether the child later does or does not make statements about a previous life that appear to explain precisely why he happens to have the defect his parents noticed when he was born.

REFERENCES

Gibbon, E. (1907). *Autobiography*. London: Oxford University Press. (First published in 1796)

Pope, A. (1966). *An Essay on Man*. London: Oxford University Press. (First published in 1733)

TWENTY-FIVE

Birthmarks and Birth Defects Corresponding to Wounds on Deceased Persons

1993[1]

Almost nothing is known about why pigmented birthmarks (moles or nevi) occur in particular locations of the skin. The causes of most birth defects are also unknown. About 35% of children who claim to remember previous lives have birthmarks and/or birth defects that they (or adult informants) attribute to wounds on a person whose life the child remembers. The cases of 210 such children have been investigated. The birthmarks were usually areas of hairless, puckered skin; some were areas of little or no pigmentation (hypopigmented macules); others were areas of increased pigmentation (hyperpigmented nevi). The birth defects were nearly always of rare types. In cases in which a deceased person was identified the details of whose life unmistakably matched the child's statements, a close correspondence was nearly always found between the birthmarks and/or birth defects on the child and the wounds on the deceased person. In 43 of 49 cases in which a medical document (usually a postmortem report) was obtained, it confirmed the correspondence between wounds and birthmarks (or birth defects). There is little evidence that parents and other informants imposed a false identity on the child in order to explain the child's birthmark or birth defect. Some paranormal process seems required to account for at least some of the details of these cases, including the birthmarks and birth defects.

INTRODUCTION

Although counts of moles (hyperpigmented nevi) have shown that the average adult has between 15 and 18 of them (Pack & Davis, 1956), little is known about their cause—except for those associated with the genetic disease neurofibromatosis—and even less is known about why birthmarks occur in one location of the body instead of in another. In a few instances a genetic factor has been plausibly suggested for the location of nevi (Cockayne, 1933; Denaro, 1944; Maruri, 1961); but the cause of the location of most birthmarks remains unknown. The causes of many, perhaps most, birth defects remain similarly unknown. In large series of birth defects in which investigators have searched for the known causes, such as chemical teratogens (like thalidomide), viral infections, and genetic factors, between 43% (Nelson & Holmes, 1989) and 65–70% (Wilson, 1973) of cases have finally been assigned to the category of "unknown causes."

Among 895 cases of children who claimed to remember a previous life (or were thought by adults to have had a previous life), birthmarks and/or birth defects attributed to the previous life were reported in 309 (35%) of the subjects. The birthmark or birth defect of the child was said to correspond to a wound (usually fatal) or other mark on the deceased person whose life the child said it remembered. This paper reports an inquiry into the validity of such claims. With my associates I have now carried the investigation of 210 such cases to a stage where I can report their details in a forthcoming book (Stevenson, 1997). This article summarizes our findings.

Children who claim to remember previous lives have been found in every part of the world where they have been looked for (Stevenson, 1983, 1987), but they are found most easily in the countries of South Asia. Typically, such a child begins to speak about a previous life almost as soon as it can speak, usually between the ages of two and three; and typically it stops doing so between the ages of five and seven (Cook [Kelly], Pasricha, Samararatne, Win Maung, & Stevenson, 1983). Although some of the children make only vague statements, others give details of names and events that permit identifying a person whose life and death corresponds to the child's statements. In some instances the person identified is already known to the child's family, but in many cases this is not so. In addition to making verifiable statements about a deceased person, many of the children show behavior (such as a phobia) that is unusual in their family but found to correspond to behavior shown by the deceased person concerned or conjecturable for him (Stevenson, 1987, 1990).

Although some of the birthmarks occurring on these children are "ordinary" hyperpigmented nevi (moles) of which every adult has some (Pack & Davis, 1956), most are not. Instead, they are more likely to be puckered and scarlike, sometimes depressed a little below the surrounding skin, areas of hairlessness, areas of markedly diminished pigmentation (hypopigmented macules), or port-wine stains (*nevi flammei*). When a relevant birthmark is a hyperpigmented nevus, it is nearly always larger in area than the "ordinary" hyperpigmented nevus. Similarly, the birth defects in these cases are of unusual types and rarely correspond to any of the "recognizable patterns of human malformation" (Smith, 1982).

METHODS

My investigations of these cases included interviews, often repeated, with the subject and with several or many other informants for both families. With rare exceptions, only firsthand informants were interviewed. All pertinent written records that existed, particularly death certificates and postmortem reports, were sought and examined. In the cases in which the informants said that the two families had no previous acquaintance, I made every effort to exclude all possibility that some information might nevertheless have passed normally to the child, perhaps through a half-forgotten mutual acquaintance of the two families. I have published elsewhere full details about methods (Stevenson, 1975, 1987[2]).

I did not accept any indicated mark as a birthmark unless a firsthand witness assured me that it had been noticed immediately after the child's birth or, at most, within a few weeks. I enquired about the occurrence of similar birthmarks in other members of the family; in nearly every instance this was denied, but in seven cases a genetic factor could not be excluded.

Birth defects of the kind in question here would be noticed immediately after the child's birth. Inquiries in these cases excluded (again with rare exceptions) the known causes of birth defects, such as close biological relationship of the parents (consanguinity), viral infections in the subject's mother during her pregnancy, and chemical causes of birth defects like alcohol.

RESULTS

Correspondences between Wounds and Birthmarks

A correspondence between birthmark and wound was judged satisfactory if the birthmark and wound were both within an area of 10 square centimeters at the same anatomical location; in fact, many of the birthmarks and wounds were much closer to the same location than this. A medical document, usually a postmortem report, was obtained in 49 cases. The correspondence between wound and birthmark was judged satisfactory or better by the mentioned criterion in 43 (88%) of these cases and not satisfactory in 6 cases. Several different explanations seem to be required to account for the discrepant cases, and I discuss these elsewhere (Stevenson, 1997). Figure 25.1 shows a birthmark (an area of hypopigmentation) on an Indian child who said he remembered the life of a man who had been killed with a shotgun fired at close range. Figure 25.2 shows the location of the wounds recorded by the pathologist. (The circles were drawn by an Indian physician who studied the postmortem report with me.)[3]

The high proportion (88%) of concordance between wounds and birthmarks in the cases for which we obtained postmortem reports (or other confirming documents) increases confidence in the accuracy of informants' memories concerning the wounds on the deceased person in those more numerous cases for which we could obtain no medical document. Not all errors of informants' memories would have resulted in attributing a correspondence between birthmarks and wounds that did not exist; in four cases (possibly five) reliance on an informant's memory would have resulted in missing a correspondence to which a medical document attested.

Cases with Two or More Birthmarks

The argument of chance as accounting for the correspondence between birthmarks and wounds becomes much reduced when the child has two or more birthmarks each corresponding to a wound on the deceased person whose life he claims to remember. Figure 25.3 shows a

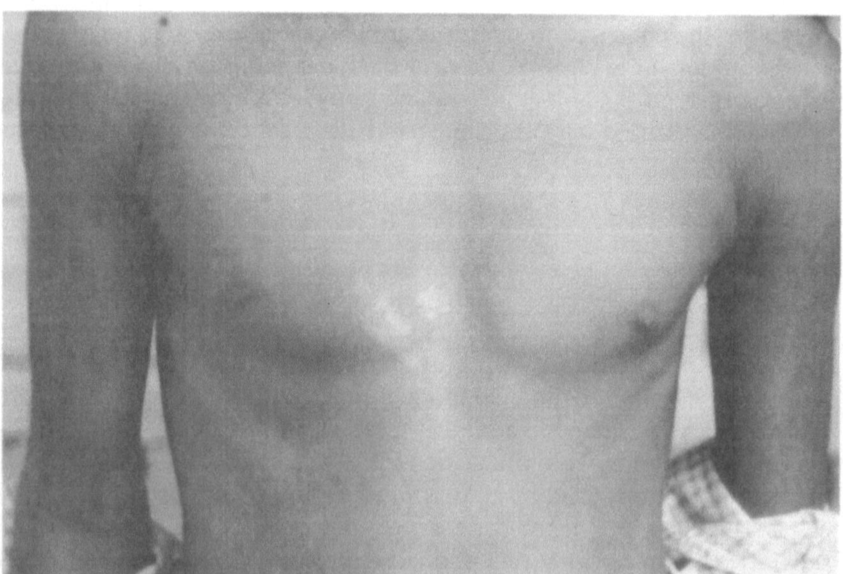

Figure 25.1. Hypopigmented macule on chest of an Indian youth who, as a child, said he remembered the life of a man, Maha Ram, who was killed with a shotgun fired at close range.

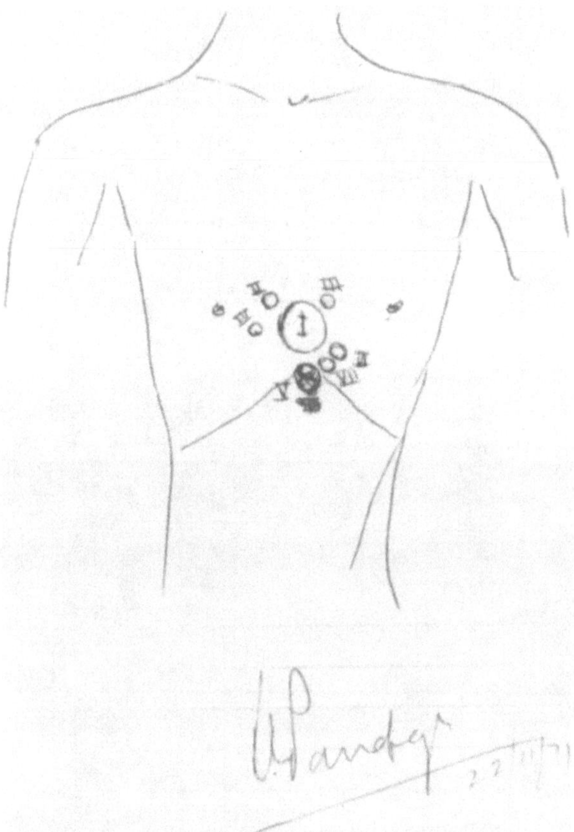

Figure 25.2. The circles show the principal shotgun wounds on Maha Ram, for comparison with Figure 2.

major abnormality of the skin (verrucous epidermal nevus) on the back of the head of a Thai man who, as a child, recalled the life of his uncle, who had been struck on the head with a heavy knife and killed almost instantly. The subject also had a deformed toe-nail of the right great toe (Figure 25.4). This corresponded to a chronic infection of the same toe from which the subject's uncle had suffered for some years before he died.[4]

The series includes 18 cases in which two birthmarks on a subject corresponded to gunshot wounds of entry and exit. In 14 of these one birthmark was larger than the other, and in 9 of these 14 the evidence clearly showed that the smaller birthmark (usually round) corresponded to the wound of entry and the larger one (usually irregular in shape) corresponded to the wound of exit. These observations accord with the fact that bullet wounds of exit are nearly always larger than wounds of entry (Fatteh, 1976; Gordon & Shapiro, 1982). Figure 25.5 shows a small

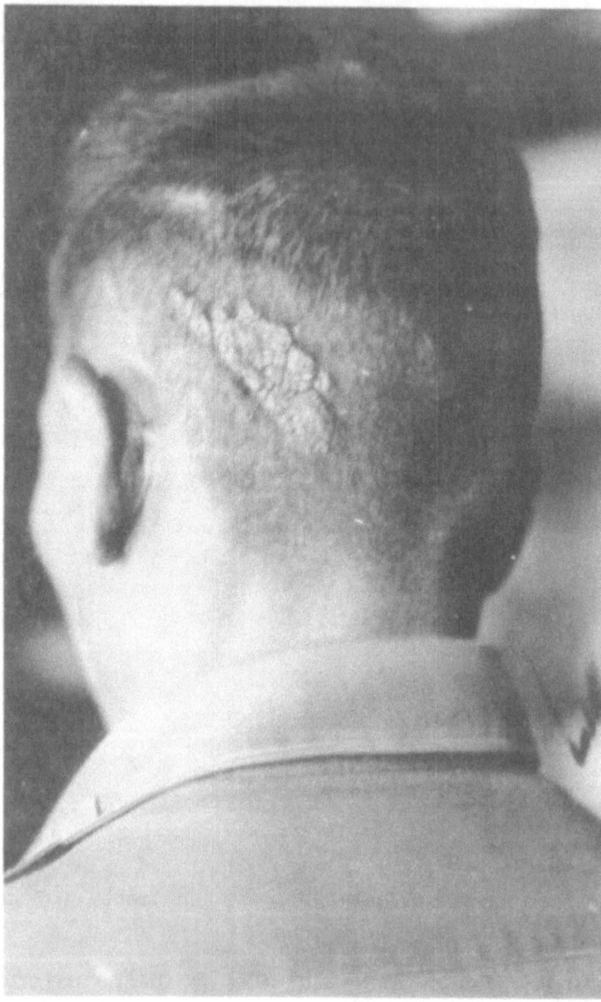

Figure 25.3. Large verrucous epidermal nevus on head of a Thai man who as a child said he remembered the life of his paternal uncle, who was killed with a blow on the head from a heavy knife.

round birthmark on the back of the head of a Thai boy, and Figure 25.6 shows a larger, irregularly shaped birthmark at the front of his head. The boy said that he remembered the life of a man who was shot in the head from behind. (The mode of death was verified, but no medical document was obtainable.)[5] In addition to the 9 cases I have investigated myself, Mills reported another case having the feature of a small round birthmark (corresponding to the wound of entry) and a larger birthmark corresponding to the wound of exit (both verified by a postmortem report) (Mills, 1989).

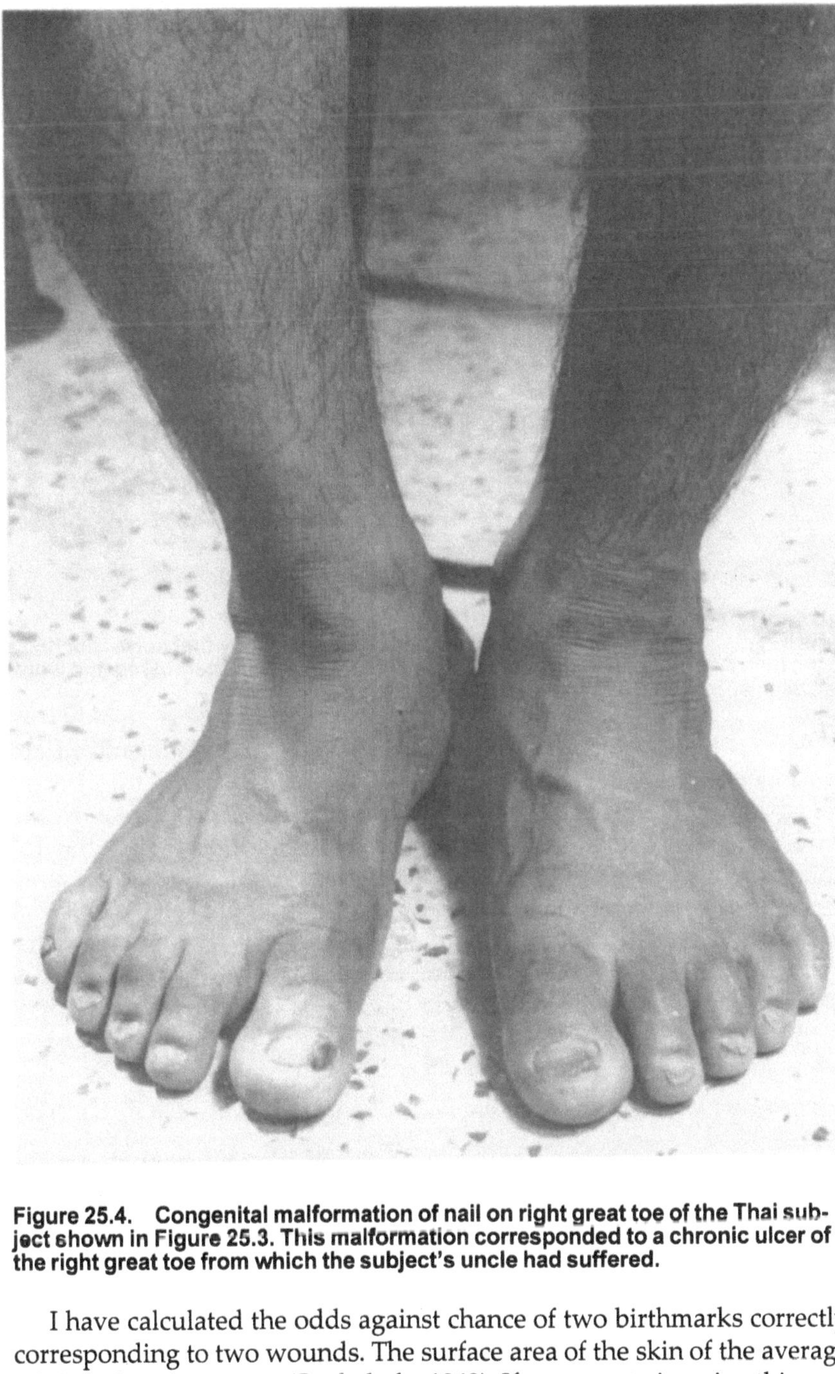

Figure 25.4. Congenital malformation of nail on right great toe of the Thai subject shown in Figure 25.3. This malformation corresponded to a chronic ulcer of the right great toe from which the subject's uncle had suffered.

I have calculated the odds against chance of two birthmarks correctly corresponding to two wounds. The surface area of the skin of the average adult male is 1.6 meters (Spalteholz, 1943). If we were to imagine this area square and spread on a flat surface, its dimensions would be approxi-

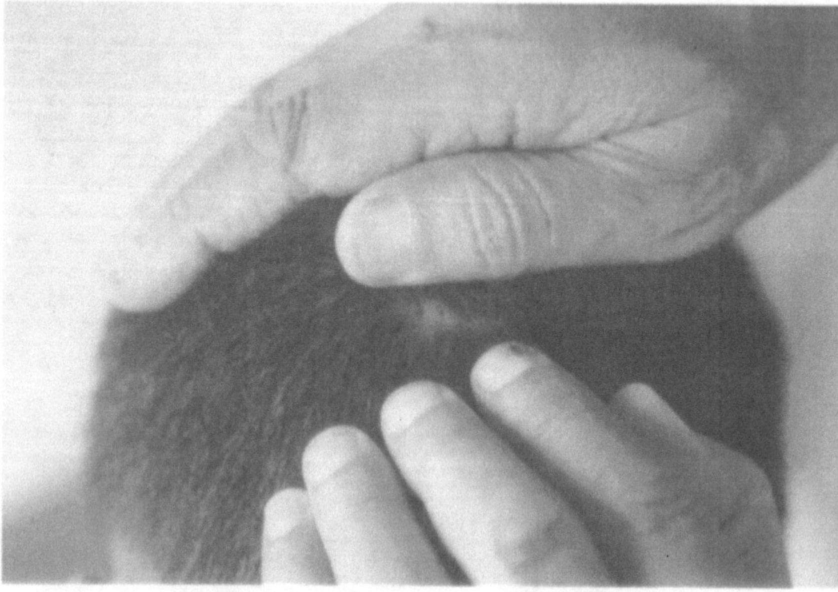

Figure 25.5. Small, round puckered birthmark on a Thai boy that corresponded to the bullet wound of entry in a man whose life he said he remembered and who had been shot with a rifle from behind.

mately 127 centimeters by 127 centimeters. Into this area would fit approximately 160 squares of the size 10 centimeters square that I mentioned above. The probability that a single birthmark on a person would correspond in location to a wound within the area of any of the 160 smaller squares is only 1/160. However, the probability of correspondences between two birthmarks and two wounds would be $(1/160)^2$, i.e., 1 in 25,600. (This calculation assumes that birthmarks are uniformly distributed over all regions of the skin. This is incorrect [Pack, Lenson, & Gerber, 1952], but I believe the variation can be ignored for the present purpose.)

Examples of Other Correspondences of Detail between Wounds and Birthmarks

A Thai woman had three separate linear hypopigmented scarlike birthmarks near the midline of her back; as a child she had remembered the life of a woman who was killed when struck three times in the back with an ax. (Informants verified this mode of death, but no medical record was obtainable.)[6] A woman of Burma was born with two perfectly round birthmarks in her left chest (Figure 25.7); they slightly overlapped, and one was about half the size of the other. As a child she said that she remembered the life of a woman who was accidentally shot and killed

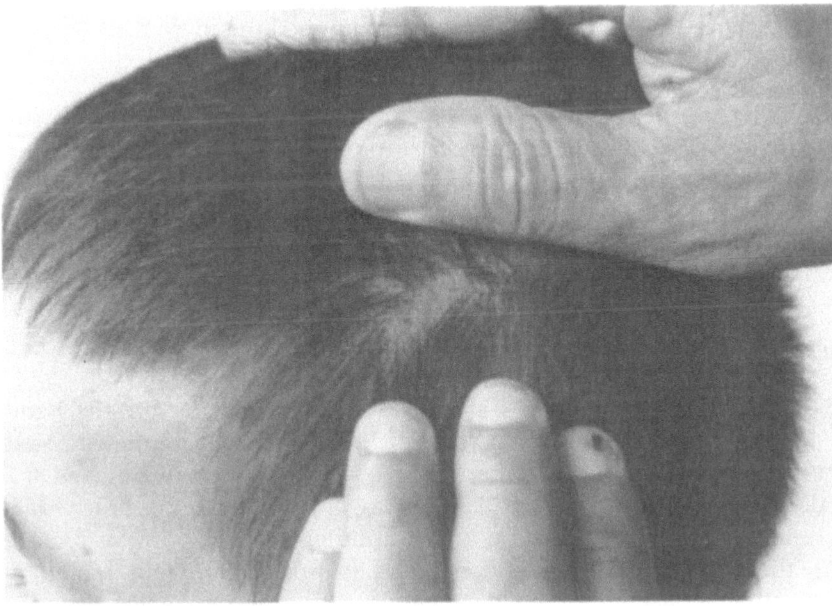

Figure 25.6. Larger, irregularly shaped birthmark on the frontal area of the head of the Thai boy shown in Figure 25.5. This birthmark corresponded to the bullet wound of exit on the Thai man whose life the boy said he remembered.

with a shotgun. A responsible informant said the shotgun cartridge had contained shot of two different sizes. (No medical record was obtainable in this case.)[7] Another Burmese child said that she remembered the life of her deceased aunt, who had died during surgery for congenital heart disease. This child had a long, vertical linear hypopigmented birthmark close to the midline of her lower chest and upper abdomen; this birthmark corresponded to the surgical incision for the repair of the aunt's heart. (I obtained a medical record in this case.)[8] In contrast, a child of Turkey had a horizontal linear birthmark across the right upper quadrant of his abdomen. It resembled the scar of a surgeon's transverse abdominal incision. The child said that he remembered the life of his paternal grandfather, who had become jaundiced and was operated on before he died. He may have had a cancer of the head of the pancreas, but I could not learn a precise medical diagnosis.[9] Two Burmese subjects remembered as children the lives of persons who had died after being bitten by venomous snakes, and the birthmarks of each corresponded to therapeutic incisions made at the sites of the snakebites on the persons whose lives they remembered.[10] Another Burmese subject also said as a child that she remembered the life of a child who had been bitten on the foot by a snake and died. In this case, however, the child's uncle had applied a burning cheroot to the site of the bite—a folk remedy for snakebite in parts of

Burma; and the subject's birthmark was round and located at the site on the foot where the bitten child's uncle had applied the cheroot.[11]

Three Examples of Birth Defects

Figure 25.8 shows the right side of the head of a Turkish boy with a diminished and malformed ear (unilateral microtia). He also had under-development of the right side of his face (hemifacial microsomia). He said that he remembered the life of a man who had been shot (with a shotgun) at point-blank range. The wounded man was taken to a hospital where he died 6 days later—of injuries to the brain caused by shot that had penetrated the right side of the skull. (I obtained a copy of the hospital record.)[12]

Figure 25.9 shows fingers almost absent congenitally on one hand (unilateral brachydactyly) in a child of India who said he remembered the life of another child who had put his right hand into the blades of a fodder-chopping machine and lost his fingers. Most cases of brachydactyly involve only a shortening of the middle phalanges. In the present case there were no phalangeal bones, and the fingers were represented by mere stubs. Unilateral brachydactyly is exceedingly rare, and I have not

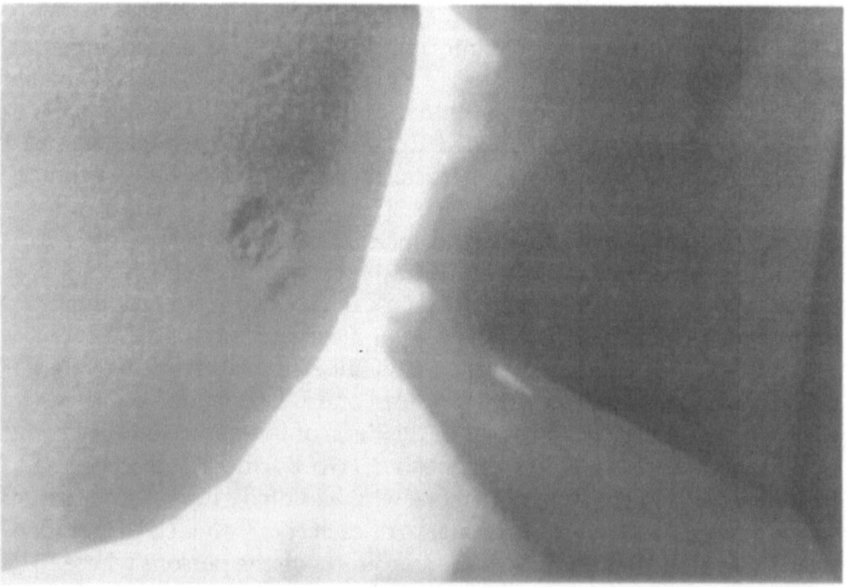

Figure 25.7. Two round, puckered, scarlike birthmarks of different sizes on the left breast of a Burmese woman who as a child said she remembered the life of a woman who was fatally wounded by a shotgun that used a cartridge containing shot of different sizes.

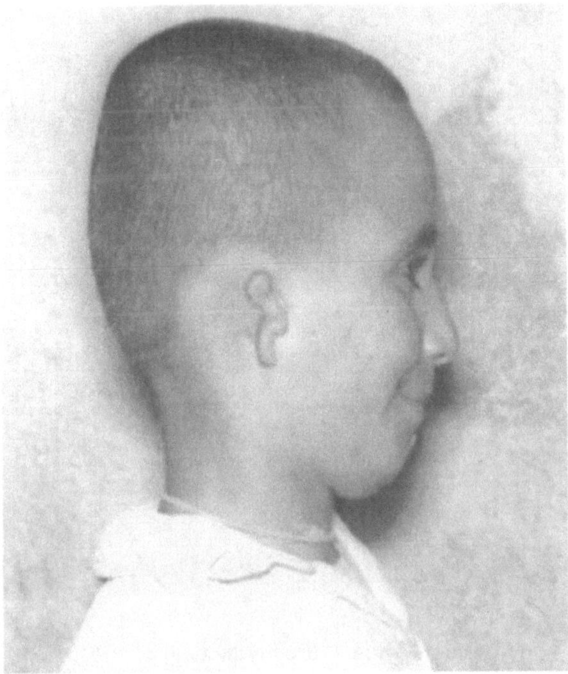

Figure 25.8. Severely malformed ear (microtia) in a Turkish boy who said that he remembered the life of a man who was fatally wounded on the right side of the head by a shotgun discharged at close range.

found a published report of a case, although a colleague (plastic surgeon) has shown me a photograph of one case that came under his care.[13]

Figure 25.10 shows congenital absence of the lower right leg (unilateral hemimelia) in a Burmese girl. She said that she remembered the life of a girl who was run over by a train. Eyewitnesses said that the train severed the girl's right leg first, before running over the trunk. Lower hemimelia is an extremely rare condition, and Frantz and O'Rahilly (1961) found it in only 12 (4.0%) of 300 cases of all congenital skeletal deficiencies that they examined.[14]

DISCUSSION

Because most (but not all) of these cases develop among persons who believe in reincarnation, we should expect that the informants for the cases would interpret them as examples according with their belief; and they usually do. It is necessary, however, for scientists to think of alternative explanations.

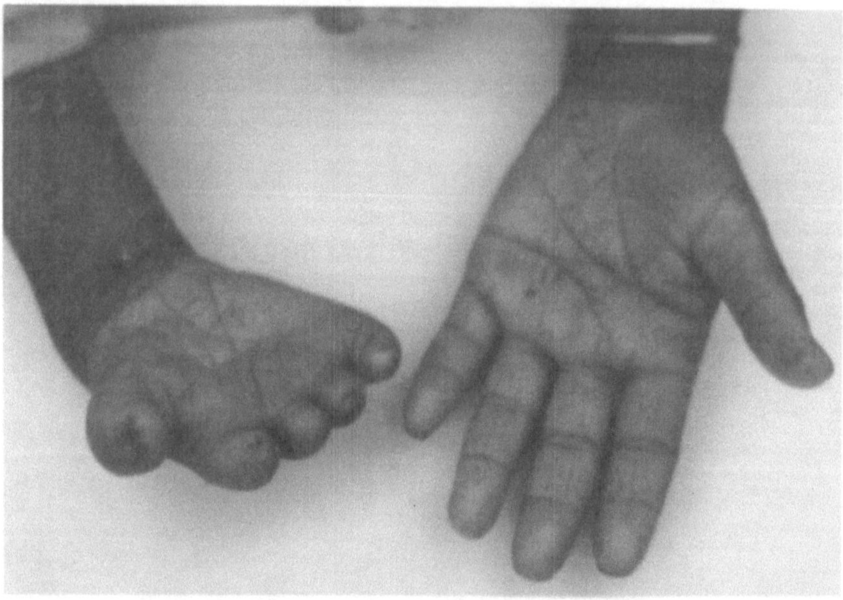

Figure 25.9. Almost absent fingers (brachydactyly) of one hand in a boy of India who said he remembered the life of a boy of another village who had put his hand into the blades of a fodder-chopping machine and had his fingers amputated.

The most obvious explanation of these cases attributes the birthmark or birth defect on the child to chance, and the reports of the child's statements and unusual behavior then become a parental fiction intended to account for the birthmark (or birth defect) in terms of the culturally accepted belief in reincarnation. There are, however, important objections to this explanation. First, the parents (and other adults concerned in a case) have no need to invent and narrate details of a previous life in order to explain their child's lesion. Believing in reincarnation, as most of them do, they are nearly always content to attribute the lesion to *some* event of a previous life without searching for a *particular* life with matching details. Second, the lives of the deceased persons figuring in the cases were of uneven quality both as to social status and commendable conduct. A few of them provided models of heroism or some other enviable quality; but many of them lived in poverty or were otherwise unexemplary. Few parents would impose an identification with such persons on their children. Third, although in most cases the two families concerned were acquainted (or even related), I am confident that in at least 13 cases (among 210 carefully examined with regard to this matter) the two families concerned had never even heard about each other before the case developed. The subject's family in these cases can have had no information with which to build up an imaginary previous life which, it later

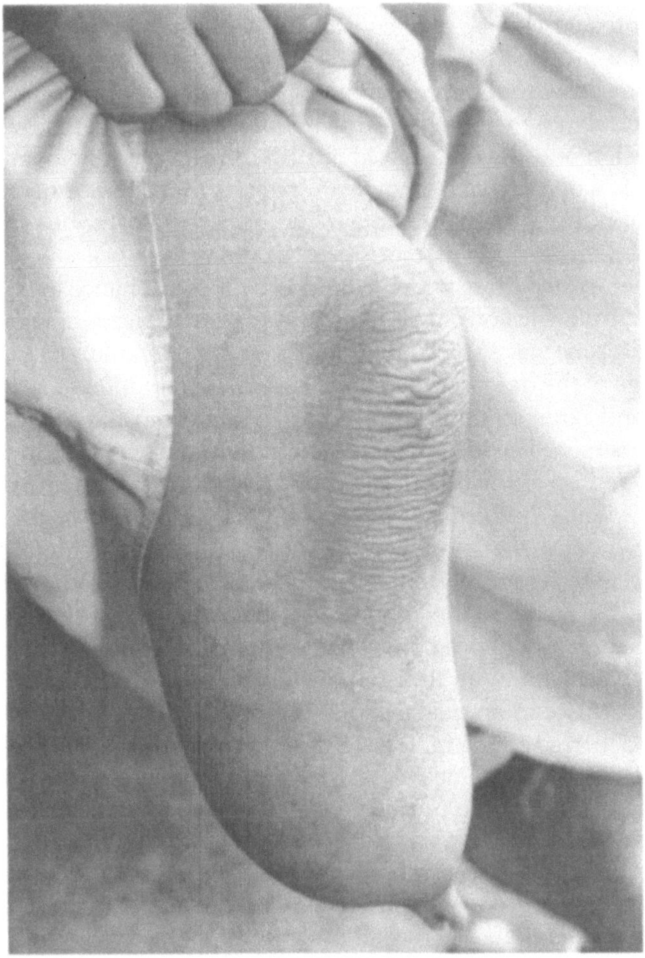

Figure 25.10. Congenital absence of lower leg (unilateral hemimelia) in a girl of Burma who said she remembered the life of a young woman who was accidentally run over by a train, with her right leg being severed first.

turned out, closely matched a real one. In another 12 cases the child's parents had heard about the death of the person concerned, but had no knowledge of the wounds on that person. Limitations of space for this article oblige me to ask readers to accept my appraisal of these 25 cases for this matter; but in my forthcoming work I give a list of the cases from which readers can find the detailed reports of the cases and from reading them judge this important question for themselves. Fourth, I think I have shown that chance is an improbable interpretation for the correspondences in location between two or more birthmarks on the subject of a case and wounds on a deceased person.

Persons who reject the explanation of chance combined with a secondarily confected history may consider other interpretations that include paranormal processes, but fall short of proposing a life after death. One of these supposes that the birthmark or birth defect occurs by chance and the subject then by telepathy learns about a deceased person who had a similar lesion and develops an identification with that person. The children subjects of these cases, however, never show paranormal powers of the magnitude required to explain the apparent memories in contexts outside of their seeming memories.

Another explanation, which would leave less to chance in the production of the child's lesion, attributes it to a maternal impression on the part of the child's mother. According to this idea, a pregnant woman, having a knowledge of the deceased person's wounds, might influence a gestating embryo and fetus so that its form corresponded to the wounds on the deceased person. The idea of maternal impressions, popular in preceding centuries and up to the first decades of this one, has fallen into disrepute. Until my own recent article (Stevenson, 1992 [reprinted in the next section]) there had been no review of series of cases since 1890 (Dabney, 1890); and cases are rarely published now (Williams & Pembroke, 1988). Nevertheless, some of the published cases—old and new—show a remarkable correspondence between an unusual stimulus in the mind of a pregnant woman and an unusual birthmark or birth defect in her laterborn child. Also, in an analysis of 113 published cases I found that the stimulus occurred to the mother in the first trimester in 80 cases (Stevenson, 1992). The first trimester is well known to be the one of greatest sensitivity of the embryo/fetus to recognized teratogens, such as thalidomide (Nowack, 1965) and rubella (Hill, Doll, Galloway, & Hughes, 1958). Applied to the present cases, however, the theory of maternal impression has obstacles as great as the normal explanation appears to have. First, in the 25 cases mentioned above, the subject's mother, although she may have heard of the death of the concerned deceased person, had no knowledge of that person's wounds. Second, this interpretation supposes that the mother not only modified the body of her unborn child with her thoughts, but after the child's birth influenced it to make statements and show behavior that it otherwise would not have done. No motive for such conduct can be discerned in most of the mothers (or fathers) of these subjects.

It is not my purpose to impose any interpretation of these cases on the readers of this article. Nor would I expect any reader to reach even a preliminary conclusion from the short summaries of cases that the brevity of this report entails. Instead, I hope that I have stimulated readers to examine the detailed reports of many cases that I am now in the process of publishing (Stevenson, 1997). "Originality and truth are found only in the details" (Stendhal, 1926).

NOTES

1. Reprinted from the *Journal of Scientific Exploration, 7*, 403–416, 1993.—Ed.
2. See also the paper "Reincarnation: Field Studies and Theoretical Issues," reprinted in part in the previous section.—Ed.
3. See the next paper in this section for the full report of this case.—Ed.
4. For the full report of this case, see Stevenson, 1997, ii:1579–1589.—Ed.
5. For the full report of this case, see Stevenson, 1997, i:300–323.—Ed.
6. For the full report of this case, see Stevenson, 1997, i:973–980.—Ed.
7. For the full report of this case, see Stevenson, 1997, i:935–946.—Ed.
8. For the full report of this case, see Stevenson, 1997, i:839–852. This child also had a second birthmark, corresponding to a mark that some friends of the previous personality had made on the back of her neck after her death. The case of Ampan Petcherat, reprinted in the previous section, also involved such an "experimental birthmark." See note 6 in that paper for a reference to other cases of this type.—Ed.
9. For the full report of this case, see Stevenson, 1997, i:514–519.—Ed.
10. For the full reports of these cases, see Stevenson, 1997, i:997–999, 1000–1005.—Ed.
11. For the full report of this case, see Stevenson, 1997, i:987–997.—Ed.
12. For the full report of this case, see Stevenson, 1997, ii:1382–1403.—Ed.
13. For the full report of this case, see Stevenson, 1997, ii:1186–1199.—Ed.
14. For the full report of this case, see Stevenson, 1997, ii:1236–1250.—Ed.

REFERENCES

Cockayne, E. A. (1933). *Inherited Abnormalities of the Skin*. London: Oxford University Press.

Cook [Kelly], E. W., Pasricha, S., Samararatne, G., Win Maung, & Stevenson, I. (1983). Review and analysis of "unsolved" cases of the reincarnation type: II. Comparison of features of solved and unsolved cases. *Journal of the American Society for Psychical Research, 77*, 115–135.

Dabney, W. C. (1890). Maternal impressions. In J. M. Keating (ed.), *Cyclopaedia of the Diseases of Children* (vol. 1, pp. 191–216). Philadelphia: J. B. Lippincott.

Denaro, S. J. (1944). The inheritance of nevi. *Journal of Heredity, 35*, 215–218.

Fatteh, A. (1976). *Medicolegal Investigation of Gunshot Wounds*. Philadelphia: J. B. Lippincott.

Frantz, C. H., & O'Rahilly, R. (1961). Congenital skeletal limb deficiencies. *Journal of Bone and Joint Surgery, 43-A*, 1202–1224.

Gordon, I., & Shapiro, H. A. (1982). *Forensic Medicine: A Guide to Principles* (2nd ed.). London: Churchill Livingstone.

Hill, A. B., Doll, R., Galloway, T. M., & Hughes, J. P. W. (1958). Virus diseases in pregnancy and congenital defects. *British Journal of Preventive and Social Medicine, 12*, 1–7.

Maruri, C. A. (1961). *La Herencia en Dermatologia*. (2nd ed.). Santander: Aldus, S.A. Artes Graficas.

Mills, A. (1989). A replication study: Three cases of children in northern India who are said to remember a previous life. *Journal of Scientific Exploration, 3*, 133–184.

Nelson, K., & Holmes, L. B. (1989). Malformations due to presumed spontaneous mutations in newborn infants. *New England Journal of Medicine, 320*, 19–23.

Nowack, E. (1965). Die sensible Phase bei der Thalidomid- Embryopathie. *Humangenetik, 1*, 516–536.

Pack, G. T., & Davis, J. (1956). Moles. *New York State Journal of Medicine, 56*, 3498–3506.

Pack, G. T., Lenson, N., & Gerber, D. M. (1952). Regional distribution of moles and melanomas. *AMA Archives of Surgery, 65*, 862–870.

Smith, D. W. (1982). *Recognizable Patterns of Human Malformation* (3rd ed.) Philadelphia: W. B. Saunders.

Spalteholz, W. (1943). *Hand Atlas of Human Anatomy* (L. F. Barker, trans.) (7th English ed.). Philadelphia: J .B. Lippincott.

Stendhal (1926). *Lucien Leuwen*. Paris: Librairie Ancienne Honoré Champion, 4, 169.

Stevenson, I. (1975). *Cases of the Reincarnation Type. Vol 1. Ten Cases in India*. Charlottesville: University Press of Virginia.

Stevenson, I. (1983). American children who claim to remember previous lives. *Journal of Nervous and Mental Disease, 171*, 742–748.

Stevenson, I. (1987). *Children Who Remember Previous Lives*. Charlottesville: University Press of Virginia.

Stevenson, I. (1990). Phobias in children who claim to remember previous lives. *Journal of Scientific Exploration, 4*, 243–254.

Stevenson, I. (1992). A new look at maternal impressions: An analysis of 50 published cases and reports of two recent examples. *Journal of Scientific Exploration, 6*, 353–373.

Stevenson, I. (1997). *Birthmarks and Birth Defects: A Contribution to their Etiology* (2 vols.). New York: Praeger.

Williams, H. C., & Pembroke, A. C. (1988). Naevus of Jamaica. *Lancet, ii*, 915.

Wilson, J. G. (1973). *Environment and Birth Defects*. New York: Academic Press.

TWENTY-SIX

The Case of Hanumant Saxena

1997[1]

SUMMARY OF THE CASE AND ITS INVESTIGATION

Hanumant Saxena was born in 1955 (probably in the month of August) in the village of Kuinya Khera, District Farrukhabad, Uttar Pradesh, India. His parents were Faujdar Saxena and his wife, Gainda Wati. Faujdar Saxena was a landless villager of extremely modest means. Hanumant was his oldest child; subsequently, another son and a daughter were born in the family.

Gainda Wati Saxena had a dream before she conceived Hanumant. In it, a man called Maha Ram Singh appeared to her. Maha Ram had been shot dead just a few weeks earlier. His assailant had shot him in the lower part of the chest at close range. When Hanumant was born, his parents noted a prominent birthmark (or group of birthmarks) on the lower part of his chest near the midline (Figure 25.1 in previous paper). Gaïnda Wati Saxena's dream and Hanumant's birthmark thus prepared his parents to believe that Hanumant was Maha Ram reborn.

Hanumant began to speak coherently when he was about a year old. He started behaving and talking as if he remembered the life of Maha Ram when he was about 3 years old. He said he was Maha Ram and, pointing to the birthmark on his chest, said that he had been shot there. He made a few other statements that were correct for Maha Ram, and he recognized some people and objects connected with him. He liked to visit Maha Ram's house and also to be with Maha Ram's mother, who lived there.

Hanumant, unlike many subjects of these cases, never seems to have become intensely involved with the memories he had of a previous life.

His mother said that he talked about the previous life until he was between 5 and 6 years of age, but his father said that he continued to visit Maha Ram's house up to the age of 10.

I first learned of the case in the summer of 1964. At that time, I penetrated into the interior of the state of Uttar Pradesh far from my base at the large city of Kanpur. I was then mainly investigating other cases already known to me; but informants told me about some others—of which this was one—and I noted down a few details about it. Although I hoped some day to return to the case, other cases seemed more accessible, and I allowed it to recede from my attention. The case was then rediscovered, so to speak, by Dr. L. P. Mehrotra (in April 1971) when he was near Kuinya Khera, also investigating other cases. He sent me notes about the case, and this stimulated me to put it on a list of cases to be investigated in the autumn of 1971. Accordingly, Dr. Mehrotra and I began to study the case systematically in November 1971. Although we made good progress, we did not finish the work to my satisfaction; and so we went back and conducted further interviews in November 1972.

In March 1979 I returned to the area with Dr. Satwant Pasricha. We had follow-up interviews with Hanumant and his father, and we also interviewed the former headman of Kuinya Khera, whom I had not met earlier. I have not met Hanumant since 1979, and so have no recent information about his later development.

An important feature in the investigation of the case was my study of the report of the autopsy on the body of Maha Ram Singh, which Dr. Mehrotra and I examined in November 1971.

PERSONS INTERVIEWED DURING THE INVESTIGATION

In or near the village of Kuinya Khera I interviewed:

Hanumant Saxena
Faujdar Saxena, Hanumant's father
Gainda Wati, Hanumant's mother
Champa, Hanumant's paternal grandmother
Bitoli, Faujdar Saxena's paternal aunt
Lov Kush Ram, Maha Ram Singh's younger brother
Ganga Devi, Maha Ram Singh's wife
Sarnam Singh, Maha Ram Singh's oldest son
Subhash Singh, Maha Ram Singh's youngest son
Devindra Kumar, villager of Kuinya Khera
Bhanwar Singh, villager of Kuinya Khera
Mauji Lal, villager of Kuinya Khera and owner of a tea shop close to which Maha Ram Singh was shot
Lov Kush, villager of Kuinya Khera
Ravindra Kumar Gangwar, former headman of Kuinya Khera

Faujdar Saxena and his wife differed on certain details of their testimony for the case. After considering the discrepancies between what they said and their somewhat different attitudes toward the case—it seems to have interested Hanumant's mother more than his father—I decided that, on the whole, the statements of Hanumant's mother seemed more reliable than those of his father. I shall mention below the most important discrepancy in their statements.

Two members of Maha Ram's family were dissident informants for the case. I shall discuss their attitudes toward it in a separate section below.

Maha Ram's mother, a potentially important informant, had died before the investigation of the case.

RELEVANT FACTS OF GEOGRAPHY AND POSSIBILITIES FOR NORMAL MEANS OF COMMUNICATION BETWEEN THE TWO FAMILIES

Both families inhabited the village of Kuinya Khera. It is a rather small village located about 20 kilometers west of the city of Farrukhabad. I estimate that its population (at the time I investigated the case) was not more than 1,000.

The houses of the families concerned in the case were approximately 250 meters from each other. They were both constructed of clay—the type of house referred to in India as *kachcha*. The Singhs were more prosperous than the Saxenas. The latter were landless, whereas the Singhs owned 6 bighas of land, the equivalent of about 2 acres. On the other hand, the Saxenas belonged to a slightly higher caste than the Singhs. Taking both factors into account, I do not think that there was much difference between their socioeconomic statuses.

The members of the families concerned knew each other before the development of the case, but Faujdar Saxena said that they were acquaintances rather than friends. At the same time, there must have been some good feeling between them beyond what is customary among acquaintances, because Faujdar attributed Maha Ram's rebirth in his family—as he saw the case—to the fact that Maha Ram "had affection for me"; and Hanumant's mother, Gainda Wati, said that Maha Ram had been a kind of village "father-in-law." She said she had known him "fairly well."

THE LIFE, DEATH, AND CHARACTER OF MAHA RAM SINGH

Maha Ram Singh was born in Kuinya Khera in about 1905. He was a peasant and agricultural laborer. He had some land, and he owned a bullock-cart that he drove for hire. He had a younger brother, Lov Kush Ram, and two younger sisters.

He married Ganga Devi, and they had three sons and two daughters.

Lov Kush Ram described his brother as a "simple, good fellow." He was not known to have any enemies.

On the evening of September 28, 1954, Maha Ram was near a tea shop that is at the crossroads less than 200 meters from his house. Someone emerged in the dark and discharged a shotgun at him from within a few meters. The assailant fled, and Maha Ram died almost immediately.

The police conducted a fruitless inquiry. They had no suspects and they made no arrests. No one could think of any reason why anyone would have wanted to kill Maha Ram. My informants conjectured that the murderer intended to kill someone else and, in the dark, mistook Maha Ram for the other person he had meant to shoot.

As happens often after a murder in an Asian village, members of the village—not just the relatives of the deceased man—came to inspect Maha Ram's body. Gainda Wati Saxena was one of those who looked at the body. She afterward thought this might have had something to do with Maha Ram's being reborn as her child.[2]

The Report of the Postmortem on Maha Ram

Maha Ram's body was taken to the Civil Hospital in Fatehgarh, where an autopsy on it was performed on September 29, 1954. The pathologist reported a major "gunshot wound," about 3.75 centimeters by 2.5 centimeters in extent, that was located in the middle and lower part of the chest. It penetrated both the chest and abdominal cavities. The lower part of the sternum and the xiphoid process were "completely fractured." Around the main wound there were six smaller wounds, five of which also penetrated both the chest and abdominal cavities. All the wounds were within an approximately circular area with a diameter of about 7.5 centimeters.

Dr. S. C. Pandeya, a staff physician at the Civil Hospital in Fatehgarh, kindly allowed me to examine the autopsy report, and we read it together. Without telling him the location of Hanumant's birthmark, I asked him to indicate (on a crude sketch of the anterior aspect of the human trunk that I made) the location of the wounds described in the autopsy report. Figure 25.2 [in the previous paper in this section] shows the completed sketch with circles that Dr. Pandeya drew in to show the location of the wounds described in the report. After Dr. Pandeya had completed the sketch reproduced in Figure 25.2, I showed him one that I had made of Hanumant's birthmark the day before. (I had photographed Hanumant's birthmark, but had not yet had my exposed film developed.)

The roman numerals written by Dr. Pandeya on the sketch of Figure 25.2 correspond to the principal wounds described by the physician who conducted the postmortem examination. Of these the most important was the one identified as Number I. The postmortem report described it as: "One gunshot wound (entry). 1½ inch x 1 inch and to the depth of the chest and abdominal cavities. In front of the chest in the middle and lower part. Margin turned inside."

The postmortem report referred to the wounds on Maha Ram as gunshot wounds. They were, however, caused by the numerous pellets of a cartridge of a shotgun (Fatteh, 1976; Gordon & Shapiro, 1982; Simpson & Knight, 1947/1985). The pellets discharged from a shotgun disperse more and more widely with increasing distance from the end of the barrel (Di Maio, 1985; Simpson & Knight, 1947/1985). An approximate formula for estimating the distance of an assailant with a shotgun from his victim states that "the spread in centimetres may be taken roughly as equal to two and a half to three times the distance in metres" (Simpson & Knight, 1947/1985, p. 81). (This formula does not take account of variations in the "choke" of the gun, which retards the dispersal of the pellets.) Applying this formula to Maha Ram's wounds, we can say that his murderer stood within 3 meters of him when he fired. . . .[3]

AN ANNOUNCING DREAM

Gainda Wati Saxena said that she dreamed of Maha Ram after his death. In the dream he appeared and said: "I am coming to you," and lay down on a cot. Gainda Wati thought she had this dream 3 weeks after Maha Ram's murder. It was not repeated.

When I asked Faujdar in 1971 whether anyone had had a dream related to Hanumant's birth, he said that he had not heard of one. However, in 1972 he remembered that his wife had had a dream about Maha Ram, which he had dismissed as insignificant. He then (in 1972) recollected that Gainda Wati told him about it just before Hanumant's birth.

Comment

The discrepancy between Faujdar's statement about the dream in 1971 and his statement in 1972 may derive from his not having understood the question put to him in 1971. I think it equally possible, however, that (as he said in 1972) he had earlier disregarded the dream as of no importance and had really forgotten it in 1971. Then in 1972, when his wife mentioned the dream, he remembered that she had told him about it when she was pregnant with Hanumant.

STATEMENTS AND RECOGNITIONS MADE BY HANUMANT

. . . Hanumant made only a few statements about the previous life. Unlike many subjects of these cases, he never mentioned, or otherwise identified, Maha Ram's murderer. (It is quite possible that the identity of this person never registered in Maha Ram's mind. He was apparently shot in the dark without any notice. The impact of the bullets hitting him may have knocked him down, and the assailant probably fled before Maha Ram, or anyone else, could see him. Maha Ram may well have died without even having time to think about who might have shot him.)

By the early 1970s, when I investigated the case, Hanumant, who was then 16 years old, had completely forgotten all the memories of the previous life that he had earlier had....

HANUMANT'S BEHAVIOR RELATED TO THE PREVIOUS LIFE

Circumstances and Manner of Hanumant's Speaking about the Previous Life

I have already mentioned that Hanumant did not make many statements about the previous life; and he does not appear to have spoken often about it. His spontaneous statements seem to have occurred either when he noticed a person (such as Ganga Devi) or something (such as the bullocks) that had been familiar to Maha Ram. He also made some statements when an older person questioned him.

Two informants mentioned that Hanumant used the present tense when he spoke about the previous life. Thus Devindra Kumar mentioned that Hanumant said: "I have three sons" .... Gainda Wati said that when Hanumant saw Ganga Devi pass in front of the Saxena house, he said: "She is my wife" .... And when he passed Maha Ram's house and bullocks, he said: "This is my house and these are my bullocks" ....

Hanumant's Attitudes toward Maha Ram's Family and Possessions

Faujdar and Gainda Wati gave somewhat different accounts of Hanumant's first visit to Maha Ram's house. Faujdar said that Hanumant had rushed into the house and had to be forcibly extracted from it. Gainda Wati did not confirm this. She said that Hanumant had wished to go into one house that belonged to Maha Ram's family, and she had not permitted him to do so. Then he had wanted to enter another house—the one by the road—and she had allowed him to do this. But (according to her) he had come away afterward quite peacefully. Since Faujdar and Gainda Wati both claimed to have been eyewitnesses of Hanumant's behavior, either one of them had misremembered the incident or they were remembering two different incidents.

Faujdar and Gainda Wati agreed that Hanumant liked to go and play at Maha Ram's house. Faujdar said that Hanumant continued to do this until he was about 10 years old.

Gainda Wati thought that Hanumant liked to go to Maha Ram's house by the side of the road because Maha Ram's mother lived there. Hanumant showed particular affection for her. Faujdar said that once when she came to their house, Hanumant, who must have been quite young then, left his mother's arms and went to Maha Ram's mother; but he does not appear to have said anything to indicate that he had recognized her. Gainda Wati said he liked to play with Maha Ram's mother, who came to visit him often. He sometimes accompanied her into the fields when she went there. Maha Ram's mother told her that once when Hanumant saw her, he wept. She asked him why he was doing that, and he replied: "You are my mother." Then she herself wept. (Gainda Wati did not witness this scene herself.) When I asked Gainda Wati about Hanumant's attitude toward Ganga Devi, Maha Ram's wife, she said that he was "very shy." Faujdar said that Hanumant had no interest in Maha Ram's wife and actually avoided meeting her.

Hanumant recognized Maha Ram's bullocks. . . . Mauji Lal said that he had heard that Hanumant used to stand in front of the bullock-cart at Maha Ram's house; but he himself had not observed Hanumant doing this, and I did not obtain a firsthand report of such behavior.

OTHER RELEVANT BEHAVIOR OF HANUMANT

Hanumant had no significant fears, such as for guns or darkness.

THE ATTITUDES OF MEMBERS OF MAHA RAM'S FAMILY TOWARD THE CASE

Lov Kush Ram, Maha Ram Singh's younger brother, had not heard Hanumant make any statement about the previous life. He nevertheless believed that Hanumant was his brother Maha Ram reborn because of the correspondence in location between Hanumant's birthmark and the wounds that Lov Kush Ram saw on his brother's chest after he was killed.

Ganga Devi, Maha Ram's wife, answered a few questions I put to her and then refused to discuss the case further. She was possibly dismayed by the crowd of moderate size that gathered as I tried to talk with her. It is more likely that she misunderstood the purpose of my visit and thought it was part of some government inquiry that she ought to avoid.

Sarnam Singh, Maha Ram's oldest son, alleged that the case was a hoax. He did not give any reason for his suspicions or indicate any possible gain the Saxenas would derive from a hoax. He said that Hanumant had said nothing about the previous life in his presence and had not recognized him. Sarnam further said that none of the members of his family accepted the case as genuine. However, this was not true, because Lov Kush Ram accepted it. When I asked Sarnam whether he had discussed the case with Lov Kush Ram, he said that he had not, and added that he and Lov Kush Ram were on bad terms. He had also not discussed the case with Faujdar Saxena.

Faujdar was not present when I talked with Sarnam. I afterwards discussed Sarnam's negative attitude toward the case with Faujdar. He thought it might have derived from a fear Sarnam might have had that Hanumant and his father would make a claim on Maha Ram's family for a share in their land. This could have led Sarnam to deny the authenticity of the case.

As I mentioned earlier, I interviewed Ravindra Kumar Gangwar, a former headman of Kuinya Khera, in 1979, when Dr. Pasricha and I went there for a follow-up interview. He remembered the case well and believed it genuine. He said that people in the village had begun saying that Hanumant was Maha Ram reborn on the basis of his birthmark alone, before Hanumant had even begun to speak about the previous life. He remembered that Hanumant had said he was Maha Ram and had pointed to the birthmark on his chest.

HANUMANT'S BIRTHMARK

Figure 25.1 [in the previous paper in this section] shows Hanumant's birthmark, which actually consisted of two main portions with some satellite marks around them. The birthmark was neither elevated nor depressed, but only an area of diminished pigmentation of the skin compared with the skin around it. It did not discharge any blood or serum after Hanumant was born. No one else in the family had a similar birthmark.

According to Faujdar, Hanumant's birthmark had become somewhat larger since his birth. (Informants for these cases sometimes remark that a birthmark has faded or become smaller since the subject's birth; they rarely say that one has become larger after the child's birth.)

In 1971 and 1972 I neglected to ask whether Hanumant's birthmark had shifted in position since his birth, as some of the birthmarks in these cases do. (The case of Nasruddin Shah [Stevenson, 1997, i:400–417] provides an example.) In 1979 I did inquire about a change of position, and Faujdar said that the birthmark was then higher on Hanumant's body than it had been earlier. (I took the photograph of Figure 25.1 in 1971.) He did not mention any lateral shift in the birthmark, which was at the same level as the wounds on Maha Ram, but somewhat more to the right side of the chest than Maha Ram's principal wound, which was reported to be in the midline. However, Hanumant himself said (also in 1979) that the birthmark used to be in his upper abdomen in the midline, so it may have shifted laterally (as well as superiorly) with his growth.

The correspondence in location between Hanumant's birthmark and the wounds that killed Maha Ram was close, but not exact. If we assume that a causal connection between them existed, the difference may be due to a lateral shift in the location of the birthmark since Hanumant's birth (as Hanumant himself suggested), to inexactitude in the pathologist's location of the wounds on Maha Ram's body (he may have described them as being more medial than they were), or to other factors of which we are ignorant.

Hanumant said that he had no pain in the area of the birthmark when he was a young child. However, beginning about 1969, he had noticed some pain in its region. This pain occurred irregularly and lasted only 10 or 15 minutes. Occasionally, the pain would awaken him from sleep. Hanumant did not know what brought the pain on. In 1972 he no longer experienced pain spontaneously in the area of the birthmark, but he still noticed some mild pain there when he lifted a heavy object.

Gainda Wati said that Hanumant had complained of pain in the area below the birthmark. Faujdar Saxena was also aware that Hanumant had occasionally had pain in the area of the birthmark. The pain had not evoked much attention in the family.[4]

COMMENTS ON THE EVIDENCE OF PARANORMAL PROCESSES IN THE CASE

Hanumant's birthmark is the most important feature of his case. The correspondence between it and the wounds on Maha Ram seems to me unlikely to have occurred by chance.

Other elements in the case are weaker and raise the question of whether Faujdar and Gainda Wati amplified or even invented statements by Hanumant in order to explain the birthmark. The refusal of Maha Ram's wife, Ganga Devi, to cooperate in our investigation and Sarnam Singh's rejection of the case made me concerned about its authenticity.

However, I am inclined to discount Sarnam's rejection of the case. His overt reason for denying its authenticity—that Hanumant could not recognize him—is a familiar one among Asian informants for refusing to accept a case. They attach much more importance to recognitions than I do.[5]

Sarnam Singh may have had other motives for rejecting the case, such as the one suggested by Faujdar—that he (Sarnam) feared Hanumant might try to claim some of the Singhs' land. I have no evidence, however, that Sarnam Singh had such thoughts, and Faujdar, who suggested that he did have them, was an interested party to the case on the other side. I regret that he and Sarnam Singh never discussed the case together.

Fortunately, the case does not depend exclusively on the statements of Hanumant's parents. Several other persons testified about it in a positive way. These included three villagers, one of them a former headman, who were not members of Hanumant's family and who had heard him make at least a few correct statements about Maha Ram's life.

The testimony of informants shows that Hanumant had a definite conviction that he was Maha Ram Singh in a previous life and that he exhibited behavior that was appropriate for such a conviction. I attach more importance to Hanumant's possessiveness toward Maha Ram's house and bullocks than I do to reports of his recognitions of them.

HANUMANT'S LATER DEVELOPMENT

Hanumant went to school for only 1 day. Consequently, the only occupation open to him was that of a village laborer, his family being landless. In 1975, at the age of 20, he married, but up to 1979 he and his wife had had no children.

In 1979, when I last met him, Hanumant's birthmark appeared to me to have faded somewhat compared with its appearance as I remembered it to have been 7 years earlier, in 1972. He was still having pain in the area of the birthmark from time to time and in fact had some pain on the day of our visit to Kuinya Khera.

NOTES

1. Excerpts from *Reincarnation and Biology: A Contribution to the Etiology of Birthmarks and Birth Defects* (vol. 1, pp. 455–467). New York: Praeger, 1997.—Ed.

2. Many Asian villagers believe that the soul of a person who dies violently stays close to his physical body after death. Women of child-bearing age are then prone to attract the discarnate person, who, wishing to be reborn, may try to "get into her body" and thus reincarnate.

In the report of the case of Maung Aye Kyaw (Stevenson, 1997, i:218) I give a partial list of cases in which the subject's mother viewed the previous personality's dead body.

In the case of Narong Yensiri (Stevenson, 1997, i:421–430) his father viewed the dead body of the person whose life Narong later remembered.

3. Other cases in which the previous personality died from the wounds of a shotgun include: Ma Mu Mu, Alan Gamble, Bhopal Singh, Semih Tutuşmuş, Pappu Singh, and Obike Nwonye (all these cases are reported in detail in Stevenson, 1997).

4. Most subjects have not complained of pain in the area of the birthmarks, but a substantial minority of them have done so. These include Chanai Choomalaiwong, Alan Gamble, Derek Pitnov, Sunita Khandelwal, Susan Wilson, Maung Win Aung, Patricia Fairley, and Dellâl Beyaz (all these cases are reported in detail in Stevenson, 1997).

5. I have elsewhere discussed why, in general, I regard the evidence from a subject's recognitions as less valuable than some other types of evidence found in these cases (Stevenson, 1975, pp. 39–42; 1987, pp. 111–113).

REFERENCES

Di Maio, V. J. M. (1985). *Gunshot Wounds: Practical Aspects of Firearms, Ballistics and Forensic Techniques*. New York: Elsevier.

Fatteh, A. (1976). *Medicolegal Investigation of Gunshot Wounds*. Philadelphia: J. B. Lippincott.

Gordon, I., & Shapiro, H. A. (1982). *Forensic Medicine: A Guide to Principles*. 2nd ed. Edinburgh: Churchill Livingstone.

Simpson, K., & Knight, B. (1985). *Forensic Medicine*. 9th ed. London: Edward Arnold. (First published in 1947)

Stevenson, I. (1975). *Cases of the Reincarnation Type. Vol. 1. Ten Cases in India*. Charlottesville: University Press of Virginia.

Stevenson, I. (1997). *Reincarnation and Biology: A Contribution to the Etiology of Birthmarks and Birth Defects* (2 vols.). NY: Praeger.

4g

Maternal Impressions

EWK

For some cases there is an alternative way of explaining some of the birthmarks and birth defects in CORT, rather than as some kind of influence of a deceased person on the developing fetus. Throughout history, cases have been reported of pregnant women who have seen someone with a disfiguring mark or injury and have later given birth to a child with a similar mark. Ian reviewed 50 such "maternal impression" cases, chosen from several hundred published accounts that he identified (Stevenson, 1992 [reprinted in part in this section], 1997, i:104–175). He chose these 50 for review primarily because (1) they had been reported in medical journals by a reliable observer, often the attending physician; (2) they involved unusual kinds of marks, thus making it less likely that the marks corresponded by chance; and (3) the correspondence between the defect observed and the subsequent birth defect was close.

In addition to the further evidence that these cases provide for the influence of mind on the body—in these instances, of the mother's mind on the developing fetus—Ian was interested in such cases because they illustrate that ideas can become discredited, not because of lack of good evidence but because of their incompatibility with prevailing theoretical assumptions. As long as physicians believed that there were nervous and circulatory system connections between the mother's body and the fetus that might potentially explain the birthmarks, cases were frequently reported, especially during the 19th century. After it became clear that there were in fact *not* sufficient connections to explain the marks, journals stopped publishing cases and doctors stopped reporting them. Ian also conjectured that, when scientists firmly dismissed such cases as "old wives' tales," the belief that they could happen may have begun to die away in the general public, and with the belief went the cases themselves. On the other hand, it is equally possible that such cases *do* continue to occur, but that mothers do not talk about them for fear of being thought superstitious or even crazy. In fact, such cases are still reported occasionally, Ian himself having investigated some (two of these are reported in the two papers reprinted in this section).

Another reason for his interest in them was that, as mentioned above, the phenomenon of maternal impressions potentially provides an alternate explanation for some of the birthmarks and birth defects in CORT. In many cases, the mother knew about the wound on the deceased person. In Hanumant's case, reprinted in the previous section, his mother had even seen the wound on Maha Ram. The close correspondence between such an unusual mode of death and the even more unusual birthmark, both occurring in the same village and within a short period of time, makes it exceedingly unlikely that this occurred by chance; but many people might think it more likely that the mother's shock at seeing the wound caused the birthmark, rather than that Hanumant was Maha Ram reborn. The former explanation at least involves the influence of living people only, not deceased ones.

The case of S. P. (Sampath Priyasantha) that I reprint in this section also illustrates the difficulty in choosing between the explanation of influence by a living person and influence by a deceased one. It also reminds us of a point that Ian made frequently: It is unlikely that there is a single explanation that works for all cases. Phenomena that appear similar may have different explanations, or even combinations of explanations. For example, some hallucinations may be caused by alcohol poisoning, some by fear of being in a "haunted" house, some by ESP of a distant accident to a friend, some by the actual return and appearance of that deceased friend to loved ones. Similarly, whatever explanation may seem best to fit CORT in general, individual cases may still have different explanations, or combinations of explanations.

REFERENCES

Stevenson, I. (1992). A new look at maternal impressions: An analysis of 50 published cases and reports of two recent examples. *Journal of Scientific Exploration, 6*, 353–373.

Stevenson, I. (1997). *Reincarnation and Biology: A Contribution to the Etiology of Birthmarks and Birth Defects* (2 vols.). New York: Praeger.

TWENTY-SEVEN

A New Look at Maternal Impressions: An Analysis of Fifty Published Cases and Reports of Two Recent Examples

1992[1]

The idea that a pregnant woman may be so frightened by the sight of some deformity on another person that her baby will be affected by a similar defect is widely believed in most parts of the world today; it was also generally believed in the West until the early years of this century. The skepticism that then developed may have derived from lack of an explanatory principle and not from lack of evidence for a significant correspondence between stimulus and birthmark or birth defect. The present paper summarizes the main features of 50 published cases in which an unusual stimulus to a pregnant woman was followed by the birth of a baby with unusual birthmarks or birth defects that nearly always corresponded closely to the stimulus the pregnant mother had received. Two[2] *recent cases that the author investigated are presented. The author concludes that in rare instances maternal impressions may indeed affect gestating babies and cause birth defects. Almost nothing is known about why such effects occur in some pregnancies, but only rarely, or about the implementing processes involved. These may be paranormal.*

INTRODUCTION AND REVIEW OF EARLIER REPORTS

The belief that a shock or other strong impression in a pregnant woman can produce a mark or other defect in her baby has been held for centuries; although it is less common now in Western countries, it is still widely accepted in other parts of the world.

In a typical reported case of this type a pregnant woman sees on the street a person with a serious deformity, such as feet that have been partly amputated. She becomes distressed and fears afterward that her baby will be similarly malformed. When the baby is born, parts of its feet are absent, the defects corresponding to the defective feet its mother saw (Montgomery, 1857). Cases of this type are usually called "maternal impressions." In most instances the stimulus is a visual one perceived by the pregnant woman, but sometimes a vivid verbal description of a defect the mother has not herself seen may act as an apparently causal factor.

Writers on reproduction and embryology in ancient Greece and Rome assumed the reality of maternal impressions, and so did their successors, at least up to the 16th century, when Paré (1573/1982) cited cases of the type and endorsed the idea that maternal impressions could cause birth defects.[3]

In the 17th century Gervase Markham expressed skepticism and even scoffed at the belief in maternal impressions (Glenister, 1964). Opposition to the belief became stronger in the 18th century. In the early years of that century two English authors buffeted each other with alternate publications on the subject. One of them, Turner (1714/1731), defended the reality of maternal effects on the fetus, while the other, Blondel (1729), decried the idea as a crude superstition (Wilson, 1992). Later in the same century William Hunter (1718–1783) railed against it in his lectures on obstetrics (Hall, 1785). Elliotson (1852), referring to his medical education in the first decades of the 19th century, stated: "All my medical teachers dismissed the idea with contempt."

Controversy about maternal impressions was equally vigorous among French scientists. Buffon, the greatest French biologist of the 18th century, severely criticized the idea (Buffon, 1830, vol. 4, pp. 480–482), but it had at least one fervent defender, Bablot (1788).

Some physicians of the 18th and 19th centuries who continued to believe in maternal impressions supposed that small nervous connections would be found between the uterus and the placenta and that these could somehow convey a mother's mental impression to her fetus. Advances in anatomy and physiology removed all basis for such conjectures and also for an equally imaginative suggestion that exchanges of blood between mother and fetus somehow transmitted the mother's impression to the fetus.

In the 1830s the German physiologist Johannes Müller (1834–1840/1840–1842, vol. 2, pp. 1404–1406) stated three reasons why he disbelieved in the effect of maternal impressions on a fetus: (a) the already mentioned lack of physical connections capable of mediating communications between the mother and fetus; (b) the frequent occurrence of negative instances in which pregnant women had been frightened and had expected to have a marked or malformed baby but had not; and (c) the lack of correspondence between the frightening stimuli that the mothers mentioned and the common types of birth defects, such as cleft lip and absent extremities. (Müller emphasized the repetitive forms—what we might today call the recognized syndromes—of congenital anomalies, which studies of embryology and teratology were then just beginning to elucidate.) Müller concluded his dismissal of maternal impressions with derisive allusions to "animal magnetism," from the study of which developed both what we today call hypnotism and also the investigations of the phenomena that are today considered paranormal. It is important to note here that although Müller was familiar with birth defects, he was writing about reports he had read of cases attributed to maternal impressions; he seems to have had no direct experience of them himself.

Müller's high reputation did not suffice to extinguish interest in maternal impressions on the part of physicians, and during the 19th century at least several hundred reports of exemplifying cases were published in medical journals and books. Moreover, the belief in maternal impressions continued to receive support among some scientists of competence and eminence. For example, Müller's contemporary, von Baer, who is justly regarded as the founder of modern embryology, reported the case of his own sister. She had been much perturbed by a fire that she saw in the distance and feared was that of her own house burning. She was then 6 or 7 months pregnant and long afterward

> declared that the flame was constantly before her eyes. Two or three months after the fire she gave birth to a daughter, who had a red mark on her forehead which went to a point at the top in the shape of a blazing flame. It did not fade until she was seven years old. (Burdach, 1837, vol. 2, p. 127; my translation)

The extensive writings on maternal impressions in the 19th century show the varying fortunes of the belief in them among physicians. If an exponent of the belief published a series of cases and supported the idea of maternal impressions, within a few years or sooner another author would publish a critique and raise again the familiar objections.

In 1865 Meadows published a defense of the concept, and, acknowledging the absence of any neural connections between mother and fetus, he suggested a process indistinguishable from modern ideas of paranormal communications. He believed the data "force upon us the conviction that mind does in some mysterious way operate across matter" (Meadows, 1865, p. 89).[4] A few years later Fisher (1870), a skeptic, again emphasized negative instances in which women had been frightened during pregnancy (and expected to have deformed children) without any ill effects on their babies. Fisher reported having made a prospective study of over 1200 children he had delivered and of whose mothers he had enquired before their deliveries "in regard to their apprehensions of deformity in their offspring" (p. 258). He found that "by far the larger number" of the mothers expressed such fears and frequently specified the nature of the deformity they expected their child might have. Yet among this group of babies he found only three cases of birth defects.[5]

Taking the opposing view, Barker (1887) published a long paper in which he cited numerous examples of correspondences between an unusual stimulus to a pregnant woman and a subsequent birthmark or birth defect on her child. In the discussion of Barker's paper, Busey (1887), in the course of reviewing 41 additional cases, addressed the familiar question of chance as an explanation for them:

> Upon the common doctrine of chance, the coincidence [between maternal impression and subsequent defect] is too remarkable to be explained so readily, and, if one [case] is suggestive, a second adds great weight, and a third is almost conclusive. The element of chance is eliminated by the great variety of causes with corresponding effects; that is, in each of the foregoing cases the circumstance producing the impression is different; yet in each case the effect is, to a greater or less degree, in correspondence with the causal circumstance. (Busey, 1887, p. 186)

In 1890 Dabney published one of the longest and most thorough reviews of this subject. He summarized reports of 90 cases published between 1853 and 1886. The series was large enough to permit an analysis of various features. He concluded that in 69 (77%) of the 90 cases there was "quite a close correspondence" between the impression upon the mother and her baby's defect. Dabney drew some other conclusions from his data. For example, he found that defects related to errors of embryological development tended to be associated with maternal impressions received early in pregnancy; in contrast, birthmarks and other abnormalities of the skin and hair tended to be associated with maternal impressions occurring later in pregnancy. Dabney also noted instances in which the mother-to-be seems to have been little or not at all consciously affected by the stimulus and had no expectation that her child would be defective. He attached little weight to what a mother said about the kind of baby she expected to have. He emphasized that maternal impressions account for few of all cases of birth defects, and his main conclusion was "that they are one of the causes of defects or deformities, but by no means the only cause" (Dabney, 1890, p. 214). Dabney was undaunted by ignorance concerning the process, psychophysiological or other, that could mediate between the maternal impression and the related birthmark or birth defect.

Skeptics remained unquelled, and they sometimes even inveighed against the publication of reports of cases of alleged maternal impressions (Murdock, 1888). Conant (1863), Morland (1853), and Rich (1891) each published instances of a pregnant woman who had been frightened, expected to have a malformed baby, and nevertheless had a normal one.

Ballantyne, who in the 1890s wrote a series of papers on this subject with reports of additional cases, adopted a stance similar to that of Dabney:

> The apparently extraordinary character of the phenomena witnessed is in itself no argument against their truth if the sources of information are reliable. . . . We are not so much concerned at present with the question, How are the effects produced? but rather with the primary inquiry whether, in conjunction with certain definite circumstances, certain clearly marked phenomena occur so frequently and so persistently as to compel the belief that there is more than the element of chance or coincidence in their association. (Ballantyne, 1890–1891, p. 625)

Ballantyne engaged himself in a cause that was, by his time, rapidly losing ground. After the beginning of this century the number of reports of maternal impressions published in medical journals declined markedly, and they eventually became sporadic (Farkas & Farkas, 1974; Formijne, 1915; Leclerc-Montmoyen, 1949; Williams & Pembroke, 1988). Historians of teratology reviewing various theories of birth defects in the second half of this century dismissed and sometimes derided the belief in maternal impressions (Barrow, 1971; Glenister, 1964; Warkany, 1959; Warkany & Kalter, 1962).

Dabney (1890, p. 191) suggested that "thinking men came to doubt the truth of those things which they could not understand." A future historian of medicine disposing of more space than I can allow myself here might connect the decline (at the end of the 19th century) in the belief in maternal impressions to the rise among members of the medical profession of an increasingly materialistic view of human nature. The failure to identify a process for the action of maternal impressions eventually led to denial that there were any phenomena to be explained. Yet there may be.

I mentioned earlier Meadows's (1865) endorsement of maternal impressions with the idea that "mind does in some mysterious way operate across matter." We are certainly not in a better position to say today what this "mysterious way" may be; but evidence developed from more than a century of systematic research has made the belief that mind can act upon matter more plausible than it seemed to be earlier. Accordingly, I believe that we should reopen the question of maternal impressions. However, we can only expect the concept to gain new adherents if we take into account two important facts.

First, we must acknowledge that major birth defects and birthmarks (of say more than a centimeter in diameter) are not common. For example, Wilde (1843) studied the incidence of congenital malformations among 23,413 births during 8 years (1832–1840) at the Imperial Lying-in Hospital of Vienna and found an incidence of 1 in 266, which is less than 0.4%. He was admittedly counting only major malformations, which he called "monstrosities"; and the incidence of congenital defects of some kind is much higher, perhaps as high as 2% today (Kennedy, 1967). However, for the purpose of the substantial birthmarks and birth defects usually associated with a maternal impression I think we are justified in saying—as I did above—that such anomalies are not common.

Second, it has been argued that if the fears of pregnant women could produce important morphological changes in their fetuses, medical reports of birth defects related to maternal impressions would be more frequent than they now are or, to return to the 19th century, than they were then. However, we can also note that reports of such correlations are (and have been) few in relation to all the births and also in relation to all the babies with congenital anomalies that have been born. Accordingly, we can say that maternal impressions can at best account for only a small portion of all congenital anomalies. It follows that if maternal impressions have any effect on fetuses, the effect occurs only among mothers and fetuses who are especially susceptible—either at a psychological level or a physical one. I agree with such predecessors as Elliotson, Dabney, and Ballantyne in believing that an unusual stimulus to a pregnant woman has sometimes caused an unusual birth defect (less often an unusual birthmark) in her baby. Taylor (1876) succinctly emphasized the importance of not allowing negative instances to bias our appraisal of the positive examples, rarer though these may be. He wrote:

> It is said that many mothers are apprehensive during their pregnancy of some impending evil to themselves or their offspring, and may even be exposed to shocking sights, which produce *no* effect on the foetus, for there is no nervous connection between the mother and her unborn babe; but all mothers and babies are not equally susceptible to such influences, therefore this proves nothing in the special cases which *cannot* be explained. (p. 73)

This is a matter that readers should judge for themselves. This requires, however, an acquaintance with reports of actual cases. Selecting 50 cases from a much larger group I will next present summaries of their principal features.

PRINCIPAL FEATURES OF 50 SELECTED CASES

In many of these cases a physician (usually the author of the report) had both seen the wounded or disfigured person who had impressed the pregnant woman and examined the later-born baby; he was thus in a position to testify to the correspondence between the stimulus and the birth defect or birthmark. I selected cases in which the correspondence between the stimulus and baby's defect was exact or at least close. Also, in order to reduce the likelihood of a chance correspondence between stimulus and birth defect I selected only cases with unusual birth defects or birthmarks. Accordingly, I did not include any case of clubfoot, and the series has only one case of cleft lip, which occurred with a cleft palate. I did, however, include a few of the common types of birthmarks—hyperpigmented macules and "port-wine" marks (nevus flammeus). I believe that these 50 cases provide substantial evidence of some paranormal process linking the stimulus received by the pregnant woman to the defect in her later-born baby.[6]

The Types of Stimuli Figuring in the Cases

In Table 27.1 I have grouped the stimuli to the pregnant woman according to their association with violent events or ones that included wounds, such as surgical operations. In 22 cases (Groups 1 and 2 summed together) the mother either was an eyewitness of another person's mutilation (criminal, accidental, or surgical) or saw the afflicted person soon after the mutilation.

In another 3 cases (Group 3) the mother heard about the mutilation of another person; and in 6 (Group 4) she was herself wounded (accidentally or surgically). In 3 more cases (Group 5) amputations accompanied or followed injuries. Thus violence—surgery is a kind of violence, but one to which the involved parties agree—figured in 34 (68%) of these 50 cases.

Duration of Pregnant Woman's Exposure to the Stimulus

The duration of the apparent stimulus for the maternal impression varied widely. In several cases the pregnant mother had the stimulus under view throughout much or all of her pregnancy. This would naturally be true in those instances where a stimulating injury with a resulting scar or deformity occurred to a member of the mother's own family, say her husband, another child, or a close neighbor. Suringar (1927) reported a case in this group. He learned about it from the mother of the affected child. When she was in the 6th month of her first pregnancy, a neighbor became seriously ill, and in order to help this person she brought one of the neighbor's children—a 10-year-old girl—to stay in her house. This child had had her hand caught in a laundry mangle and had lost part of one of the middle fingers of the left hand. The mother-to-be often worked alongside the child when there was housework to do, and she thus frequently had occasion to see the child's mutilated hand. Her son of this pregnancy was born with the middle finger of the left hand absent. Suringar's informant believed that her frequent viewing of the child's mutilated hand—over a period of some time—was the cause of her son's defect, all the more because no other member of her or her husband's family had had any such defect.

However, in some cases the mother seems to have had only a fleeting glance at the stimulating lesion. This was true in the case of a pregnant

Table 27.1. Types of Stimuli Figuring in 50 Cases of Maternal Impressions

Nature of Stimulus to Pregnant Woman in This Group	*Number of Cases*
1. Woman an eyewitness of another person's being wounded	7
2. Woman saw an injured (or operated upon) person soon after the wounding [a]	15
3. Woman heard about the mutilation of (or operation on) another person	3
4. Woman was mutilated herself or underwent surgery	6
5. Woman saw a person with a birth defect or major postnatal defect, e.g., the stump of an amputated arm	15
6. Woman saw a person with a lesion that was not congenital, accidental, or postoperative	1
7. Other kinds of stimuli	3

Note: [a] Unless the report of the case explicitly states that the pregnant woman was an eyewitness of the wounding, I have assumed that she saw the wound only soon afterward.

woman who just briefly saw in the street a woman with a "port-wine" birthmark (Liébeault, 1892). It was true in another case in which the pregnant woman barely glimpsed the scene where another woman was being operated on for a large umbilical hernia (Lacambre, 1906). In another case a young man who was run over by a cart must have been quickly transported from the scene, so that the pregnant woman who saw the accident would have seen his wounds only briefly (Moore, 1886). Carreras (1910) described a case in which a young boy was knocked down by a cart and his head wounded so that his scalp required extensive stitching. His mother, then less than 2 months pregnant, later accompanied her son to the hospital and was present when his wound was dressed. She wanted to keep her eyes closed so that she would not see the wound, but could not prevent herself from taking a quick glance at it. The sight profoundly disturbed her. When, 7 months later, she gave birth to her baby, a daughter, it was immediately noticed that the baby had an area of hairlessness on the left parietal region of the scalp at the site where the brother had been wounded. Carreras, who examined the girl, stated that the affected hairless area measured 1 centimeter in width and about 6 centimeters in length; it closely resembled the residue of a healed wound.

The duration of the mother's exposure to the stimulus, therefore, seems to be less important than its effect on her and also less important than any tendency she may have to dwell on the memory of the stimulus later. I discuss this third feature next.

Emotional Reaction of the Pregnant Woman to the Stimulus

In most instances the woman was described as "frightened" or "shocked," and where such adjectives are missing in the reports they can often be reasonably conjectured by considering the usual feelings that a woman would have when someone like her husband or child is seriously injured.

Some of the women became obsessed with the stimulus and could not stop thinking about it. In the case reported by Liébeault (1892) the woman affected actually hallucinated the original stimulus (a "port-wine" birthmark) appearing on other persons whom she saw in the street. However, other women seemed to have dismissed the stimulus from their minds and related it to a lesion in the baby only after the baby was born.

Curiosity appears to have been the dominant condition in three women who figured in a small epidemic of cleft lip that occurred in Belgium in the late 19th century (Theyskens, 1881). A woman who was in the first weeks of a pregnancy happened to see someone with an unrepaired cleft lip. She was greatly disturbed by the sight of this person and went to see Theyskens, telling him that she was firmly convinced that her baby would have a cleft lip. Theyskens tried unavailingly to reassure her. In fact, her baby was born with a cleft lip. The matter was much discussed in the area, and several pregnant neighbors came to see the new baby for themselves. As a result, according to Theyskens, some months later he had to repair three more cleft lips of babies born to these curious neighbors of the first affected baby. A similar, although less numerous spread of a birth defect of the forearm attributed to maternal impressions occurred in two cases cited by Elliotson (1852).

The Mother's Expectation of an Effect from the Stimulus

The beliefs of the pregnant women as to the effects of the stimuli on the babies varied widely. Some were unshakeably convinced that their babies would be damaged, others equally sure that there would be no effect from the stimulus.

In 8 of the 50 cases the mother did not expect to have a defective baby after she had an apparently affecting impression; in other cases the report does not state whether the mother expected the baby to be affected, and I think we can assume that in some, perhaps in most, of these cases the mother also had no such fear.

In 3 cases the woman feared having a baby with a birthmark and tried, with apparent success, to divert it from an exposed part of the body to a place where it would not ordinarily be seen.

On the whole, the 50 cases here analyzed support Dabney's (1890) judgment (based on a larger sample) that the mother's opinion about whether the baby will be affected indicates poorly what will in fact happen to the baby.

Pertinent Observations about the Pregnant Woman's Personality

The authors of the reports of the cases that I have studied concerned themselves almost exclusively with the correspondences in time and appearance (mainly anatomical location) between the stimulus and the mark or defect on the later-born child. Most of them obviously, and probably all of them, believed that a maternal impression could affect an embryo or a fetus; otherwise they would not have taken the trouble to record the cases they reported. Only a few of them seemed aware of the possibility—and commented on it—that certain women might be more susceptible to maternal impressions than others. Their reports, therefore, contain almost no discriminating information on this aspect of the cases. In a few of the reports we are told, for example, that the woman was "known to be, at all times, very nervous and easily alarmed" (Montgomery, 1857) or that she had been diagnosed as having hysteria (Lagache, 1908). These, however, are exceptional; most of the reports convey little or nothing pertinent to this topic.

Period of the Pregnancy When the Stimulus Occurred

For an analysis of the trimester of pregnancy when the stimulus occurred I increased the size of the sample by adding an additional 85 cases to the 50 cases just reviewed. These additional cases were drawn (with a few exceptions) from the same sources—medical journals and monographs—as the first 50. They included some of the commoner birth defects, such as simple cleft lip, which I had excluded from the 50 selected cases. For 113 of the 135 cases information was available concerning the trimester of the pregnancy when the pregnant woman was exposed to the attributed stimulus. The results of the analysis are shown in Table 27.2. The difference in the incidences of the stimuli among trimesters is statistically significant ($p < .001$). I think it is also medically significant, because we can safely assume that a pregnant woman would be equally likely to encounter a stimulus of the kind we are considering in one trimester as in either of the others. The 1st trimester is that in which the main features of the limbs and organs are developed. During it the embryo-fetus is more sensitive to the teratogenic influence of infections and noxious drugs or toxins than it is in later trimesters. One would expect the 1st trimester to be also the period of greatest sensitivity to psychical influences.

However, several of the birthmarks and six of the birth defects corresponded to stimuli experienced by the mother in the 2nd or 3rd trimester

Table 27.2. Trimester of Pregnancy during which Mother-to-be Received Stimulus of Maternal Impression (N = 135)

	1st Trimester	*2nd Trimester*	*3rd Trimester*	*Not Stated*
No. of instances of stimulus occurring during this trimester	80	20	13	22

$X^2 = 71.9$, df = 2, $p < .001$.

Note: Cases for which the stimulus was noted as occurring "early in pregnancy" were counted in the 1st trimester, as were two cases in which the stimulus occurred before the woman became pregnant. When estimates crossed the boundaries between trimesters, the cases were assigned to the later trimester, e.g., an estimate of "3–4 months" was assigned to the 2nd trimester.

of her pregnancy (Lagache, 1908; Thompson, 1878). In these cases, by the time of the mother's receiving the stimulus the organ in the baby that corresponded to the stimulus would, in ordinary embryological development, have been fully formed.

It has been suggested that a woman who has just learned that she is pregnant (and therefore is in the 1st trimester of her pregnancy) may be more apprehensive and hence more attentive to unusual stimuli than she is in the later phases of the pregnancy. If this is true—but I do not know of any evidence suggesting that it is—pregnant women might be led retrospectively to attribute significance to events of the 1st trimester more than to those of the later 2 trimesters. A retrospective false memory, however, seems excluded in those numerous cases in which, as I mentioned earlier, the physician reporting the case had seen both the stimulus to the mother and the defect in the later-born baby.

Unusualness of the Birth Defects and Their Correspondence to the Stimuli

As I mentioned earlier, I deliberately selected many of the 50 cases for this analysis because the lesions were *not* those commonly occurring as birth defects. I wished thereby to neutralize, at least for these cases, Müller's (1834–1840/1840-1842, vol. 2, pp. 1404–1406) objection that the lesions attributed to maternal impressions belong to the common types of birth defects and correspond little to the stimuli alleged to be their causes.

The correspondence between stimulus and lesion seems to be exact or extremely close in 46 (92%) of the 50 cases. This is an even higher proportion of correspondences than Dabney (1890) found; as I mentioned earlier, he considered that stimulus and lesion corresponded closely in 69 (77%) of 90 cases.[7]

In two cases a limb of the baby was affected in a manner corresponding to the stimulus, but on the side opposite to that of the stimulus. (This may have happened in several other cases, for which the reports do not specify the side of an injury or defect on the person seen by the woman.)

In one case, the pregnant woman's hand was seriously injured by her husband, but there was apparently no residual defect, such as occurred in her baby's brachydactyly. In another case, the man who impressed the pregnant woman had a stump of an arm, presumably from an amputation; her baby had no forearm and rudimentary fingers developing from the upper arm.

Nearly all the lesions of the babies are rare, and a small number are extremely so. Indeed, a few may be unique among birth defects. I include among the group of extremely rare congenital lesions: a case of a tracheal (thyroglossal) sinus; a case of birthmarks corresponding to marks of four bloody fingers on a face; a case of absent middle digits and metacarpal bones; a case of an unusual syndrome comprised of constrictions of the legs, a raw cicatrized area of the groin, and red marks on the backs of the hands; a case of the absence of the penis; and a case of the absence of a single metacarpal bone.

For some of the birth defects figuring in these cases we have reports of their incidence that seem to me adequately reliable. In Table 27.3 I give figures for several of the pertinent incidences. Readers can see that with the exception of cleft lip all the listed birth defects are rare, and most are extremely rare. The incidence of cases may be somewhat higher than the available figures suggest, because some cases of ordinarily hidden birth defects, such as absence of the penis, may never come to medical attention and hence would not figure in counts of medical reports. However, Wilde (1843) included information from all (or nearly all) births in the Imperial Lying-In Hospital of Vienna over a period of 8 years; and Birch-Jensen (1949) included in his survey of defects of the upper limbs the entire population of Denmark.

Rare as many of the pertinent birth defects are, their infrequency is only part of what we need to consider in appraising the likelihood that a maternal impression has caused a birth defect (or birthmark). We need also to consider how common is the mother's experience to which the defect is attributed. For the frequencies of this side of the cases I can offer no figures. However, although some of the stimulating experiences, such as seeing on the street someone with a "port-wine" birthmark, are fairly common, others are surely extremely rare. It must be most unusual for a woman to examine the site where a man's penis has been surgically amputated; this was the stimulating event in the case reported by Owen (1863) of a congenital absence of the penis. It is surely also unusual for a person to have his face and neck slapped with a bloody hand leaving the red impressions of four fingers on the face and neck; this was the stimu-

Table 27.3. Incidences of Some of the Birth Defects Figuring in Cases of Maternal Impressions

Birth Defect	*Reported Incidence at Birth*	*Source of Data on Incidence*
1. Umbilical hernia	1 in 23,413	Wilde (1843) (Austria)
2. Absence of the penis	1 in 30,000,000	Harris (1898) (USA)
	No figures of incidence, but only 15 cases reported up to 1951	Campbell (1951) (USA)
3. Unilateral absence of forearm	1 in 22,000	Birch-Jensen (1949) (Denmark)
4. Unilateral absence of hand	1 in 65,000	Birch-Jensen (1949) (Denmark)
5. Thyroglossal sinus (small opening in the neck)	"never congenital"	Bland-Sutton (1893/1903) (England)
	"rarely congenital"	Bailey (1929) (England)
	In a series of 310 cases, none had been noted at birth	Marshall and Becker (1949) (USA)
6. Anotia (absence of external ear)	No figures of incidence, but only 7 cases reported up to1948	Ružić (1948) (Yugoslavia)
7. Cleft lip with cleft palate	1 in 2,100	Wilde (1843) (Austria)
	1 in 2,100	MacMahon and McKeown (1953) (England)
8. Ectrodactyly (absence of one or more fingers)	1 in 90,000	Birch-Jensen (1949) (Denmark)
9. Brachydactyly (short fingers)	1 in 40,000	Birch-Jensen (1949) (Denmark)

lating event in the case of a baby born with a birthmark on its neck and face suggesting "four bloody fingers" (Lee, 1891).

The Pregnant Woman's State of Consciousness When Stimulated

In all 50 cases the mother of the apparently affected baby was awake when she was stimulated by the injury or deformity that corresponded to that of her later-born baby. However, two other cases have been reported in which a mother dreamed of some injury, and a corresponding malformation occurred in her later-born child. Hammond (1868) described the case of a woman who dreamed during her pregnancy—Hammond did not say how far advanced the pregnancy was—that she saw a man who had lost part of the external ear. When her child was born, "a portion of one ear was deficient, and the organ was exactly like the defective ear she had seen in her dream." Hammond added: "I have examined this child, and the ear looks exactly as if a portion had been cut off with a sharp knife" (Hammond, 1868, p. 19). In the second case of this type a baby was delivered and immediately found not to have the great toe of the right foot. On learning this the baby's mother said that during the 4th month of her pregnancy she had dreamed that a rat had bitten off the great toe of her right foot. The impression was so vivid "that she awoke screaming, and narrated the cause of her fright to her husband, who corroborated her statement" (Brydon, 1886, p. 670). . . .

THE CASE OF ASTRIDE STEVAUX

Astride Stevaux was born in Saverne, Alsace, France, on June 6, 1956. Her parents were André Stevaux and his wife, Antoinette. Astride was the first of their three children—all daughters.

When Astride was born, she was immediately found to have a major birth defect of her left hand. Its three middle fingers were markedly underdeveloped in both length and volume, although they did have small nails at their ends (Figure 27.1). The thumb and fifth finger of Astride's left hand and all the fingers of her right hand were normal.

When Astride was born, her father was about 22 years old. When he was 17, he had injured his *right* hand in an accident. He was then working on a farm and helping to operate a fodder-chopping machine. His hand became caught in the cogs that catch the stalks and feed them toward the blades. He lost much blood, and in the end it was necessary to amputate the index and middle fingers of the injured hand. The fourth and fifth fingers were saved, but could not be fully extended (Figure 27.2). Eventually he recovered almost complete use of the hand, and he became a butcher.

André and Antoinette Stevaux married on December 27, 1954. Antoinette became pregnant with Astride about 9 months later.

The congenital deformity of Astride's left hand was attributed by at least some persons in her community to an impression on her mother from her father's deformed hand. Information about the case circulated in the community until it eventually reached Dr. Bernadette Chauvin (a native of Alsace), and she informed me about it.

Having learned of the case and obtained the agreement of the Stevaux family, I went to their home in the village of Haegen, near Strasbourg, on November 28, 1987. I was able to interview André and Antoinette Stevaux as well as Astride herself.

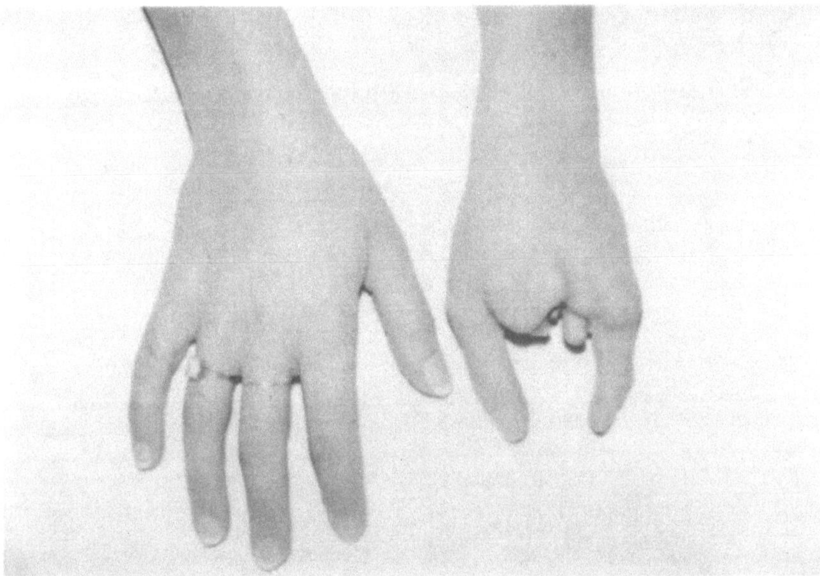

Figure 27.1. Hands of Astride Stevaux. The middle three fingers of the left hand were markedly malformed, although each had a rudimentary nail. The other fingers were all normal.

Antoinette Steveux's Condition during Her Pregnancy

Antoinette Stevaux said that she paid no attention whatever to the deformity of her husband's hand during her pregnancy. Neither she nor anyone else in their circle predicted that her baby would be deformed. It was only after Astride's birth that some persons of the area began to conjecture that Astride's deformity derived from the impression that her mother must have had during her pregnancy when she would have had the deformed hand of her husband in view every day.

Other Relevant Information

André and Antoinette Stevaux were not related. Their other two daughters were entirely normal. Astride married and had a daughter who was also normal.

During her pregnancy with Astride, Antoinette Stevaux enjoyed perfect health. She took no drugs or medications during her pregnancy.

Comment

This case is not like the typical one attributed to a maternal impression. First, Antoinette Stevaux underwent no single fright or shock dur-

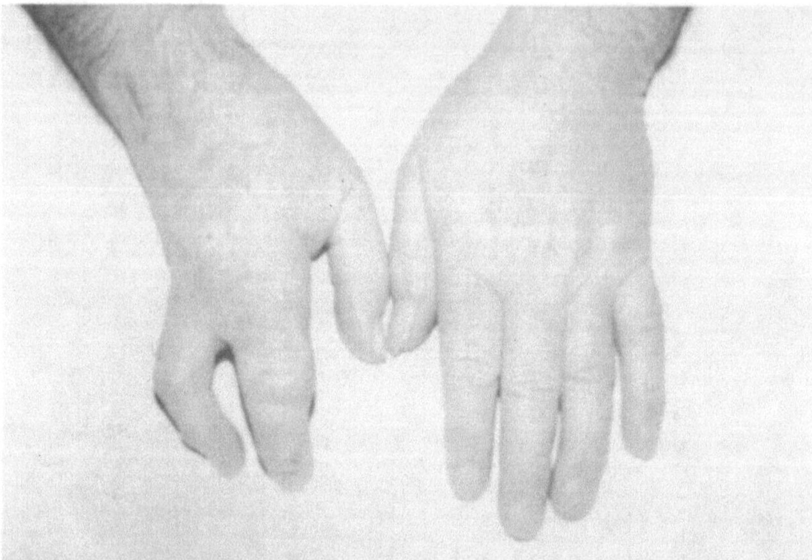

Figure 27.2. Hands of André Stevaux. The index and middle finger of the right hand were missing following their amputation. The fourth and fifth fingers of the same hand could not be fully extended.

ing her pregnancy; however, as I mentioned earlier, in some cases a pregnant woman has been frequently or constantly exposed to a deformity in a member of her family. Second, Antoinette Stevaux expected no effect on her baby from her husband's deformity; however, in at least 8 of the 50 cases earlier analyzed the pregnant woman concerned had no expectation of any effect on her baby from the stimulus she experienced. Third, André Stevaux's *right* hand was injured and he lost two fingers from it, whereas Astride's deformity was on her *left* hand; however, in 2 of the 50 cases earlier analyzed a right/left reversal of lesions occurred. The lesions of André and Astride Stevaux were not identical, but I consider them closely similar. Thus, although the case has features deviating from the standard case of a maternal impression, its exceptional features have occurred in other cases that seem to me to qualify as instances for which a maternal impression is a possible interpretation.

CONCLUDING REMARKS

I do not doubt that many women are frightened during a pregnancy without this having ill effects on their babies. Although negative cases are far less often reported than positive ones in the literature of maternal impressions, I cited some examples earlier of published cases in which a pregnant woman had been frightened, expected her baby to be deformed, and nevertheless delivered a normal baby (Conant, 1863; Morland, 1853; Rich, 1891). My question is: Does a frightening experience in a pregnant woman *sometimes* have an effect on the form of her baby? The answer to this question will depend on judgments concerning the likelihood that the correspondence between the attributed stimulus and the birth defect on the later-born baby could have occurred by chance. I have tried to reduce the likelihood of chance as a factor in the 50 cases I analyzed by selecting ones in which the stimulus was unusual and the birth defect was also unusual.

My examination of published cases and my study of the few cases that have come under my own observation have persuaded me to give an affirmative judgment on the question. I will not undertake in this paper to suggest how a woman's mental images could affect her baby. Here I am concerned to show that this may happen, not how it does. If maternal impressions do sometimes affect gestating babies, however, and if adequately explanatory physical connections between the mother-to-be and her baby cannot be identified, this may oblige us to postulate some paranormal process.

NOTES

1. Excerpts from the *Journal of Scientific Exploration*, 6, 353–373, 1992.—Ed.
2. I have omitted here the report of the case of Calvin Ewing, which has been summarized in the paper "Bodily Changes Corresponding to Another Person's Mental Images" in part 2.—Ed.
3. Readers wishing to have more information about the history of the belief in maternal impressions than I shall include in this section can find it in Barrow (1971), Glenister (1964), Gould and Pyle (1896), King (1978), and Warkany (1959). Rousseau (1982), in an essay on Tobias Smollett, reviewed ideas about maternal impressions current in 18th-century England. Smollett, a physician as well as a novelist, wittily exploited the belief for scenes in *Peregrine Pickle* (Smollett, 1751/1964).
4. Using different terms, several later authors proposed that some paranormal process would ultimately account for birth defects related to maternal impressions (Bruck, 1924; Drzewiecki, 1891; and Lowman, 1889).
5. In a paper of more than 50 pages, Fisher devoted less than 1 page to the report of his survey. He did not state how many of the women he questioned expected (as opposed to merely fearing) that they would have deformed children, although many of them did expect as well as fear such an outcome. He also did not state whether the three women who did deliver babies with anomalies had been exposed to frightening stimuli during their pregnancies.
6. In my forthcoming book (Stevenson, 1997) I give for the 50 cases (a) details of the stimulus to the mother, (b) a brief description of the birthmark or birth defect on the baby, and (c) a reference to the published report of each case.
7. Eleven of the 50 cases I selected also appeared in Dabney's (1890) inventory of 90 cases.

REFERENCES

Bablot, B. (1788). *Dissertation sur le Pouvoir de l'Imagination des Femmes Enceintes.* Paris: Royez.

Bailey, H. (1929). *Branchial Cysts and Other Essays on Surgical Subjects of the Facio-Cervical Region.* London: H. K. Lewis.

Ballantyne, J. W. (1890–1891). Maternal impressions. *Edinburgh Medical Journal, 36,* 624–635.

Ballantyne, J. W. (1891–1892). A series of thirteen cases of alleged maternal impression. *Edinburgh Medical Journal, 37,* 1025–1034.

Barker, F. (1887). The influence of maternal impressions on the fetus. *Transactions of the American Gynecological Society for the Year 1886, 11,* 152–175.

Barrow, M. V. (1971). A brief history of teratology to the early 20th century. *Teratology, 4,* 119–130.

Birch-Jensen, A. (1949). *Congenital Deformities of the Upper Extremities.* Copenhagen: Andelsbogtrykkeriet i Odense and Det Danske Forlag.

Bland-Sutton, J. (1903). *Tumours: Innocent and Malignant* (3d ed.). Chicago: W. T. Keener. (First published in 1893)

Blondel, J. A. (1729). *The Power of the Mother's Imagination over the Foetus examin'd.* London: John Brotherton.

Bruck, C. (1924). *Experimentelle Telepathie: Neue Versuche zur Telepathischen Übertragung von Zeichnungen.* Stuttgart: J. Puttmann.

Brydon, J. (1886). Maternal impressions. *British Medical Journal, i,* 670.

Buffon, G.-L. de. (1830). *Oeuvres Complètes.* Brussels: T. Lejeune.

Burdach, K. F. (1837). *Die Physiologie als Erfahrungswissenschaft.* Leipzig: Leopold Voss.

Busey, S. C. (1887). Discussion of Barker, F. The influence of maternal impressions on the fetus. *Transactions of the American Gynecological Society for the Year 1886, 11,* 176–196.

Campbell, M. (1951). *Clinical Pediatric Urology.* Philadelphia: W. B. Saunders.

Carreras, E. (1910). *Le Impressioni Materne.* Milan: Casa Editrice "Luce e Ombra."

Conant, D. S. (1863). The science, causes, and anatomical peculiarities of human monstrosities. *Transactions of the New York Academy of Medicine, 2,* 269–298.

Dabney, W. C. (1890). Maternal impressions. In J. M. Keating (ed.), *Cyclopaedia of the Diseases of Children* (vol. 1, pp. 191–216). Philadelphia: J. B. Lippincott.

Drzewiecki, J. (1891). Über den Einfluss der Eindrüke der Mutter auf den Fötus oder das sogenannte "Versehen" der Schwangeren. *Wiener Medizinische Wochenschrift, 41,* 1810–1811, 1857–1859. (Also published in 1891. The influence of maternal impressions upon the foetus. *Medical Record, 40,* 529–531; and in 1892. L'influence des impressions maternelles sur le foetus. *Revue de 1'Hypnotisme, 6,* 196–202)

Elliotson, J. (1852). An instance of the effect of maternal mental impression upon the offspring before its birth. *Zoist, 10,* 379–385.

Farkas, G., & Farkas, G., Jr. (1974). Is the popular belief about "maternal impression" in pregnancy unscientific? *Proceedings of the XXIII International Congress of the History of Medicine, 2,* 1303–1304. London: Wellcome Institute of the History of Medicine.

Fisher, G. J. (1870). Does maternal mental influence have any constructive or destructive power in the production of malformations or monstrosities at any stage of embryonic development? *American Journal of Insanity, 26,* 241–295.

Formijne, A. J. (1915). Het verzien van zwangeren. *Nederlandsch Tijdschrift voor Geneeskunde, 59,* 1876–1877.

Glenister, T. W. (1964). Fantasies, facts and foetuses. *Medical History, 8,* 15–30.

Gould, G. M., & Pyle, W. L. (1896). *Anomalies and Curiosities of Medicine.* Philadelphia: W. B. Saunders.

Hall, C. (1785). *The Medical Family Instructor: Containing a Selection of Interesting Subjects, Calculated for the Information and Preservation of Mankind. Together with the Management of Child-bed Women, and Children, to Which Is Added an Appendix, on Canine Madness.* Shrewsbury: T. Wood.

Hammond, W. A. (1868). On the influence of the maternal mind over the offspring during pregnancy and lactation. *Quarterly Journal of Psychological Medicine and Medical Jurisprudence, 2*, 1–28.

Harris, R. P. (1898). Congenital absence of the penis, the urethra making its exit into or below the rectum, and emptying the bladder by, or exterior to, the anus. *Philadelphia Medical Journal, 1*, 71–77.

Kennedy, W. P. (1967). Epidemiological aspects of the problem of congenital malformations. *Birth Defects: Original Article Series, 3*, 1–18.

King, L. S. (1978). *The Philosophy of Medicine: The Early Eighteenth Century*. Cambridge, MA: Harvard University Press.

Lacambre, J. (1906). L'imagination de la mère peut-elle agir sur le foetus? Correspondance médico-littéraire. *La Chronique Médicale, 13*, 683.

Lagache, H. (1908). À propos d'un accident de travail. Amputation de trois doigts; autoplastie de la face dorsale de la main gauche.—Curieuse coincidence d'un cas tératologique. *L'écho Médical du Nord, 12*, 66–69.

Leclerc-Montmoyen, L. F. (1949). Les anomalies foetales. *Le Concours Médical, 71*, 1405–1406.

Lee, H. B. (1891). Maternal impressions. *Medical Record, 40*, 509.

Liébeault, A. (1892). De l'influence psychique exercée par la mère sur le foetus. *Revue de l'Hypnotisme, 6*, 52–54.

Lowman, W. R. (1889). Resumé on maternal impressions. *Medical Record, 36*, 176–179.

MacMahon, B., & McKeown, T. (1953). The incidence of harelip and cleft palate related to birth rank and maternal age. *American Journal of Human Genetics, 5*, 176–183.

Marshall, S. F., & Becker, W. F. (1949). Thyroglossal cysts and sinuses. *Annals of Surgery, 129*, 642–651.

Meadows, A. (1865). Case of monstrosity, with remarks on the influence of maternal impressions on the foetus in utero. *Transactions of the Obstetrical Society of London, 7*, 84–94.

Montgomery, W. F. (1857). *An Exposition of the Signs and Symptoms of Pregnancy: With Some Other Papers on Subjects Connected with Midwifery*. Philadelphia: Blanchard and Lea.

Moore, G. R. (1886). Maternal impressions. *British Medical Journal, i*, 1012.

Morland, W. W. (1853). Cases of arrest of development, blemishes, etc., in infants, attributed to strong mental action in the mother while pregnant; disagreeable sights; sudden shock, etc. Discussion upon the question whether such action of the mind be ever a cause of such observed results. *American Journal of the Medical Sciences, 25*, 356–361.

Müller, J. (1840-1842). *Elements of Physiology* (2 vols.). (William Baly, trans.). London: Taylor and Walton. (First published in German in 1834–1840)

Murdock, E. P. (1888). Maternal impressions. *Medical Record, 34*, 607.

Owen, A. P. (1863). Arrest of development in the foetus. *Lancet, i*, 25.

Paré, A. (1982). *On Monsters and Marvels*. (J. L. Pallister, trans.). Chicago: University of Chicago Press. (First published in 1573)

Rich, E. S. (1891). Maternal impressions [Correspondence]. *Medical Record, 40*, 643.

Rousseau, G. S. (1982). *Tobias Smollett: Essays of Two Decades*. Edinburgh: T. & T. Clark.

Ružić, J. (1948). Der siebente Fall kompletter Anotie. *Acta Otolaryngologica, 36*, 186–190.

Smollett, T. (1964). *The Adventures of Peregrine Pickle*. Oxford: Oxford University Press. (First published in 1751)

Stevenson, I. (1997). *Reincarnation and Biology: A Contribution to the Etiology of Birthmarks and Birth Defects* (2 vols.). New York: Praeger.

Suringar, J. V. (1927). Het Verzien. *De Tempel, 5*, 154–161.

Taylor, W. T. (1876). On maternal impressions affecting the foetus. *Philadelphia Medical Times, 7*, 73–75.

Theyskens, J. (1881). *Over Het Misbruiken van Het Bovennatuurlijke*. Ghent: J. Vuylsteke.

Thompson, A. (1878). Congenital deformity. *Transactions of the Obstetrical Society of London, for the Year 1877, 19*, 94–96.

Turner, D. (1731). *De Morbis Cutaneis: A Treatise of Diseases Incident to the Skin* (4th ed.). London: Walthoe, Wilkin, Bonwicke, Birt, Ward, and Wicksteed. (First published in 1714)

Warkany, J. (1959). Congenital malformations in the past. *Journal of Chronic Diseases, 10,* 84–96.

Warkany, J., & Kalter, H. (1962). Maternal impressions and congenital malformations. *Plastic and Reconstructive Surgery, 30,* 628–637.

Wilde, W. R. (1843). Statistics of deliveries, statistics of monstrosities. *American Journal of the Medical Sciences, 6,* 239–240. (Abstracted from Wilde, W. R. *Austria: Its Literary, Scientific, and Medical Institutions. With Notes Upon the Present State of Science, and a Guide to the Hospitals and Sanatory Establishments of Vienna* (pp. 222–225). Dublin: William Cuny, 1843)

Williams, H. C., & Pembroke, A. C. (1988). Naevus of Jamaica. *Lancet, ii,* 915.

Wilson, P. K. (1992). "Out of sight, out of mind?": The Daniel Turner-James Blondel dispute over the power of the maternal imagination. *Annals of Science, 49,* 63–85.

TWENTY-EIGHT

A Case of Severe Birth Defects Possibly Due to Cursing

1989[12]

For centuries it was widely believed that a strong unpleasant shock to a pregnant woman could cause birth defects in her baby. Medical books and journals published numerous cases of this type up to the early decades of the present century. The idea of "maternal impression" gradually lost ground during the 18th and 19th centuries, mainly because it seemed to conflict with the facts of physiology. In cases of "maternal impression," the pregnant mother was usually reported to have viewed someone with a shocking deformity that her baby was said to reproduce. It has also been thought that cursing, verbally inflicted and without a visual stimulus, could produce birth defects. Three cases of this type, one published by a pediatrician in 1960, are briefly reviewed, and then a new case is reported. In both of the modern cases, the commonly recognized etiological factors in birth defects could not be identified.

Children who claim to remember previous lives are often born with birthmarks and birth defects that correspond to wounds or other marks on a person whose life the child later remembers. In many cases the evidence of such correspondence depends on the memories of informants who saw the deceased person's body; but in some 30 cases, medical documents, usually postmortem reports, have provided the stronger evidence of a contemporaneously written record of the wounds. I have reported a few cases of this type (Stevenson, 1966/1974) and am preparing to publish reports of a much larger number of cases with fuller documentation, including photographs of the birthmarks and birth defects (Stevenson, 1993, 1997). The birthmarks and birth defects occurring in these cases are not, for the most part, of the commonly recognized types; and it has been possible to exclude in most cases all the recognized physical causes of birthmarks and birth defects, such as genetic factors and illness of the mother during her pregnancy.

In many cases of the type just mentioned the child's mother had seen the dead body of the person her child later claimed to have been. In others she had not seen the body, but had heard descriptions of its wounds. Under these circumstances it could be supposed that images in her mind of the dead person's wounds had somehow affected the body of her child and produced in it birthmarks or birth defects corresponding to the images in the mother's mind and thus also to the dead person's wounds. As I continued my investigations of these cases I learned that the hypothesis of maternal impression—to give the process I have just described its usual name in English—was a serious rival to other interpretations of these cases, including reincarnation.

The principal case reported in this paper illustrates the competition between the hypothesis of maternal impression and that of reincarnation, if we decide from the evidence that some paranormal process seems to have been involved. I hope to facilitate appraisal of the case report by first giving a brief account of the hypothesis of maternal impression and summaries of published cases in which cursing provided the source of the possibly causative imagery in the mind of a pregnant woman who gave birth to a defective child.

THE CONCEPT OF MATERNAL IMPRESSION AS A CAUSE OF BIRTH DEFECTS

It was widely believed for centuries—by laypeople and physicians alike—that strong mental impressions in a pregnant woman could cause birth defects (or birthmarks) in the baby born of her pregnancy. Authors of reports of such cases frequently drew attention to close correspondences of site and appearance between some shocking deformity seen by the pregnant woman and the birth defect of her later-born child. For example, if the sight of a man with deformed feet had frightened a pregnant woman, her baby's congenitally deformed feet would be attributed to this fright (Montgomery, 1857, pp. 35–36). The medical literature of the 18th and 19th centuries contained numerous reports of cases of this kind.

Even in the 18th century voices of skepticism, such as that of the famous obstetrician William Hunter,[3] were heard. These, however, did not stop the publication of reports of such cases in medical journals. In 1890 Dabney reviewed and analyzed 90 cases of maternal impression, reports of which had been published between 1853 and 1886 (Dabney, 1890). Nevertheless, by that time the hypothesis of maternal impression was steadily losing popularity, and only sporadic reports of apparently exemplifying cases occurred in the early years of the 20th century. By the middle of this century, authorities on teratology discounted and even derided the concept (Barrow, 1971; Warkany, 1959, 1971). Warkany (1959, p. 89) pointed out that the hypothesis of maternal impression lost credibility with advances in anatomy and physiology during the 19th century. "It was known," he wrote, "that the maternal and fetal circulations were separated. How could images be transmitted through the placenta?"

One possible answer to this question is that the influence might be transmitted through some paranormal process as yet not recognized, let alone understood. A careful study of the published reports of cases of maternal impression and the investigation of a few cases that have come under my direct observation have convinced me that the hypothesis of maternal impression deserves renewed attention. I do not expect any reader to agree with my judgment on this matter until he or she has studied the extensive review of reported cases that I have included in my mentioned forthcoming work (see also Stevenson, 1992 [previous paper in this volume]). This will provide summaries of about 50 cases in which a pregnant woman, after seeing (or occasionally after hearing about) an unusual injury or deformity, gave birth to a baby with birthmarks or birth defects corresponding closely to the apparently stimulating injury or deformity that the woman had seen or learned about.

Cursing as a Generator of Maternal Impressions

In the standard case of a birth defect attributed to a maternal impression (as published in the 19th century and the first decades of this one), the mother had nearly always been directly exposed to the sight of some shockingly deformed person. However, a few cases have been reported in which the mother was said to have imagined (and caused) a congenital deformity in her child without any visual experience to guide her. In these cases the mother-to-be would only have heard a description of wounds or defects narrated by someone else who had seen them, such as her husband.

A subgroup of cases without direct visual stimulation of the woman's mental imagery is that occurring with a curse. When one person curses another, the cursing person evokes in the cursed one mental images of some unpleasant and even fatal event that is to happen.

The medical literature on cursing is sparse. There is now widespread skepticism in the West about the efficacy of cursing, and one is surprised to find an occasional educated Western person who believes in its power (Raine, 1977, p. 73). Reports of the effects of cursing, moreover, rarely mention that the curse had specified a particular penalty that the cursed person was to endure; he or she should suffer or die, but was usually not told how (Burrell, 1963; Mathis, 1964). However, I have found 3 published reports of cases in which the cursing person predicted birth defects in a child of the person cursed. I shall summarize them next.

Readers may think that the first 2 of these cases deserve only the status of legends because, although reports of them were published in the 19th century, their origins lay much farther back. This means, however, that the cursing occurred during a period when people believed in the power of cursing, and such a belief may be necessary for a curse to be effective.

The birth defect in both these cases was that of hereditary brachydactyly, which, by the time of the proband's life, had already afflicted in one case nine generations of the family (Kellie, 1808), in the other six generations (Mackinder, 1857). These cases occurred in different parts of England (Uxbridge and Gainsborough), but both were said to have begun, generations earlier, in the cursing of a pregnant woman by her husband and for the same offense. (Perhaps the families were distantly related and the same account became transmitted in two lines of descent.) In each case, the husband of the unfortunate woman had cultivated fruit trees with great solicitude, and, when the time came to pluck the fruit, he had strictly forbidden anyone else in his household to take the first fruit. The fruit nevertheless disappeared. The enraged man then cursed the thief. In the earlier of these two accounts the man "with dreadful rashness wished, that if she [his wife] was guilty, the child which she was then with might be born without fingers" (Kellie, 1808, p. 253). In the second case the angry man was said to have "cursed the thief, and prayed, for so heinous an offence, that the fingers which touched the apple might all be chopped off. His wife, enceinte, feared much . . . , but dared not confess the crime . . . a child was born; but, sad to tell, the fingers which its father had wished to be amputated had strangely forgotten to grow" (Mackinder, 1857, p. 846).[4]

The next case known to me occurred in Australia and in modern times (Turner, 1960). It is that of an infant with almost complete amelia that followed a cursing of the baby's mother by her mother. The former, a 16-year-old Australian girl, had become illegitimately pregnant in the hope of forcing her parents to allow her to marry a Maltese man of whom they strongly disapproved. The girl's mother, instead of consenting to the marriage, became angry, roundly cursed her daughter, and said that if she continued with the pregnancy the baby would be born "without arms and legs, and blind" (p. 502). (The mother first cursed her daughter during the 5th or 6th week of the pregnancy.) Several persons witnessed the cursing, and the mother repeated it every 2 or 3 weeks in letters to her daughter during the remainder of the pregnancy. The pregnancy ran to term, and the daughter was delivered of a gravely deformed male baby. Both the infant's legs were absent, and of the right arm only the proximal half of the upper part was present. The left arm was normal down to the hand, but it had only two fingers. The infant seemed otherwise normal and was probably not blind. It was cared for in the.hospital of its birth for 6 months and then transferred to a babies' home, where it died at the age of 7 months.

Dr. Elizabeth Turner (a pediatrician), who reported this case, found no evidence that any of the commonly recognized etiological factors in birth defects had occurred in it. Since Turner published her report before excessive consumption of alcohol had been clearly identified as a factor in causing birth defects, I corresponded with her about this possibility. She assured me that alcohol could not have been a causative agent in the case. (She mentioned in her letter to me of October 27, 1978 that she had become aware of the teratogenic effects of alcohol before other pediatricians had published papers bringing this factor in birth defects to widespread attention.) So far as she could tell, the stress of the cursing by the pregnant woman's mother was the only causative factor identified in the case. After briefly reviewing some evidence from pharmacological experiments bearing on the role of stress in causing reduction deformities of limbs, Turner concluded her report by expressing the "hope that it may stimulate others with experience of similar cases to document and record them" (p. 503).

CASE REPORT

A research assistant of mine in Sri Lanka (Tissa Jayawardene) noticed in a newspaper a photograph of a male infant, S.P., who had been born (on August 13, 1980) without arms and with deformed legs. Knowing of my interest in unusual birth defects, he went to the village where the baby lived and photographed the baby himself, afterward sending me a photograph of the baby, who was then 4 months old (see Figure 28.1). When I was next in Sri Lanka (in October 1982), I went to the village of the baby's family, but learned that he had died (of "some urinary trouble") in April 1982, at the age of about 20 months. He was then just beginning to speak.

The photograph showed almost all that I could learn about the baby's birth defects. There was complete absence of the arms. A finger nubbin was visible at the left shoulder; I do not know whether there was one at the corresponding site of the right shoulder. Both legs were morphologically normal, but both feet were deformed and turned medially; plaster casts (visible in the photograph) had been applied in the hope of correcting the deformities. At the time of his death, the baby could crawl, but could not walk well because of his deformed feet.

I inquired of the child's father whether he knew of anyone in his family or circle of acquaintances who had lost his arms before dying.[5] It turned out that he did. The person in question was someone whom the father (with his brother) had murdered in February 1974. The father then narrated the following history, which I corroborated (in its essential features) from the baby's mother, its uncle, and other villagers, particularly members of the murdered man's family.

The murdered man, Y.S., was, at the time of his death, 25 years of age and married. He had been in his village what the Sinhalese call a "chandiya," by which they mean someone who is rough, tough, and given to bullying other people. He had a record of violent behavior, as had other members of his family. His older brother told me, *en passant*, that he (the informant) had himself killed three men; and their father had died when he had nervously dropped a bomb that he was preparing for use against his enemies in the village. Y.S.'s older brother also told me that Y.S. had been "ruthless," and he compared him to the German soldier Field Marshal Erich Rommel.

A quarrel over Y.S.'s dog, which had entered the house of one of his adversaries and eaten a cooked curry, began with the womenfolk and spread to the men. The baby's father and uncle decided to finish with Y.S. They arranged somehow for him to be made drunk with alcohol and lured over to their side of the village. They then cut off his arms and legs with a sword. Other villagers, angry at Y.S., came, like the lesser senators at Caesar's murder, and inflicted additional wounds.

I obtained a copy of the postmortem examination of Y.S.'s body. With regard to both legs and the right arm, the report confirmed that the distal portions of these limbs were almost fully severed from their proximal parts. It described three deep wounds of the right arm. However, although it mentioned numerous other wounds including one of the left wrist, it did not mention any wound that nearly severed the distal part of the left arm. The principal murderer and his brother, as well as four members of Y.S.'s family who had seen the body, all agreed that all the limbs had been nearly cut off so that the distal parts remained dangling. Discounting the testimony of the principal murderer and his brother, who were themselves drunk when they killed Y.S., and that of one of Y.S.'s relatives (who may compliantly have agreed with his mother), there remain the concordant statements on this detail of three other members of Y.S.'s family whom I happened to interview independently of each other. It is possible that, when the pathologist described the left arm, he slipped and wrote "right" when he should have written "left." It is also possible that my informants, remembering events of 8 and a half years earlier and aware of S.P.'s birth defects, harmonized their memories to accord with the birth defects.

The principal murderer (S.P.'s father) and his brother (who had helped him) were arrested, tried, and sentenced to 3 years in prison. The prison permitted the murderer to have frequent day-long passes when he would visit his wife, and they were therefore able to continue having children.

Y.S.'s death sorely affected his mother, and she believed that the punishment imposed by the terrestrial court was insufficient retribution for

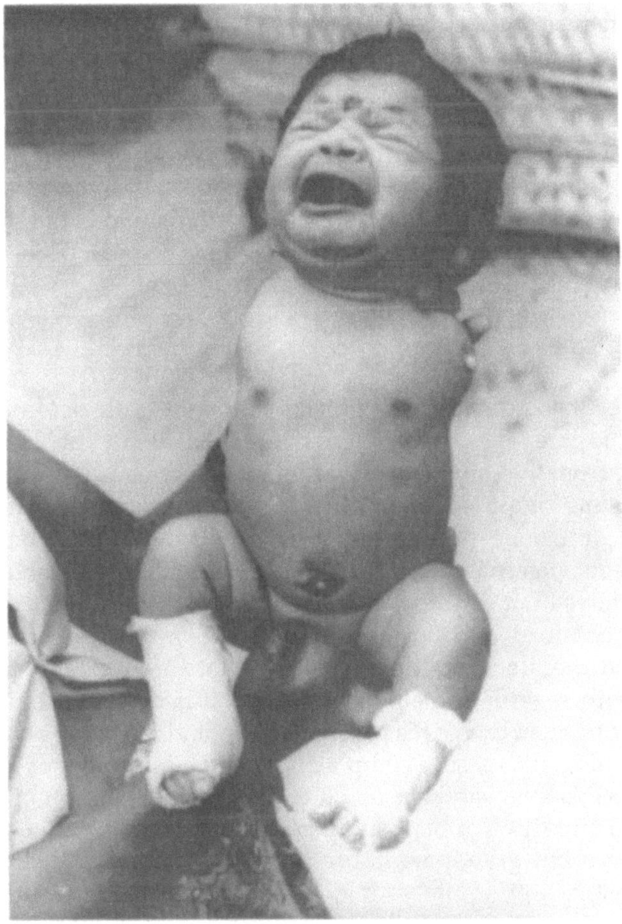

Figure 28.1. S.P. at the age of 4 months. There is complete absence of both upper limbs. Both feet have the defect known as talipes equinovarus and plaster casts have been applied with a view to correcting the deformities.

her son's murder. S.P.'s mother told me that Y.S.'s mother several times said to her publicly: "For killing my son, you will have a deformed child." (Even though the murderer's wife had not participated directly in the murder, the wrath of Y.S.'s mother fell on the entire family.) Y.S.'s sister corroborated to me that their mother had had the habit of cursing the murderer's family whenever she went by their house; but she did not recall the specific detail of her wishing the family to have a deformed child. Y.S.'s mother, whom I also interviewed, denied that she had made such a specific curse against the family. She said that she had merely called on the gods—Kataragama and Vishnu—to punish the murderer in some way. (I do not believe she would have admitted to me that she had cursed the mother, and I think that S.P.'s mother was speaking the truth about the nature of the curse.)

Both the murder itself and the subsequent curse troubled the murderer's wife. She recalled mentioning to her husband that Y.S. might be reborn as their son, and when she became pregnant she feared that her baby might be deformed. Then a daughter was born and was normal. The murderer's wife relaxed, thinking that the curse had somehow been neutralized. She and her husband were dismayed, therefore, but not entirely surprised, when her next pregnancy ended in the birth of the badly deformed male infant, S.P.

Excluding Known Causes of Birth Defects

None of the ordinarily recognized causes of birth defects are identified in this case. The parents were not related, at any rate closely; since they came from the same village they might have had some remote common ancestor. I inquired about other birth defects in the family and was told there were none. (The several members of the family whom I saw—S.P.'s parents, paternal uncle, and one sister—had no limb defects.) After my interviews I felt dissatisfied with the completeness of the family history I had obtained, and at my request Tissa Jayawardene returned to the village and inquired about every member of the two families of S.P.'s parents with regard to their having had birth defects. His informants were S.P.'s mother, one of his paternal aunts, and the latter's husband. He drew genealogies to assure completeness of the information. This survey included S.P.'s three siblings, all 20 of his cousins, all eight of his uncles and aunts, and three of his grandparents. Information could not be furnished about one grandparent, presumably because she had died when the informants were quite young. None of these persons suffered from any birth defect known to the informants. The only abnormality they recalled for any of these persons was "mental weakness" in one of S.P.'s cousins.

S.P.'s mother told me that she had enjoyed good health during her pregnancy with S.P., and that she had taken no drugs or alcohol. After my interview with S.P.'s mother, Godwin Samararatne (my senior assistant in Sri Lanka) had a further interview with her concerning the medical care she had received during her pregnancy with S.P. He learned the following details: When her pregnancy was at 5 months, she attended a clinic in a nearby town and was told her pregnancy was normal. She returned to the clinic at 6 months, was examined by the medical officer, and was again told the pregnancy was normal. She was given some tablets, probably vitamins. At the 8th month she again attended the clinic and was told the pregnancy was normal. She was examined this time by the head nurse, but not by the doctor, apparently because the pregnancy was still judged normal. Records of these visits were not obtainable, but we did obtain a copy of the record of S.P.'s delivery at a nearby hospital. The delivery was described as taking place normally at full term. The hospital report noted the absence of the upper limbs of the baby and talipes equinovarus of the feet. The baby was also noted to have a hydrocele.

DISCUSSION

I shall first describe the interpretations of this case favored by the informants and then offer my own opinion.

The idea that some events happen by chance is a Western notion and a relatively recent one (in its widespread acceptance) even in the West. The majority of men and women have believed, and the majority of them still believe, that we can find causes for everything that happens to us, as individuals, if only we seek well enough. Moreover, causes are, ultimately, due to the conduct or misconduct of persons. Accordingly, my informants considered that some personal factor had entered into the causation of the birth defects in S.P.

All the informants were Theravadin Buddhists and believed in reincarnation. (Their everyday religion is syncretistic, not pure Buddhism, and permits appeals during life's crises to Hindu gods, such as Visnu and Kataragama.) S.P.'s parents believed that S.P. was the murdered Y.S. reborn, with congenital deformities corresponding to the wounds on Y.S. On the other hand, Y.S.'s mother and older brother could not accept that Y.S.,who had, after all, been the victim in the murder, could be reborn as a deformed child. Why should he suffer, they reasoned, for another's crime? They believed that S.P.'s birth defects were a punishment of his parents for the crime of murdering Y.S.

Although most Sinhalese people believe in maternal impressions, none of my informants mentioned a maternal impression as a possible cause of the birth defects. S.P.'s mother had not viewed Y.S.'s dead body (although she must have heard the descriptions of the wounds); nor was she pregnant at the time of the murder. These features are usually present in "standard" cases of maternal impression, and their absence in this case may have led the informants to set this interpretation aside.

However, the members of Y.S.'s family who believed that S.P.'s birth defects punished his family for the murder must also have believed that the cursing (whatever specific words were used) had been successful. Sorcery is widely practiced in Sri Lanka and its efficacy generally believed in. In sorcery the complainant hires a priest to invoke the supernatural powers of gods in order to punish—with injury, illness, or death—a person who has seriously offended him. The act of sorcery is a kind of vicarious cursing. It appears to be much commoner than face-to-face cursing, because Obeyesekere (1975, p. 16) found that only 10% of surveyed clients at three Sri Lanka sorcery shrines had engaged in personal confrontation with their adversaries. Only 4% (included in the mentioned 10%) had engaged in physical or verbal abuse, which might, we could suppose, have included a direct cursing.

In offering my own opinion of the case I must first disclaim any intention to suggest that we can draw a firm conclusion from this single case. My only purpose in presenting it is to bring to readers' attention the possibility that images in a pregnant woman's mind may influence the form of her baby's body.

We now know a great deal more about the causes of birth defects, in medical terms, than was known 100 or even 50 years ago. Genetic factors, excessive alcohol and certain drugs taken by a pregnant woman, and some illnesses, especially rubella (German measles), occurring during pregnancy have all been clearly identified as factors in birth defects. Older maternal age also predisposes to the occurrence of some birth defects, particularly Down syndrome. All these factors should be considered and excluded before we entertain other possibilities. Having done that, however, we are entitled to consider other explanations. All the known causes of birth defects together explain only 30-35% of them (Wilson, 1973). There remain 65–70% in which physicians must acknowledge that they have no explanation. I believe that in Turner's case and in the one reported here we can exclude the known causes of birth defects. For these cases we can, therefore, consider other possible causative factors.

Although not excluding chance as firmly as my informants did, I believe that there was some causal connection between the wounds on Y.S. (which were highly unusual) and the birth defects of S.P. (which were also unusual[6] and corresponded with satisfactory closeness to Y.S.'s wounds).

Bodily changes that correspond to mental images may occur through psychosomatic processes as in cases of stigmatism (Thurston, 1952) and the reproduction of wounds during the revival of memories of traumatic experiences (Moody, 1946 [see Figure 7.1 earlier in this volume]). However, the placental connections between mother and embryo include no nervous pathways and permit the passage of few proteins from mother to embryo. It is therefore difficult to understand how the mother's thoughts could influence the embryo through normal processes.

A direct psychokinetic effect of the cursing woman on the embryo is theoretically possible, but lacks the support of a case parallel to the present one in which the mother did not know that her baby had been the object of a cursing. At least I do not know of any such case. Accordingly, in order to account for the correspondence between the curse and S.P.'s birth defects, I favor other paranormal explanations: a maternal impression and reincarnation.

S.P.'s mother was not pregnant at the time of Y.S.'s murder, and although she had probably not entirely forgotten the curse when she became pregnant with S.P., it seems to have sunk into the lower levels of her mind. It certainly did not preoccupy her in the manner usually described by women figuring in cases of maternal impressions. These considerations make me slightly favor the hypothesis that S.P. was Y.S. reborn. I need hardly add that, considered as an instance of reincarnation, the case is much weaker in evidence than the many cases in which the subject, when old enough to speak, made numerous verified statements about the previous life he then claimed to remember. S.P. died before he had begun to speak coherently, and we do not know whether he would have expressed any memories of a previous life if he had lived. I have investigated a few other cases (to be published) in which a birth defect was the only (or almost the only) item of evidence linking a subject with a particular deceased person.

If we seriously consider either maternal impression or reincarnation as an explanatory hypothesis for this case (and similar ones) we are bound to ask how images in the mind of one person (respectively, in this case, the pregnant mother-to-be or the murdered man) can influence the form of an embryo. This question leads to conjectures about an intermediate vehicle that somehow acts as a template for the communication of physical form from one body to another. I intend to discuss this possibility in the larger work from which I have extracted this case report. To do so here would carry me beyond my stated intention in presenting this case and also far beyond the warrant for such conjectures that a single case can provide.

NOTES

1. Reprinted from the *Journal of Scientific Exploration*, *3*, 201–212, 1989.—Ed.

2. A report of the case here presented will be included in a work now in progress that will describe a large number of cases suggestive of reincarnation the subjects of which had birthmarks and birth defects possibly deriving from previous lives they remembered (Stevenson, 1997). A much abbreviated report of the case has been published elsewhere (Stevenson, 1985). I am publishing the present report in the hope of stimulating discussion of this case (and similar other ones) and of their best interpretation.

3. Authors skeptical about maternal impressions sometimes state that William Hunter conducted a prospective study of pregnant women who claimed they had been frightened but who nevertheless gave birth to normal babies. Charles Darwin (1868) stated that Hunter described this study and its negative results to his father, Dr. Robert Darwin. However, such an investigation was never published and probably was never carried out. Two authorities on William Hunter whom I consulted knew nothing about it. It remains true, however, that Hunter inveighed against the belief in maternal impressions in his lectures (Hall, 1785).

4. In this case the husband (and father) did not aim his curse at the unborn baby as did the husband (and father) of the first case. However, one may suppose that both the women cursed had somewhat similar mental images after being cursed.

5. I asked this question with the hypothesis of reincarnation in mind and from my experience with children having severe birth defects that corresponded to fatal

wounds in a person whose life the child later remembered. As mentioned, full details of such cases will be published in a forthcoming book (Stevenson, 1997).

6. Birch-Jensen (1949) stated that the incidence of amelia of the upper arm at birth was 1 in about 270,000. Frantz and O'Rahilly (1961) found that among 13 cases of amelia of the upper arm, 7 (54%) were bilateral. Combining these data we can estimate that the incidence of bilateral amelia of the upper arm is about 1 in 500,000 births. The condition is so unusual that it is not even mentioned in the usual inventories of the incidences of common congenital deformities. (Amelia did occur more commonly during the brief epidemic of thalidomide intoxication, but that drug was not in question in the present case.)

REFERENCES

Barrow, M. V. (1971). A brief history of teratology to the early 20th century. *Teratology, 4*, 119–130.

Birch-Jensen, A. (1949). *Congenital Deformities of the Upper Extremities*. Copenhagen: Andelsbogtrykkeriet i Odense and Det Danske Forlag.

Burrell, R. J. W. (1963). The possible bearing of curse death and other factors in Bantu culture on the etiology of myocardial infarction. In T. N. James & J. W. Keyes (eds.), *The Etiology of Myocardial Infarction* (pp. 95–100). Boston: Little, Brown.

Dabney, W. C. (1890). Maternal impressions. In J. M. Keating (ed.), *Cyclopaedia of the Diseases of Children* (vol. 1, pp. 191–216). Philadelphia: J. B. Lippincott.

Darwin, C. (1868). *The Variation of Animals and Plants under Domestication* (2 vols.). New York: Orange Judd.

Frantz, C. H., & O'Rahilly, R. (1961). Congenital skeletal limb deficiencies. *Journal of Bone and Joint Surgery, 43-A*, 1202–1224.

Hall, C. (1785). *The Medical Family Instructor: Containing a Selection of Interesting Subjects, Calculated for the Information and Preservation of Mankind, Together with the Management of Child-bed Women, and Children*. Shrewsbury: T. Wood.

Kellie, G. (1808). Case of defect in the fingers. *Edinburgh Medical and Surgical Journal, 4*, 252–253.

Mackinder, D. (1857). Deficiency of fingers transmitted through six generations. *British Medical Journal, ii*, 845–846.

Mathis, J. L. (1964). A sophisticated version of voodoo death: Report of a case. *Psychosomatic Medicine, 26*, 104–107.

Montgomery, W. F. (1857). *An Exposition of the Signs and Symptoms of Pregnancy*. Philadelphia: Blanchard and Lea.

Moody, R. L. (1946). Bodily changes during abreaction. *Lancet, ii*, 934–935.

Obeyesekere, G. (1975). Sorcery, premeditated murder, and the canalization of aggression in Sri Lanka. *Ethnology, 14*, 1–23.

Raine, K. (1977). *The Lion's Mouth*. London: Hamish Hamilton.

Stevenson, I. (1974). *Twenty Cases Suggestive of Reincarnation* (2nd ed.). Charlottesville: University Press of Virginia. (First published in 1966)

Stevenson, I. (1985). Birth defects from cursing? A case report. *British Medical Journal, 290*, 1813.

Stevenson, I. (1992). A new look at maternal impressions: An analysis of 50 published cases and reports of two recent examples. *Journal of Scientific Exploration, 6*, 353–373.

Stevenson, I. (1993). Birthmarks and birth defects corresponding to wounds in deceased persons. *Journal of Scientific Exploration, 7*, 403–410.

Stevenson, I. (1997). *Reincarnation and Biology: A Contribution to Their Etiology*. (2 Vols.). New York: Praeger.

Thurston, H. (1952). *The Physical Phenomena of Mysticism*. London: Burns Oates.

Turner, E. K. (1960). Teratogenic effects on the human foetus through maternal emotional stress: Report of a case. *Medical Journal of Australia, 47*, 502–503.

Warkany, J. (1959). Congenital malformations in the past. *Journal of Chronic Diseases, 10,* 84–96.

Warkany, J. (1971). *Congenital Malformations: Notes and Comments*. Chicago: Year Book Medical Publishers.

Wilson, J. G. (1973). *Environment and Birth Defects*. New York: Academic Press.

4h

Possession

EWK

In addition to maternal impression, there is yet another possible explanation for some CORT that must be taken seriously. Many cultures have believed in some form of "possession," a situation in which a deceased person, or at least some aspect of a deceased person's mind, takes over either temporarily or permanently a living person's mind and body. Cases of "possession," particularly in the context of shamanistic rituals, are frequently reported in the anthropological literature. In the psychical research literature, one of the most well-investigated and famous cases is that of Lurancy Vennum, who temporarily took on the personality and exhibited memories of a recently deceased girl named Mary Roff (references to this case are given in the following paper). Cases of this type were of interest to Ian not only as an interpretation of CORT alternative to that of reincarnation but also because of their kinship to other phenomena involving extreme personality changes, namely, multiple personality and mediumship.[1]

Ian had early become aware of some cases in which the deceased person had died *after* the child's birth. In one, first reported in 1966 (Stevenson, 1966/1974, pp. 34–52), a three-year-old boy named Jasbir became quite ill and was thought to have died. When he recovered, he began to speak as if he were recalling the life of a man who had died during Jasbir's illness. The case of this type that I have reprinted in this section more closely resembles those of multiple personality, in that the subject was an adult, but with one notable exception: Unlike most alternate personalities, which seem to be fictitious creations of the patient, the alternate personality in this case was an actual person who had died at a time when, like Jasbir, the subject had been ill.

NOTE

1. In addition to the cases of mediumship that Ian published, he also published a case of multiple personality (Congdon, Hain, & Stevenson, 1961).

REFERENCES

Congdon, M. H., Hain, J., & Stevenson, I. (1961). A case of multiple personality illustrating the transition from role-playing. *Journal of Nervous & Mental Disease, 132,* 497–504.

Stevenson, I. (1974). *Twenty Cases Suggestive of Reincarnation* (2nd rev. ed.) Charlottesville: University Press of Virginia, 1974. (Original work published in 1966)

TWENTY-NINE

A Case of the Possession Type in India with Evidence of Paranormal Knowledge

1989[1]

A young married woman, Sumitra, in a village of northern India, apparently died and then revived. After a period of confusion she stated that she was one Shiva who had been murdered in another village. She gave enough details to permit verification of her statements, which corresponded to facts in the life of another young married woman called Shiva. Shiva had lived in a place about 100 km away, and she had died violently there—either by suicide or murder—about two months before Sumitra's apparent death and revival. Subsequently, Sumitra recognized 23 persons (in person or in photographs) known to Shiva. She also showed in several respects new behavior that accorded with Shiva's personality and attainments. For example, Shiva's family were Brahmins (high caste), whereas Sumitra's were Thakurs (second caste); after the change in her personality Sumitra showed Brahmin habits that were strange in her family. Extensive interviews with 53 informants satisfied the investigators that the families concerned had been, as they claimed, completely unknown to each other before the case developed and that Sumitra had had no normal knowledge of the people and events in Shiva's life. The authors conclude that the subject demonstrated knowledge of another person's life obtained paranormally.

The word *possession* designates a wide variety of conditions that psychiatrists, psychologists, and anthropologists describe. It indicates that a person has undergone such a marked change of behavior that other persons seem no longer to be in contact with the ordinary personality of the affected person.

Possession states occur widely in India (Carstairs & Kapur, 1976; Teja, Khanna, & Subrahmanyam, 1970).[2] Most psychiatrists, psychologists, and anthropologists have emphasized the similarities between cases of the possession type and diagnostic entities recognized in the West, such as multiple personality and hysteria. Accordingly, they tend to use phrases such as "possession syndrome" and "hysterical possession." They also, in varying degrees, offer motivational explanations of the condition that depict it as beneficial to the affected person in improving his status and perhaps resolving internal and external conflicts. However, Claus (1979) cautioned against psychological and sociological interpretations for *all* cases until we have more information. Along the same line, Lewis (1971, pp. 178–179) wrote: "Nothing after all is easier than leaping to conclusions and projecting our own psychological assumptions and interpretations onto exotic evidence which may correspond only in superficial detail with apparently similar data in our own culture."

The question arises of whether some ostensibly possessed persons show knowledge about the life of a deceased person that they could not have obtained normally. We think that in a small number of cases the subjects do show such knowledge. Cases of this kind are rare, and yet sufficiently well known in India so that the Hindi word *parakayapravesh* ("entering into another body") exists for designating them. One of us (I.S.) has studied several cases of the type with evidence of paranormal knowledge[3] and has published reports of two of them (Stevenson, 1966/1974, 1983a). Their occurrence and that of occasional other cases of ostensible possession with evidence of paranormal processes, such as the case of Uttara Huddar (in which the subject spoke a language she had not learned and assumed the personality of a deceased woman completely unknown to her family) (Stevenson & Pasricha, 1979 [reprinted in the next section]; Stevenson, 1984), have encouraged us to search for new cases of the possession type with evidence of paranormal processes.

Such evidence is not easily obtained. The ostensibly possessing personalities (when not gods or godlings) are usually persons known to the subject or about whom the subject may easily have learned normally. In cases of this type it is difficult to obtain satisfactory evidence of the subject's having knowledge paranormally acquired. We believe we have satisfied this criterion in the case we now report. It involves two completely unrelated and unacquainted persons. Their families lived in widely separated towns and villages, and the informants' testimony warrants believing that they had had no contact with each other before the case developed.

CASE REPORT

Summary of the Case and Its Investigation

When this case developed, the subject, Sumitra Singh, was a young married woman of about 17. She was living with her husband and their one child in her husband's family home (according to the custom in India) in the village of Sharifpura, in the Farrukhabad District of the State of Uttar Pradesh, India. Early in 1985 she began to develop episodes of loss of consciousness with eye-roll movements and clenching of the teeth. Sometimes she would speak during these trance-like states, and one day in July she predicted that she would die three days later. When the predicted day (July 19) came, she seemed to die. At least members of her family and other villagers considered her dead, because she was pulseless and apneic, and her face was drained of blood like that of a dead person. They had begun grieving and also preparing for Sumitra's funeral, when she unexpectedly revived.

Following a brief period of confusion Sumitra began to behave like a different person. She did not recognize the people around her and said that her name was Shiva and that she had been murdered by her in-laws at a place called Dibiyapur. She rejected Sumitra's husband and child and asked to be taken to Shiva's two children. She stated many details that were subsequently found to correspond with the life of another young married woman, Shiva Diwedi, who had died violently—whether from murder or suicide is still unclear—at Dibiyapur on the night of May 18–19, 1985, that is, two months before Sumitra's apparent death and revival. Shiva's parental family believed that her in-laws had murdered her and then attempted to simulate suicide by laying her body on railway tracks nearby. Her father, Ram Siya Tripathi, filed a complaint, and this instituted a judicial inquiry. Reports of Shiva's death and of the legal proceedings appeared in newspapers published in Etawah, the district town where Ram Siya Tripathi lived.

Sumitra's in-laws said that they knew nothing of a Shiva who had died at a place called Dibiyapur. At first they thought that Sumitra had gone mad and later that she had become possessed by a discarnate spirit; but they made no attempt to verify what she was saying. It was about a month before Ram Siya Tripathi learned about Sumitra's statements. This occurred, almost accidentally, when he heard a rumor, while he was visiting Dibiyapur, that his deceased daughter had taken possession of a girl in a distant village. Nearly two more months elapsed before he was able to verify this information by having someone from a village called Murra, which is close to Sharifpura, visit Sumitra and her family.

The information gathered corresponded to facts in the life of Ram Siya's deceased daughter, Shiva, and so on October 20, 1985, Ram Siya went himself (accompanied by a relative) to Sharifpura, where Sumitra recognized him and said she was his daughter. Sumitra also recognized in Sharifpura and Etawah (where she visited Ram Siya during the following days) at least 13 members of Shiva's family and circle of friends.

In addition to Sumitra's statements about the life of Shiva and her recognitions of persons Shiva had known, she showed a marked change in behavior. Sumitra's family belonged to the Thakur caste and they were villagers with almost no education; Sumitra herself had had no formal education, although she could read and write a little. The Tripathis, on the other hand, were Brahmins and middle-class urbanites. Ram Siya was a lecturer in a college, and Shiva had been educated up to the level of earning a B.A. degree. After her revival, Sumitra's behavior changed from that of a simple village girl to that of a moderately well-educated woman of higher caste and more urban manners, who could now read and write Hindi fluently.

The case came to our attention soon after the first exchanges of visits between the families concerned. The *Indian Express* published a report of the case on October 26, 1985. One of I.S.'s correspondents in India noticed this and sent a copy of the report to him. At about the same time a correspondent in northern India sent to S.P. a copy of a report of the case in a Hindi newspaper, *Dainik Jagran,* that had appeared on October 23, 1985.

Methods of Investigation

Our principal method of investigation was interviews with informants, particularly firsthand witnesses of the apparent death of Sumitra and the change in her personality that followed her revival; but we spent almost as much time interviewing the members of Shiva's family.

We were able to begin our interviews within three weeks of learning about the case. In November 1985, S.P. conducted a series of interviews with some of the principal informants for it. These included Sumitra and her mother-in-law, Shiva's parents, and one of Shiva's maternal uncles.

In February and March 1986, we worked together on the case for seven days. We interviewed again all but one of the persons S.P. had interviewed earlier. In addition, we interviewed numerous other informants for the case, especially in Sumitra's village of Sharifpura. We met her father in his village, Angad ka Nagla. We had to seek out other informants in four other towns and villages of the Farrukhabad District and the neighboring districts of Etawah, Mainpuri, and Hardoi.

In November 1986, February 1987, and October 1987 two of us (I.S. and S.P.) spent another 10 days on fieldwork for the case. During these three periods we interviewed (in Dibiyapur) Shiva's husband and father-in-law, whom we had not met earlier. We also interviewed informants who had connections through marriage or trade with more than one of the communities involved in the case; we intended these interviews to help us to assess the likelihood that information about Shiva's life and death could have reached Sumitra's family along normal lines of communication. We also, during this later phase of the investigation, had new interviews with some previous informants, including Sumitra and her husband and Shiva's parents.

By the end of our investigation in October 1987 we had interviewed 24 members of Sumitra's and Shiva's families, and we had interviewed all the more important witnesses among these persons two or more times. In addition, we had interviewed another 29 persons who were able to furnish background information, especially that mentioned above concerning communications between the communities involved in the case.

During the interviews S.P. made notes, mostly in Hindi, and also acted as principal interpreter for I.S. and N.McC-R., both of whom made notes in English, as nearly verbatim as possible. During a few special interviews we made tape recordings only, or in addition to making notes.

In our interviews we gave particular attention to the following aspects of the case: the preceding illness, apparent death, and revival of Sumitra; the possibilities for normal communication of information about Shiva's life and death to Sumitra and her family; and the circumstances under which Sumitra, after her revival, identified Shiva's family in person and in photographs.

In addition to our interviews we obtained copies of newspaper reports (published in Etawah) of Shiva's death and of Ram Siya Tripathi's allegations that her in-laws had murdered her. We also obtained copies of the photographs of Shiva's family in which Sumitra had correctly identified persons normally unknown to her before the change in her personality.

One of us (I.S.) has published elsewhere further details of the methods followed (Stevenson, 1966/1974, 1975).

Relevant Facts of Geography and Possibilities for Normal Communication between the Families Concerned

This case occurred in the Farrukhabad and Etawah Districts of the State of Uttar Pradesh. Etawah is a small city of about 100,000 inhabitants located approximately 500 km southeast of Delhi. It is a district town on the main line of the railway that joins Delhi to Kanpur (about 250 km east of Etawah) and, ultimately, to Calcutta. Shiva's parents lived in Etawah from the time she was three years old until the case developed.

After her marriage Shiva moved to the home of her in-laws at Dibiyapur, which is about 55 km east of Etawah. Almost adjoining Dibiyapur is the railway station of Phaphoond, which is on the main railway line linking Etawah and Kanpur.

Sharifpura, the village where Sumitra was living when the case developed, is just outside the Etawah District in the Farrukhabad District, about 65 km north of Etawah and about 100 km (in a direct line) from

Dibiyapur. Some of Sumitra's in-laws lived in the town of Sikandarpur, which is about 30 km farther north and west from Sharifpura, in the Farrukhabad District.

Angad ka Nagla, where Sumitra's father lived, is about 15 km east of Sharifpura and perhaps slightly south.

Informants for Sumitra's side of the case said that they had no previous acquaintance with Shiva's family, and members of Shiva's family similarly said they were completely ignorant of Sumitra's family before the case developed. Apart from the long (for India) geographical distances between the families, they were further separated by significant differences of caste, education, and economic position.

Strong support for the informants' denial of prior acquaintance (or knowledge about each other) comes from the slow and roundabout manner in which Shiva's family learned about the personality change in Sumitra. Sumitra's father and her in-laws made no attempt to verify her statements about Shiva. Word about them first reached the neighboring village of Murra, which is 2 km from Sharifpura. From there it traveled to Dibiyapur apparently conveyed by women of Murra who had married and were living there. Ram Siya Tripathi, on a visit to Dibiyapur, heard a rumor that his dead daughter had taken possession of a girl in a distant village called Sharifpura. However, he had never been to Sharifpura and did not even know where it was located. After another two weeks he learned about a man called Ram Prakash Dube, a native of Murra who was living in Etawah, but whom he had not previously known. He asked Ram Prakash Dube to inquire in Murra about the truth of the account he had heard in Dibiyapur. The monsoon rains led to further delays. When Ram Prakash Dube next visited Murra, he looked into the story and confirmed its main outlines to Ram Siya Tripathi, who, as we have mentioned, then went to Sharifpura and had his first meeting with Sumitra on October 20, 1985. This was exactly three months after Sumitra's apparent death and revival. We believe that if the families concerned had been previously acquainted or had had any lines of communication through mutual acquaintances, they would have exchanged information about Sumitra's change of personality much sooner than they did.

If Ram Siya Tripathi had not complained to the police about the unseemly haste with which his daughter's body had been cremated (as we shall describe below), few persons outside those immediately concerned would have heard about her death. However, when the police began to investigate the matter, the newspapers of Etawah took notice and published accounts of Shiva's death and of the judicial inquiry. Some of the newspapers carrying these reports reached Sikandarpur, where persons who might have come in contact with the family of Sumitra's mother-in-law read them. At least one newspaper with a report also reached a reader of Sharifpura. The brother of the headman of Sharifpura said that he had read about Shiva's death in a newspaper before the change in

Sumitra; but he gave the matter little attention at the time. The headman himself, a schoolteacher, said that he learned about Shiva's death only after Sumitra's changeover. In addition, we learned of two traders who went regularly between Sharifpura and Etawah on business. After the case developed one of them became acquainted with Ram Siya Tripathi, but had not known him earlier.

Members of Sumitra's family said that they had heard nothing about Shiva's death before Sumitra's death, revival, and personality change. However, in view of the circulation of some newspapers in their area, and of some trading between Sharifpura and Etawah, it is best to assume that they might have learned of Shiva's death and perhaps also learned about some of the allegations of suicide and homicide that figured in the newspaper reports. (There was no radio station in the area. Some television had been introduced at Etawah only [Sharifpura had no electricity], but it only relayed programs from Delhi and broadcast no local news.) The newspaper reports included some of the names of Shiva's parental family and in-laws. The important question remaining is, therefore, whether Sumitra, after the change in her personality, demonstrated knowledge and behavior corresponding to Shiva's life that went beyond the information available in the newspapers reporting the death of Shiva and the related judicial inquiry.

The Life, Last Illness, Apparent Death, and Revival of Sumitra

Sumitra was born in (probably) 1968[4] in Ahmedabad, Gujarat, where her father, Chotte Singh, had gone for employment in one of the many textile mills there. He was a native of Angad ka Nagla, a village of the Etawah District. He and other members of his family belonged to the Thakur caste.

Sumitra's early life was unusual in the degree to which she lived separated from one or both of her parents. The separations reflected her father's efforts to break out of the life of a village cultivator and become a steady wage-earner.

Because of her parents' movements Sumitra lived for about eight years with an older cousin, Phool Mala, in the village of Birpur, in the neighboring district of Mainpuri. Sumitra never attended school, but Phool Mala taught her the elements of reading and writing. Phool Mala herself had gone to a primary school only for a year or two, and she had mainly learned to read and write at home. She taught Sumitra as much as she knew. She said that Sumitra could read the *Ramayana* and was able to write a letter. Sumitra's father told us (incorrectly) that she could not write at all, and her husband said that she could write "a very little like a child in kindergarten." He thought that she was (when he knew her) unable to write a letter, but we learned that she had occasionally done this.

Sumitra's mother, Ganga Devi, died in 1979, when Sumitra was about 11.

In childhood Sumitra enjoyed good physical health. When she was about 13 (in 1981), she was married (in the Indian style of arranged marriages) to Jagdish Singh and moved to her husband's village of Sharifpura, which is about 15 km from Angad ka Nagla, where her father was then living. Sumitra's marriage to a considerable extent repeated the pattern of separations that she had experienced in childhood, because her husband, like her father, went to a city (in his case, Delhi) trying to obtain regular employment, and he was often away from Sharifpura for months at a time. After three years of marriage, Sumitra gave birth to a baby boy in December, 1984. A month or two later, early in 1985, she began to suffer from periods of loss of consciousness or trance in which her eyes would roll upwards and she would clench her teeth. She seemed not to have fallen suddenly in any of these episodes. The spells lasted varying times—from a few minutes to a whole day. Sometimes Sumitra would say afterward that Santoshi Ma[5] had possessed her. On two occasions she was seemingly possessed briefly by discarnate personalities. One of these communicating personalities said that she had been a woman of Sharifpura who had drowned herself in a well; the other (a male) said that he had been a man of another state in India. She gave some particulars about this latter life that have not been verified and are probably unverifiable.

During these episodes of apparent possession, Sumitra's condition sufficiently troubled her family so that they consulted local healers. Of these the most prominent was a man called Vishwa Nath. He was a distant relative of the family, a cultivator regularly, and without experience in other cases like Sumitra's. Nevertheless, he seemed to have a pacifying influence on her. He himself at times went into trances when he would be possessed, as he would say afterward, by the Hindu god Hanuman.

Vishwa Nath's intervention did not arrest Sumitra's episodes of trance; and, as we described earlier, she predicted her death, and three days later (on July 19, 1985) she lost consciousness and seemed to die. We questioned several eyewitnesses of this event. Her respiration and pulse stopped and her face became drained of blood like that of a dead person. A considerable group of persons surrounding Sumitra were convinced that she had died, and some began to cry. It was proposed to put her body on the ground (a Hindu ritual performed for persons who are thought about to die or who have died). Sumitra seemed to be dead for a period estimated by her father-in-law and brother-in-law as about five minutes. Some other informants thought that she had been dead for much longer than five minutes before she revived, but we think they may have estimated the onset of death from a time when her breathing became shallow and barely perceptible. No doctor was in or near the village, so Sumitra's heart was not auscultated, and we have reported the villagers' judgment that Sumitra was dead without asserting ourselves that she was.

When Sumitra revived she did not recognize her surroundings including the people of her husband's family. She said little or nothing for a day after her revival. Then she began to say that she was Shiva and to describe details of the life and death of Shiva. We shall summarize her statements about Shiva's life in a later section of this report, after we describe what we could learn about Shiva's death.

Upon hearing Sumitra's statements about Shiva's life and death, her in-laws thought first that she had gone mad and then that she had become possessed by a wandering discarnate personality who could be exorcised away or might leave spontaneously as had the ones previously manifesting in Sumitra.

In the autumn of 1986 Sumitra became confused for a few hours and seemed to resume her ordinary personality. Then the Shiva personality resumed control and was still dominant at the time of our last interviews in October 1987. By this time the Shiva personality had been dominant—with the single brief exception just noted—for more than two years.

The Life and Death of Shiva

Shiva Tripathi was born in Sevpur in the Etawah District on October 24, 1962. Her parents were members of the Brahmin caste and her father, Ram Siya Tripathi, was a lecturer in a college. After 1965 the family lived in Etawah, and Shiva grew up there along with five brothers and sisters. She attended school and then college from which she graduated with a B.A. in Home Economics.

At the age of 18 and a half she was married to a man called Chhedi Lal, who lived in the village or small town of Dibiyapur.

Shiva gave birth to two children who became known by the nicknames of Tinku and Rinku. (Tinku was about 18 months old and Rinku less than 6 months old when Shiva died.) Shiva was living (according to the custom of joint households in India) in her in-laws' house. Friction developed between Shiva and her in-laws. It is possible that Shiva's superior education and more urban manners irritated her in-laws. They grumbled when Shiva returned to Etawah in order to write final examinations for her college degree. Shiva complained that her mother-in-law had told her to go and hang herself. At one stage her father-in-law wrote to Shiva's father and suggested that he take her back, but nothing came of this.

A more serious quarrel developed in the second half of May 1985. Shiva was invited to attend the wedding of a member of her family, and her in-laws, after at first agreeing to her absence for this function, changed their minds and forbade her to leave the house. On the evening of May 18, 1985 Shiva's maternal uncle by marriage, Brijesh Pathak, who lived in a village (Kainjari) about a kilometer from Dibiyapur, called on the family and learned from Shiva about the quarrel she had had with her in-laws. Shiva was crying and told him that her mother-in-law and one of her sisters-in-law had beaten her. She did not seem depressed, and she did not talk of suicide. Her uncle tried to calm the family members and advised them to ask Shiva's father to come and arrange a more durable peace.

The next morning Brijesh Pathak and his brothers learned that Shiva had died in an "accident." Her dead body had been found on the railway tracks, and her in-laws said that she had thrown herself in front of a train. We interviewed five persons who saw Shiva's body on the morning of May 19 before it was cremated. When discovered, it lay between two rails of a track at the railway station of Phaphoond (which adjoins Dibiyapur). The body was intact and therefore had not been run over by the wheels of a train; several trains had passed the station during the night.

Brijesh Pathak, remembering the quarrel between Shiva and her in-laws of the night before, asked them to delay cremation of the body until he could go to Etawah and bring Shiva's father (which would take only four hours, because the railway stations of Dibiyapur and Etawah are both on the main railway line). However, Shiva's in-laws ignored his pleas, obtained permission from local authorities to cremate her body,[6] and lit the fire at about 11:00 a.m. To make it burn more quickly they had poured fuel oil on the wood.

Shiva's in-laws said that they had noticed her unexpected absence from the house and had gone in search of her. Her body had been found on the railway tracks at the railway station, and they concluded that she had thrown herself in front of a train. They presented this account of Shiva's death during judicial inquiries and also in our interviews with them.

Although it is not uncommon for young married women in India who are harassed by their in-laws to commit suicide, several circumstances in the death of Shiva pointed away from suicide and raised a suspicion of murder. First, there was the history of the quarrel on the evening of May 18, when Shiva had told her uncle that her in-laws had been beating her. Second, rumors began to circulate in Dibiyapur about persons having seen Shiva's in-laws carrying her during the night to the railway station at Phaphoond (just a few hundred meters from their home). They were said to have explained that they were taking her to the hospital. Although there were people around the railway station, it was night, and at one point the lights in the station failed; it would then have been dark, so that a dead body might have been placed on the tracks unobserved. (Firsthand confirmation of this report would have been of critical importance, but we were unable to learn even the name of a firsthand informant.) Third, Brijesh Pathak, who saw his niece's body lying on the platform of the railway station before it was taken away by her in-laws, remarked that only the head was injured; he thought it suspicious that a body knocked down by a train was not more extensively damaged.[7] Fourth, although it is customary to have an inquest and autopsy after any accidental death, the *panchnama* was signed with suspicious haste, the expressed wishes of Shiva's uncle to delay the cremation until her father could arrive were ignored, and the cremation proceeded with hurriedly.

Ram Siya Tripathi arrived at Dibiyapur around 2:00 in the afternoon of May 19. By that time the cremation fire had reduced his daughter's body to ashes. After considering all that he could learn about the circumstances of her death, he complained to the police, and they began a belated inquiry. Later, he filed a formal charge of murder against Shiva's in-laws. Shiva's husband and father-in-law were arrested and then released for lack of evidence. Her mother-in-law and sister-in-law absconded and remained in hiding for some months. In 1986 they returned to their home, were arrested, and then released pending an expected trial. In October 1987 the judicial inquiry was continuing with the usual delays of such proceedings.

On the facts available to us, we must suspend judgment about how Shiva died. That she died violently and after a quarrel with her in-laws on the night of May 18-19, 1985 is established. Her in-laws may have killed her and put her body on the railway tracks to simulate a suicide; or she may have thrown herself in front of a train during a trough of depression following the quarrel with her in-laws.

Sumitra's Statements about the Life and Death of Shiva

Sumitra's statements made after her revival may be divided into three groups. The first group consists of names of persons and places that the newspaper accounts of Shiva's death and her father's lawsuit had published. We think it extremely unlikely that anyone communicated even the fact of Shiva's death, to say nothing of its details, to Sumitra or her family. However, as we have mentioned, some newspapers were circulated in the general area of Sharifpura, and so we must assume that Sumitra's family might have learned about Shiva's death normally. This means we cannot count as paranormally derived any of the names Sumitra stated that had appeared in newspaper accounts.

A second group of Sumitra's statements remains unverified. We refer to her account of Shiva's final quarrel with her in-laws and of how her sister-in-law had hit her on the head with a brick, after which her body was laid on the tracks at the railway station to simulate suicide. Nothing refutes these statements, but they remain unverified and may be wrong.

A third group of statements, those concerned with nicknames and private affairs not published in the newspapers, includes statements that we think contain information Sumitra could not have obtained normally. We learned of 19 items that we felt justified in placing in this, the most important group. These showed that Sumitra had knowledge of: a particular yellow sari that Shiva had owned, a watch that had belonged to Shiva and the box (in the Tripathi home) in which it was kept, the respective order of birth of Shiva's maternal uncles (although one who was younger actually looked older than one of the older uncles), one of Shiva's nicknames familiarly used in the home (Shiv Shanker), the names of two educational institutions where Shiva had studied (Sarvodya College and Sorawal Intermediate College), the pet names of Shiva's two children (Rinku and Tinku), the names of two friends of Shiva who happened to have the same name, and the names of Shiva's two brothers, two of her sisters, two of her maternal uncles, a maternal aunt (by marriage), and a nephew.

Sumitra's Recognitions of Shiva's Family Members and Friends

Observers of recognitions in cases suggestive of reincarnation—of which the present case may be considered a variant—frequently vitiate them by asking leading questions or by cueing the subject with glances directed toward the person to be recognized (Stevenson, 1975, pp. 39-40). Nevertheless, there remain several circumstances in which recognitions may occur that deserve credit as showing paranormal knowledge on the part of the subject. These are: recognitions that the subject makes spontaneously without anyone's having asked him or her to identify another person[8]; recognitions that occur when the subject is confronted with a person and asked a question like: "Do you know who this person is?" or "Tell me who I am"; and recognitions in which the subject immediately afterward adds a statement about some intimate detail, perhaps a nickname, not known outside a small circle of family and friends. We learned of 12 members of Shiva's family and circle of friends whom Sumitra recognized under conditions that we believe excluded cueing. We shall describe the circumstances of seven of Sumitra's recognitions, including one in which cueing might have played a part and six in which we think it did not.

1. Ram Siya Tripathi, Shiva's father. When he first went to Sharifpura, he introduced himself outside the house and someone told Sumitra, who was then inside, that "her father" (that is, Shiva's) had come to the house. We therefore attach no significance to Sumitra's telling Ram Siya Tripathi what his name was. However, she called him "Papa" (as Shiva had) and wept. Also, when Ram Siya Tripathi asked her, Sumitra immediately stated two pet names by which Shiva was sometimes called in her family: Aruna and Shiv Shanker. The first of these names, Aruna, had been published in a newspaper report of Shiva's death, but the second had not.

2. Baleshwar Prasad Chaturvedi, Shiva's maternal uncle by marriage. Sumitra recognized him at the time he accompanied Ram Siya Tripathi to Sharifpura. Asked who he was, Sumitra at first said he was Arvind's father. (Arvind was one of Shiva's maternal uncles.) Asked to try again, Sumitra then said that Baleshwar Prasad Chaturvedi was the father of Arvind's wife. This was correct.

3. Ram Rani, Shiva's mother. This recognition occurred at the time of Sumitra's first visit to Etawah. Ram Siya tried to mislead Sumitra by telling her that her (Shiva's) mother was standing in a group of other women at the Tripathi house. In fact, Ram Rani had gone inside the house and was not in this group of women. Sumitra insisted that her (that is, Shiva's) mother was not among the group of other women; she then went into the house and searched for Shiva's mother whom she found and embraced tearfully. (Attempts were also made in another instance to mislead Sumitra deliberately, but failed.) In connection with this recognition we should note that Ram Siya Tripathi had already shown Sumitra a photograph of Ram Rani (see below).

4. Ram Naresh, another of Shiva's maternal uncles. This recognition occurred at the time of Sumitra's first visit to Etawah. Ram Naresh presented himself to Sumitra and said: "Who am I?" Sumitra said: "You are my mother's brother." He said: "Which one?" She replied: "Ram Naresh of Kanpur." He had formerly lived in Kanpur, and had moved to Etawah after Shiva's death.

5. Ram Prakash Dixit, another of Shiva's maternal uncles. He went to Sharifpura (at the end of October, less than 10 days after Ram Siya Tripathi had first met Sumitra). He had grown a beard, which Shiva had never seen. When Sumitra first saw him, he was sitting in front of her and remained silent. She recognized him as Shiva's mother's brother, but was at first unable to give his name. He then spoke a few words, and she immediately recognized his voice and stated his name.

6. Manish, Shiva's nephew (the son of her sister Uma). This recognition occurred in Etawah on November 22, 1985. Sumitra was at the Tripathi house on an upstairs terrace. One of Shiva's brothers, noticing Uma and Manish approaching, drew Sumitra's attention to them. Sumitra looked down and said "Manish has come." Sumitra went down from the terrace, hugged Uma, and called her "sister." However, this cannot count as a flawless recognition, because Ram Siya Tripathi had already shown Sumitra a photograph of Uma (see below).

7. Krishna Devi Dube, a friend of Shiva's youth. This recognition occurred at Sikandarpur when Sumitra visited her mother-in-law's family,

in February 1986. More than eight years earlier, Krishna Devi and Shiva had known each other when Shiva used to visit one of her maternal uncles (Brijesh Pathak) in the village of Kainjari, Krishna Devi's native place. When Krishna Devi married, she moved to Sikandarpur and had not met Shiva for more than eight years prior to Shiva's death. When Sumitra saw Krishna Devi, she said: "Jiji! How come you are here? I died and have come into a Thakur's family and am helpless." Shiva would have known normally that Krishna Devi had married and moved to Sikandarpur; nevertheless, the Shiva personality of Sumitra—if we may use that expression here—seemed surprised to meet Krishna Devi in Sikandarpur. Shiva, when alive, had called Krishna Devi "Jiji." This word means "sister," and although Shiva and Krishna Devi were not real sisters, close female friends in India may use this form of address with each other.

In addition to the above mentioned and other recognitions of living persons, Sumitra was able to recognize 15 members of Shiva's family in photographs. When Ram Siya Tripathi first met Sumitra in Sharifpura, he showed her eight photographs in an album that he had brought. One was of his wife and children that was taken in 1967, that is, about 18 years earlier. Sumitra correctly identified all six persons in the photograph: Ram Siya Tripathi, his wife, his mother, his daughter Uma, his son Raman, and his daughter Shiva. Of the last, Sumitra said: "This is me." Shown another photograph, this one of five of the Tripathi children, Sumitra correctly identified and named all the persons in the photograph. (Some of these persons figured in the previous photograph and in others shown to Sumitra.)

Another photograph showed three adult women, two of them holding infants. Sumitra identified Shiva's mother in it and said the child on her lap was Shiva's brother Raman. She then said that one of the other women was a maternal aunt. She said the third woman was possibly another aunt, but she was unsure of this, and she could not recognize the child on this woman's lap.

Upon seeing a photograph of Shiva's young son Tinku, Sumitra began to cry, said the photograph was of Tinku, and asked where Tinku and Rinku then were.

When a photograph of Shiva's sister-in-law Rama Kanti was shown to Sumitra, she said: "This is Rama Kanti who hit me with a brick." (Ram Siya Tripathi said Sumitra's recognition of this photograph dispelled his remaining doubts about whether his daughter Shiva was possessing her.)

In showing the photographs to Sumitra, Ram Siya Tripathi's attitude appears to have been one of keen interest mixed with skepticism. He said that as he showed Sumitra the photographs in the album, he asked her to identify the persons in them and gave her no cues. She gave the name of each person and usually the relationship of the person to Shiva. The villager, Lal Man Dube, who escorted Ram Siya Tripathi and his relative Baleshwar Prasad Chaturvedi to the house of Sumitra's in-laws in Sharifpura, witnessed Sumitra's recognitions of the photographs as Ram Siya Tripathi showed them to her. He confirmed that her recognizing statements about them were entirely spontaneous and not cued by any remarks the visitors made. We have described only a portion of the photographs she recognized, and we have examined the photographs ourselves. Excluding repetitions—of the same person appearing in more than one of the photographs—Sumitra was asked to identify 17 persons in the photographs. She unhesitatingly identified 12 of them, identified another three after some hesitation, and failed to recognize two persons.

Ram Siya Tripathi showed the album of photographs to Sumitra when he first met her on October 20, 1985. Although he did not give her cues before she recognized each photograph, he did tell her after she had finished that she had recognized all the people in them correctly. We think it likely also that he communicated to her, if only nonverbally, that she was correct after her statements about each photograph, if not about each person in a photograph. Under these circumstances, Sumitra had some advantage in recognizing persons she met later in Etawah whose faces she had already seen in the photographs. (We have referred to two of these persons above, Shiva's mother and sister.) However, Sumitra was credited with recognizing and identifying (usually by name) eight members of the family or their circle of friends whose photographs she had not seen.

Some of the newspaper accounts of the death of Shiva and of the subsequent judicial inquiry included photographs of Shiva, but these were taken in 1979. The photographs of her as a child (which Sumitra recognized) and the photographs of other members of the Tripathi family had not been published.

In sum, Sumitra recognized 23 members of Shiva's family and acquaintances either in person or in photographs, some of them in both ways.

Sumitra's Failure to Recognize People and Places Familiar to Her

After her revival from apparent death Sumitra could not recognize the people around her in Sharifpura, such as her husband and her in-laws; they all seemed complete strangers to her. Similarly, when her father came from Angad ka Nagla to see her, she did not recognize him. Ordinarily, she would have greeted him and called him "Father," but instead she said of him: "I do not know him." She was persuaded to go to Angad ka Nagla, and somewhat reluctantly agreed to do so. She said that she had no connections there and no interest in the place. In the village she recognized no one and seemed not to recognize any of the places with which Sumitra would have been familiar.

Similarly, when Phool Mala, Sumitra's older cousin who had in effect raised her from the age of five, went to see her in Sharifpura, she did not recognize her; nor did she recognize Phool Mala's husband, Risal Singh.

Sumitra, after her revival, showed no interest in her husband and child. She refused her husband's amatory advances for some time and did not acknowledge that her child was hers. Instead, she asked about Shiva's two children. Over a period of some days and weeks, she gradually came to accept her husband and son and to respond appropriately to them. Of her child she said (while still insisting that she was Shiva, not Sumitra): "If I look after this child [meaning Sumitra's son] God will take care of them [meaning Shiva's children]. If I neglect this child, would God not punish me?"

Under this heading we may mention also Sumitra's disorientation for place. For example, when her mother-in-law took her out to the fields for natural functions—the usual site for these in Indian villages—she seemed nonplussed and asked what they were doing in the fields. When her mother-in-law explained, she said: "We have a latrine inside the house [meaning in Etawah and Dibiyapur]." This was correct for both the house of Shiva's parents and that of her in-laws.

Sumitra's Changed Behavior after Reviving

We have already described Sumitra's initial failure (after her revival) to recognize the people around her in Sharifpura, and how, after neglecting her husband and child, she gradually resumed more or less normal relations with them. However, she said that her son was Jagdish Singh's child from his first marriage. Her attitude toward members of the family of her in-laws was that they were good people and, as she was thrust among them, she would be as gracious about the necessary adjustment as she could be. Nevertheless, there remained important differences in her behavior compared with that before her apparent death and revival. We shall now describe some of these changed behaviors.

Sumitra's Different Identification of Herself and Modes of Addressing Other Persons

Sumitra obstinately insisted that she was Shiva and sometimes would not respond or carry out a request unless she was called Shiva. She addressed her husband, Jagdish Singh, as "Thakur Sahib," showing respect, but distance. Previously she had called him (with the indirection Indian wives commonly use) "Guddi's brother." (Guddi was Jagdish's sister.) Formerly Sumitra had called her father-in-law by a Hindi word "chacha," meaning an uncle; now she called him "Father." Formerly she had called her mother-in-law by a word, "Amma," for mother; now she addressed her by another, more respectful word for mother, "Mataji."

In the month following Sumitra's apparent death and revival, a particularly poignant episode occurred. At that season (August) it is customary in northern India for women to show their loyalty to their brothers by tying a short length of string around a brother's wrist. This is known as the *rakhi* ceremony, and Hindus attach great importance to it. When Sumitra's brother came to Sharifpura and asked her to return with him to Angad ka Nagla for the rakhi ceremony, she refused saying she knew no one at Angad ka Nagla. The brother began weeping and begged her to tie the rakhi string on him. She still refused and began to weep herself saying that she had no brothers near her to whom she could tie the rakhi string. (We have our account of this episode only from Sumitra and have not learned about it from Sumitra's family.)

Different Style of Dress

Sumitra changed her style of dress. She wore her sari in a different manner and put on sandals, which Sumitra, like most village women, had rarely worn. Her new habits of dressing accorded with Shiva's style.

Caste Snobbery

After her revival Sumitra showed, for a time, a definite hauteur toward her in-laws, the Singhs. Thinking of herself as Shiva, a Brahmin, she regarded them, Thakurs, as inferior.

On the occasion of Sumitra's first journey to Etawah with Shiva's father, Ram Siya Tripathi, and her husband, Jagdish Singh, the group stopped at the home of Baleshwar Prasad Chaturvedi in the village of Umrain. After they had eaten a meal, Sumitra told Jagdish Singh: "Please wash the plates and utensils you used. You are a Thakur and they are Brahmins. It does not matter for me [meaning about her plates and utensils], because I am one of them."

Sumitra's Increased Literacy

Sumitra could read a little, and she was able to write letters and occasionally did so. However, the testimony of informants was concordant that she had never attended school and had attained only a very limited knowledge of reading and writing. After her revival she showed a marked improvement in her ability to read and write. We observed her in both of these activities and found her able to read and write Hindi with great facility. However, we wish to emphasize that the significant change in Sumitra's literacy was not in her basic ability to read and write but in her fluency in these activities and in her interest in writing. Whereas formerly she only wrote a letter occasionally, after the change in her personality she wrote letters and postcards often to Shiva's family in Etawah.

Other Unusual Behavior

Ram Siya Tripathi said that he noticed in Sumitra some behavior that he regarded as characteristic of Shiva, such as a certain boldness and a tendency to joke. Her husband said that Sumitra, before her apparent death and revival, would usually get up at about 6:00 a.m.; after her death and revival she got up much earlier, at about 4:00 a.m. Shiva had been an early riser; her father said that she used to get up at 5:00 to 5:30 a.m. and even earlier in the summers. One of her uncles commented to us that Shiva used to go to bed earlier and get up earlier than other members of the family. However, we recognize that traits such as we have mentioned in this section are difficult to appraise, and we think they are less important than the others we have mentioned.

DISCUSSION

We propose to discuss what we believe are the four principal interpretations of the case: fraud; cryptomnesia (source amnesia) with secondary personality; secondary personality having paranormal knowledge; and possession of Sumitra's body by the deceased Shiva.

Fraud

We think we can exclude a hoax perpetrated by Sumitra alone. A barely literate village woman in India could not have obtained detailed accurate information about another woman who lived 100 km away without assistance. If there was a hoaxing team, who composed it? Sumitra's husband, as a man, could move around more easily than Sumitra, but he was not in a position to go to places like Dibiyapur and Etawah in order to search out unpublished details about the life of Shiva. It has been suggested that the exorcist Vishwa Nath, who had access to Sumitra (although probably never alone) before and after her apparent death and recovery, might have obtained information about Shiva and coached Sumitra with the details of which he had knowledge. However, this suggestion also, in our view, fails to take account of the information Sumitra had of the private life of the Tripathi family, and it fails to explain her ability to recognize 23 strange persons in person or in photographs.

Shiva's in-laws at Dibiyapur had all the information included in Sumitra's statements about Shiva's life and death, but they were already incriminated in Shiva's death and had an interest, therefore, in Sumitra's silence. Sumitra's "Shiva personality" was saying publicly that Shiva's in-laws had murdered her, and the in-laws could not be suspected of promoting this view of Shiva's death.

Shiva's parental family also had the information included in Sumitra's statements. Ram Siya Tripathi might have collaborated in a hoax. In talking with us, he himself mentioned this possibility. When we asked him whether he thought Sumitra might have learned normally about Shiva he said: "No. If she had done that how could she recognize me and members of my family?" Then he spontaneously added: "People say I have made this case up, but why would I do that? I am gaining nothing, and my [legal] case [against Shiva's in-laws] will not be improved. Sumitra cannot be a witness. I am not getting my daughter back." We think he is correct on these points.

Sumitra and her in-laws might have gained a little status from the change in her behavior and from the social elevation of a "new" family member from the Thakur caste to the Brahmin one. In addition, her husband, who had been away a lot prior to the change, was staying at home more than he had before and presumably giving her more attention. However, all these possible gains seem to us minuscule.

Cryptomnesia

The interpretation of cryptomnesia with secondary personality suggests that Sumitra somehow obtained information about Shiva's life normally without being aware that she had done so and also without her family being aware of this. She would then have used the information in the construction of a secondary personality (Stevenson, 1983b). As mentioned, information published in the newspapers about Shiva's death may have reached persons in Sharifpura, even though we found no evidence that it had. The next steps are, however, difficult to imagine. How could the published information—and much else besides—have been passed on to Sumitra without others being aware that this had happened? Moreover, how could information in a verbal form have enabled Sumitra to recognize many members of Shiva's family in person and in old photographs? Such recognitions depend on tacit knowing that cannot be conveyed in words (Polanyi, 1966).[9]

Apart from the newspapers there were the traders who went between Sharifpura and Etawah and the women of the neighboring village of Murra who were married in Dibiyapur or nearby. The latter group particularly drew our attention. If one or two of them had brought the news of Sumitra's death, revival, and changed personality to Dibiyapur, could they not also have been conduits for information from Dibiyapur about Shiva's death and other details of her life? We spent considerable time both at Dibiyapur and Murra in probing for ways in which this might have happened, and we cannot see any way in which it could. Although Murra and Sharifpura are only 2 km apart by road (and closer across the fields), there is little intercourse between the villages except on special occasions. Because they are so close, they are considered twin villages and each is inside the other's boundaries for acceptable exogamy; therefore, there are no marriages between the two villages. At the same time, the villages are far enough apart so that the inhabitants of one do not meet those of the other when they are at work in their fields. One informant of Sharifpura, who lived less than 60 m from Sumitra's house (and was distantly related to her), assured us that it would have been "impossible" for women of Murra to have told or taught Sumitra what she knew about Shiva's family. Again, even supposing that the women of Murra had brought back and somehow conveyed to Sharifpura some news of Shiva's death, such knowledge as they may have had would not have accounted for all of Sumitra's knowledge of Shiva's private life and for her ability to recognize so many persons known to Shiva, but whom Sumitra had never seen before.

Secondary Personality with Paranormal Knowledge

Most secondary personalities do not demonstrate paranormal knowledge;[10] but a few exceptions have occurred, and the case of Doris Fischer (Prince, 1915–1916, 1926) belongs in this small group. There is no evidence that Sumitra had any powers of extrasensory perception before her apparent death and revival. However, if she somehow acquired such powers she might conceivably have obtained information paranormally about the life and death of Shiva and then developed a secondary personality with that information. The sudden enhancement of Sumitra's ability to read and write makes the case parallel to that of Pearl Curran; she was a person of extremely modest education whose secondary personality, "Patience Worth," wrote a series of remarkable historical novels that seemed far beyond the normal capacities of Mrs. Curran (Litvag, 1972; Prince, 1927). However, "Patience Worth" showed little evidence of telepathy and certainly nothing like what Sumitra demonstrated, if we attribute her knowledge of details of Shiva's life to that process.

Possession

The evidence that Sumitra's case provides of paranormally acquired information invites comparison between it and the cases of Lurancy Vennum (Hodgson, 1901; Stevens, 1887) and Maria Talarico (Giovetti, 1985; Scambio, 1939). However, these were cases in which the change of personality was so marked that the term *possession* seemed applicable to them. And this is the fourth interpretation we wish considered for the present case.

If the other interpretations we have mentioned should be set aside as inadequately accounting for all the facts of the case, we are led to consider that a drastic change of personality occurred. When personality becomes altered unrecognizably, taking on the attributes and the knowledge a deceased personality was known to have, it may be best to speak of the change as a type of possession or reincarnation. Although we do not dogmatically assert that this is the correct interpretation of this case, we believe much of the evidence makes it the most plausible one.

NOTES

1. Reprinted from the *Journal of Scientific Exploration*, 3, 81–101, 1989 (co-authors S. Pasricha & N. McClean-Rice).—Ed.

2. Possession states occur in many other countries, one might almost say in all of them. However, we think it unnecessary to review the unmanageably extensive literature on this subject, all the more so since adequate reviews with further references have been published elsewhere (Bourguignon, 1976; Lewis, 1971; Pattison, Kahan, & Hurd, 1986). We should like to record our agreement with Lewis (1971, pp. 29–30), who warned against the futility of trying to find a single interpretation that will fit all cases of ostensible possession. The word *possession* labels many conditions of various types and different origins and processes.

3. Although we shall refer to knowledge ostensibly obtained without the known sensory organs as *paranormal knowledge*, we do not mean thereby to beg the question of how such knowledge is communicated. However, the important question in any specific case, including the one of this paper, is *whether* such knowledge has been obtained, not *how* it was obtained.

4. The absence of adequate written records in the villages makes some of the dates and ages that we give in this report approximate only. However, we know precisely the dates of Shiva's death and of Sumitra's later apparent death and revival.

5. Santoshi Ma is a Hindu goddess regarded as the special protector of pious and faithful women. She was little known until this century and is not even mentioned in some standard works of reference for Hinduism, such as Walker (1968/1983). An immensely successful moving picture film about her in the 1970s both expressed and promoted the cult of Santoshi Ma in regions of northern India. Villagers of Uttar Pradesh would regard apparent communications from Santoshi Ma and seeming possession by her as unusual, but not pathological.

6. The legal formalities for cremation of a body in a village of India require that five notables of the village sign a document (called a *panchnama*, which means "five names") authorizing cremation. Although some of the persons forming such committees are honest and incorruptible, many of them, at least in small villages, are likely to be friendly with the family of a deceased person and will do the family's bidding with and without bribery. Not surprisingly, observers give no credence to a *panchnama* if other evidence points to suspicious circumstances.

7. However, if a train strikes a living person the head alone may be damaged either by impact with the train itself or if the body is lifted, thrown away from the train, and falls so that the head strikes the ground first. A more suspicious circumstance to us in this case is the location of the dead body within the rails of a single line. We find it difficult to believe that a person intending to commit suicide could have thrown herself so neatly in front of a train as to remain, after the train had passed, within the two rails of a track. We should have expected the train either to have thrown the body away from the line or to have run over it and severed it in two or more parts.

8. See the case of Ampan Petcherat (reprinted earlier in part 4 of this volume) for an example of such a recognition.—Ed.

9. Readers interested in a fuller discussion of this point—here asserted axiomatically—can find it in Stevenson (1974, 1984).

10. It would be more accurate to say that secondary personalities are not observed or not reported often to demonstrate paranormal knowledge. This may be partly due to the failure of observers to examine open-mindedly the evidence that some cases, such as the present one in our view, provide.

REFERENCES

Bourguignon, E. (1976). *Possession*. San Francisco: Chandler and Sharp.

Carstairs, M., & Kapur, R. L. (1976). *The great universe of Kota: Stress, change and mental disorder in an Indian village*. London: The Hogarth Press.

Claus, P. J. (1979). Spirit possession and spirit mediumship from the perspective of Tulu oral traditions. *Culture, Medicine, and Psychiatry, 3*, 29–52.

Giovetti, P. (1985). Lo storico caso di possessione di Siano (Catanzaro). *Luce e Ombra, 85*, 5–59.

Hodgson, R. (1901). Report of meeting of S.P.R. *Journal of the Society for Psychical Research, 10*, 98–104.

Lewis, I. M. (1971). *Ecstatic Religion: An Anthropological Study of Spirit Possession and Shamanism*. Harmondsworth, Middlesex: Penguin Books.

Litvag, I. (1972). *Singer in the Shadows: The Strange Story of Patience Worth*. New York: Macmillan.

Pattison, E. M., Kahan, J., & Hurd, G. S. (1986). Trance and possession states. In B. B. Wolman & M. Ullman (eds.), *Handbook of States of Consciousness* (pp. 286–310). New York: Van Nostrand Reinhold.

Polanyi, M. (1966). *The Tacit Dimension*. Garden City, NY: Doubleday.

Prince, W. F. (1915–1916). The Doris case of multiple personality. *Proceedings of the American Society for Psychical Research, 9–10*, 1–1419.

Prince, W. F. (1926). *The Psychic in the House*. Boston: Boston Society for Psychic Research.

Prince, W. F. (1927). *The Case of Patience Worth*. Boston: Boston Society for Psychic Research.

Scambio, G. (1939). Strano fenomeno di personalità indotta in una giovane di Siano. *La Ricerca Psichica (Luce e Ombra), 39*, 349–362.

Stevens, E. W. (1887). *The Watseka Wonder: A Narrative of Startling Phenomena Occurring in the Case of Mary Lurancy Vennum*. Chicago: Religio-Philosophical Publishing House.

Stevenson, I. (1974). *Twenty Cases Suggestive of Reincarnation* (2d rev. ed.). Charlottesville: University Press of Virginia. (First published in 1966)

Stevenson, I. (1974). *Xenoglossy: A Review and Report of a Case*. Charlottesville: University Press of Virginia.

Stevenson, I. (1975). *Cases of the Reincarnation Type. I. Ten Cases in India*. Charlottesville: University Press of Virginia.

Stevenson, I. (1983a). *Cases of the Reincarnation Type. IV. Twelve Cases in Thailand and Burma*. Charlottesville: University Press of Virginia.

Stevenson, I. (1983b). Cryptomnesia and parapsychology. *Journal of the Society for Psychical Research, 52*, 1–30.

Stevenson, I. (1984). *Unlearned Language: New Studies in Xenoglossy*. Charlottesville: University Press of Virginia.

Stevenson, I., & Pasricha, S. (1979). A case of secondary personality with xenoglossy. *American Journal of Psychiatry, 136*, 1591–1592.

Teja, J. S., Khanna, B. S., & Subrahmanyam, T. B. (1970). "Possession states" in Indian patients. *Indian Journal of Psychiatry, 12*, 71–87.

Walker, B. (1983). *Hindu World: An Encyclopedia Survey of Hinduism* (2 vols.). New Delhi: Munshiram Manoharlal Publishers. (First published in 1968)

4i

Xenoglossy

EWK

As readers will have noted, the debate recurring with regard to all the types of phenomena examined in part 4—from apparitions to mediumship to various kinds of CORT—is whether explanations involving only living persons are adequate or whether there are situations in which the activity of a surviving deceased person seems to be involved. In the running debate between "super-psi" and "survival" interpretations, Ian often pointed to one feature that he thought tipped the scales in favor of survival. Following Ducasse (1962), he argued that, whereas cognitive information such as names or events may be accessible through some process we call ESP or "psi," skills that require training and practice are *not*. One such skill is language. It usually takes long periods of time to acquire fluency in a language, whether one's primary language or another. How can acquisition of the specific and complex vocabulary and syntax of a language, normally requiring long-term exposure and practice, be accomplished by a process such as telepathy or clairvoyance that seems to be one of short-term perception or information transfer?

The importance of cases in which a person shows the ability to speak a language that he or she did not learn normally cannot be overemphasized. In particular, it is the ability to speak fluently and responsively, that is, to understand what is being said and to respond appropriately. Some people have simply uttered, parrot-like, words, phrases, or sentences in a language they did not know, but such cases almost always prove to be ones in which the person was merely reciting, from memory only and without understanding, something they had heard or seen but not consciously remembered (Stevenson, 1983). In contrast, the cases in which someone has actually conversed in a language he or she did not know are as rare as they are important. As far as I know, only three such cases have been thoroughly investigated and reported—all three by Ian (see appendix).

By far the most important of these is known as the Sharada case. It is unique because, in addition to the immensely important fact that the subject in an altered state of consciousness spoke fluently and responsively an archaic form of a language that she had not learned normally, she also had specific knowledge about people, places, and customs dating to more than 150 years before the subject was born, knowledge that Ian and his colleagues laboriously verified as accurate. The case is so important that Ian devoted most of a full-length book to it (Stevenson, 1984). As an introduction, I have reprinted here a short summary published earlier in the *American Journal of Psychiatry.*[1]

NOTE

1. Ian also published a longer paper describing this case (Stevenson & Pasricha, 1980).

REFERENCES

Ducasse, C. J. (1962). What would constitute conclusive evidence of survival after death? *Journal of the Society for Psychical Research, 41,* 401–406.

Stevenson, I. (1983). Cryptomnesia and parapsychology. *Journal of the Society for Psychical Research, 52,* 1–30.

Stevenson, I. (1984). *Unlearned Language: New Studies in Xenoglossy.* Charlottesville: University Press of Virginia.

Stevenson, I., & Pasricha, S. (1980). A preliminary report on an unusual case of the reincarnation type with xenoglossy. *Journal of the American Society for Psychical Research, 74,* 331–348.

THIRTY

A Case of Secondary Personality with Xenoglossy

1979[1]

Early in 1974, Ms. A, a 32-year-old unmarried woman, who lived in Nagpur, Maharashtra, India, began to undergo marked changes of personality. A new personality, who called herself Sharada, manifested behavior startlingly different from Ms. A's normal conduct. The most remarkable aspect of this unusual behavior was Sharada's complete inability to speak Marathi, which is Ms. A's native language. Instead, Sharada spoke fluent Bengali, a language Ms. A denied knowing how to speak. Because Ms. A's family understood no Bengali, they initially had great difficulty communicating with Sharada. Some Bengali-speaking persons of Nagpur identified the language Sharada spoke and also acted as interpreters for her.

The Sharada personality has taken control at least 30 times, for periods lasting from 1 day to 7 weeks. We began investigating the case in the summer of 1975 and continued to do so at intervals over the next 3 years.

Characteristics of the Sharada Phases

The Sharada phases usually came on gradually, with the transition lasting several hours. Some of the transitions occurred overnight while Ms. A slept. The Sharada personality tended to appear particularly on the eighth (ashtami) day of the waxing or waning moon.

Sharada dressed, acted, and spoke like a married Bengali woman. Unlike Ms. A, who taught at a university and helped her mother with housework, Sharada spent her days in a room, occupied almost exclusively in devotional activities and singing.

Sharada gave a circumstantial account of her life, with details that corresponded accurately to conditions in the villages of Bengal during the early 19th century. She had no knowledge of any inventions of the industrial revolution or of later technology. She had a marked preference for the foods of Bengal and a knowledge of them that one would not expect in a woman—even an educated one—of west central India. She showed an equally surprising familiarity with the names of small towns and villages in Bengal and with their location in relation to rivers.

Sharada gave details of the family in Bengal of which she claimed to be a member, including the family name and the names of male family members. A family of this name was found in Bansberia, one of the towns in (West) Bengal that Sharada mentioned. The head of this family has a genealogy that goes back to the early 19th century. It lists six of the men Sharada mentioned, in the relationships that she claimed they had to her. The genealogy is exclusively male, so we cannot say that we have traced Sharada directly, although we have verified many of her statements. From the genealogy, Sharada's life can be dated to the years between 1810 and 1830.

Sharada said that she had married and gone to live with her husband in another part of Bengal. She also said that on a later visit to her own family she had been bitten by a snake and had "fainted." She did not remember dying and could not explain how, after "fainting," she came to Nagpur, more than 1200 km west of Bengal.

Sharada and Ms. A (in her normal state) claim to know nothing about each other. We believe, however, that neither one is completely amnesic for the other.

We have interviewed Ms. A on several occasions when she has been in her normal state, but our knowledge of Sharada derives almost exclusively from the reports of other persons. During one visit to Nagpur, however, one of us (S.P.) spent a few hours with Sharada.

Sharada's Bengali

Five Bengali-speaking persons we interviewed gave concordant testimony about Sharada's ability to speak fluent Bengali. Her fluency contrasted with the lack of this quality in two other persons who have demonstrated responsive xenoglossy (the ability to speak an unlearned foreign language), both of whom conversed haltingly and imperfectly in the foreign languages they spoke (Stevenson, 1974b, 1976). Sharada's Bengali was free of English, whereas the vocabulary of modern Bengali includes about 20% of English loan-words. This feature of the case accords with other evidence indicating a life in Bengal in the early 19th century.

Relevant Information About Ms. A's Background

Ms. A and her family have always lived in Maharashtra, which is in west central India. She has never visited Bengal. Marathi is the principal language spoken by her family, and none of the family can speak Bengali. Her mother speaks only Marathi and some Hindi. Other members of the family (including Ms. A) can speak some English and some Hindi. Although Ms. A's father had a few Bengali friends (there are Bengali residents in Nagpur), none of them ever spoke Bengali with him—during Ms. A's childhood or later—because he himself understood and spoke no Bengali. Ms. A, her parents, and two of her older sisters denied that she had ever learned or tried to learn to speak Bengali or had ever had an opportunity to do so. She had studied Sanskrit when younger and retained some knowledge of it, and during her high school years she had taken a few lessons (at most) in reading the Bengali script. Our extensive interviews with Ms. A, members of her immediate family, and other persons in a position to have relevant information have convinced us that she had no normal knowledge of spoken Bengali.

Discussion

The marked alterations of personality in this case have some resemblance to mediumistic trances, but the differences are greater than the similarities. Mediumistic trances are almost always induced voluntarily, whereas Ms. A's personality changes occurred quite involuntarily. Mediumistic trances usually last an hour or two at the most; Sharada remained "in control" for days, sometimes for weeks.

The case also has some resemblance to cases of secondary personality, but the usual secondary personality claims to be more or less contemporary and co-local with the primary personality, whereas Sharada described a life in another part of her country and about 150 years earlier. Furthermore, the usual secondary personality has no paranormal powers, although there have been rare exceptions (Prince, 1915, 1916). Sharada's ability to speak fluent Bengali constitutes, in our opinion, a paranormally acquired skill (Stevenson, 1974b).

The case also resembles in some respects cases suggestive of reincarnation (Pasricha & Stevenson, 1977; Stevenson, 1974a, 1975), but in such cases the subject usually begins to speak about the previous life he or she claims to remember between the ages of 2 and 5. Moreover, such a child's ordinary personality is rarely suppressed completely (as was Ms. A's) during the narration of his or her claimed memories.

NOTE

1. Originally published in the *American Journal of Psychiatry, 136,* 1591–1592, 1979 (with S. Pasricha).—Ed.

REFERENCES

Pasricha, S., & Stevenson, I. (1977). Three cases of the reincarnation type in India. *Indian Journal of Psychiatry, 19,* 36–42.

Prince, W.F. (1915). The Doris case of multiple personality. Part 1. *Proceedings of the American Society for Psychical Research, 9,* 9–700.

Prince, W.F. (1916). The Doris case of multiple personality. Part 2. *Proceedings of the American Society for Psychical Research, 10,* 701–1419.

Stevenson, I. (1974a). *Twenty Cases Suggestive of Reincarnation.* Charlottesville: University Press of Virginia.

Stevenson, I. (1974b). *Xenoglossy: A Review and Report of a Case.* Charlottesville: University Press of Virginia.

Stevenson, I. (1975). *Cases of the Reincarnation Type. Vol 1: Ten Cases in India.* Charlottesville: University Press of Virginia.

Stevenson, I. (1976). A preliminary report of a new case of responsive xenoglossy: The case of Gretchen. *Journal of the American Society for Psychical Research, 70,* 66–77.

5

Implications

EWK

The central theme toward which all of Ian's work in medicine, psychiatry, and psychical research converged was that human personality involves more than genetic makeup, the workings of the brain, the influence of early childhood environment, and the experiences of one postnatal, pre-mortem span of time. In addition to these influences, the development of the individual self may begin before birth and continue after death.

It is extremely important, however, to remember the principle that guided Ian as well as those predecessors whom he admired most, such as William James, Frederic Myers, and Edmund Gurney. As I mentioned in the General Introduction, this is the principle of tertium quid, that is, that an adequate understanding of any phenomenon is more likely to come from an inclusive "both/and" approach than from an exclusive "either/or" approach. Whether the phenomenon is a disease, an apparition, or the nature of human consciousness, multiple factors contribute to it, and an adequate understanding of it must incorporate all those factors. As we saw in part 2, Ian believed that we can have a medical science that is both technologically advanced and humanly caring, that brings together the best of the new and the old medicine (1985, p. 581). In a paper reprinted here in part 5, he similarly argued that religion and psychiatry are not contradictory but complementary. In the same vein, he frequently insisted that "The Explanatory Value of Reincarnation" (Stevenson, 1977, 2000; see also 1997, i:5–6 [reprinted in ch. 24]) lies not in replacing the undeniable influences of genetics and environment—"nature" and "nurture"—but in offering an additional factor to help explain what the first two alone cannot and what is thus usually attributed to "chance." Finally, for Ian as well as his predecessors in psychical research, the importance of psychical research is that it offers a point at which the usual antitheses of science/religion and matter/mind can come together in a broader view—as he put it, psychical research is "the liberal center" or "third force" between naive credulity and destructive skepticism (Stevenson, 1984, p. 100; 1990, p. 160 [reprinted in part 3]).

If human personality is more than a product of the physical body—a "self" transcending that body's particular genetic and environmental influences—the resulting conclusion would seem to be that the ultimate responsibility for one's conduct, character, and happiness lies within oneself. In the remainder of this part, I include some of what Ian had to say about the implications of a wider outlook on the many factors contributing to our uniqueness as individual selves.

REFERENCES

Stevenson, I. (1977). The explanatory value of the idea of reincarnation. *Journal of Nervous and Mental Disease, 164,* 305–326.

Stevenson, I. (1984). Guest editorial: Are parapsychology journals good for parapsychology? *Journal of the American Society for Psychical Research, 78,* 97–104.

Stevenson, I. (1985). The end of patient abuse in medical care. *Virginia Quarterly Review, 61,* 565–583.

Stevenson, I. (1990). Thoughts on the decline of major paranormal phenomena (Presidential Address). *Proceedings of the Society for Psychical Research, 57,* 149–162.

Stevenson, I. (1997). *Reincarnation and Biology: A Contribution to the Etiology of Birthmarks and Birth Defects* (2 vols.). Westport, CT: Praeger.

Stevenson, I. (2000). The phenomenon of claimed memories of previous lives: Possible interpretations and importance. *Medical Hypotheses, 54,* 652–659.

THIRTY-ONE

"The Explanatory Value of the Idea of Reincarnation"

1977[1]

Most psychiatrists and psychologists today believe that infancy and childhood are more important periods in the formation of personality than any later periods; but this idea is only an assumption, as I mentioned some years ago (Stevenson, 1957). Cases of the reincarnation type challenge it and suggest that although personality is indeed being formed in childhood, its development actually begins much earlier in other terrestrial lives anterior to the child's present life. If we allow ourselves to think of the formation of human personality as extending further back in time than conception and birth, we may be able to explain better than we now can a number of anomalies in child development and human personality.[2] . . .

Here I need to offer a disclaimer. . . . I think it is essential to emphasize strongly that I am not offering reincarnation as a comprehensive system capable of explaining everything we need to know about child development and human personality; nor do I think of it as replacing present knowledge derived from genetics, other branches of biology, and the study of environmental influences in the development of personality. The idea of reincarnation is offered as a supplement only, not as a substitute for knowledge in these areas. It suggests a third factor, in addition to genetic and environmental factors, for understanding the problems it touches on.

In inviting readers to consider reincarnation as having explanatory value, I am therefore not questioning any acknowledged facts; but I am questioning some assumptions. The most important of these is that human personality consists of nothing but the expressions of the molecules and cells of which our physical bodies are built. The corollary of this assumption, that human personality could have no existence before or after the physical body of its current manifestation, is equally in question. I am fully aware of the gravity of challenging these assumptions and I do not wish to make this challenge to anyone unwilling to examine the evidence that I believe justifies it; nor am I presenting that evidence without appreciation and acknowledgment of its many imperfections. It is far from compelling toward any conclusion except that of the importance of further investigations of the type of case that has provided it.

NOTES

1. Excerpts reprinted from the *Journal of Nervous and Mental Disease, 164,* 305–326, 1977.—Ed.

2. The poorly explained phenomena that Ian goes on to discuss in this paper include phobias, philias and unusual animosities manifesting in early childhood; unusual skills not learned normally; abnormalities in child-parent relationships; gender confusion; birthmarks and birth defects; differences in personality and physical characteristics in monozygotic twins; and unusual pregnancy cravings.

REFERENCE

Stevenson, I. (1957). Is the human personality more plastic in infancy and childhood? *American Journal of Psychiatry, 114,* 152–161.

THIRTY-TWO

Comments on "Is Outcome for Schizophrenia Better in Nonindustrial Societies? The Case of Sri Lanka"

1979[1]

A central corollary of the belief in rebirth is acceptance of personal responsibility for one's own condition whatever that may be. Sinhalese Buddhists naturally practice their religion with varying degrees of conviction and fervor. But to the extent that they believe in rebirth—as most of them do—they cannot blame anyone but themselves for their misfortunes, including a mental illness. They cannot turn on their families—or on that larger, abstract family, society—and attribute their troubles to the faults of others. It follows also that neither the families of patients nor society manifesting through government dispensaries and agencies feel any responsibility for causing mental illness. These attitudes contrast markedly with those generated by the one-life eschatology pronounced on us so confidently in the West by many scientists and most theologians. The Western systems which allow for only one life and yet which cannot ignore the most widespread inequities at birth leave us with only two ways of accounting for unfavorable conditions at birth or later: either an unjust God (or an arbitrary fate) assigned them to us, or our parents (and their extension, society) caused them. On either explanation, the individual himself is not encouraged to accept responsibility and, on the contrary, families and society are. This is not the place to debate the merits of these opposing views of man's nature. I merely wish to draw attention to the different results that follow from different assumptions about the nature of man.

NOTE

1. Excerpts from Dr. Stevenson's comments (*Journal of Nervous and Mental Disease, 167*, 159–160, 1979) on a paper by Nancy E. Waxler ("Is Outcome for Schizophrenia Better in Nonindustrial Societies?" *Journal of Nervous and Mental Disease, 167*, 144–158, 1979).—Ed.

THIRTY-THREE

The Significance of Survival for Our Present Life

1969[1]

Many persons believe that if we could demonstrate a proof of survival, a moral transformation of mankind would automatically follow. I once believed this myself, but no longer do so. My enthusiasm for this theory was first shaken in 1961 when I called on the Ramakrishna Swami Mukherjee in Chandigarh at the time of my first visit to India. When the Swami asked me what I was doing in India, I enthusiastically expounded my search for evidence bearing on reincarnation. After I concluded, a long silence followed and then the Swami replied, and I think I can remember his exact words, which sank into me deeply: "Yes, we here in India know that reincarnation occurs. But you see, it does not make any difference. We have just as many rogues and villains in India where everyone believes in reincarnation as you have in the West." The Swami's remark might have applied to other places and periods also. During the Middle Ages in Europe everyone—or almost everyone—believed in a life after death with merited rewards and punishments; and yet life was hardly less vicious then than it is today. Thinking about such examples has considerably reduced my confidence in the influence on human conduct of a belief in survival, even one supported by much better evidence than we now have. Nevertheless, I still think the belief and the evidence make some difference, and I hope it will be worth while to examine the implications of the belief in survival a little further.

One often hears it said that only a belief in survival can confer meaning to life. This I think very much overstates the case and by rash generalization keeps us from realizing the one area in which a belief in survival should significantly change the meaning of life for us. Materialists or physical monists who believe in one life with its complete extinction at death can still find abundant meaning in life. Many, of course, use their conviction of the absence of a life after death to pursue selfish pleasures which have only the most local and personal interest. Others, however, have found life rich and enjoyable and have contributed much to make it even more so for their children, their contemporaries, and their successors. We can enjoy and share the pleasures of art, literature, music, beautiful scenery, and many other riches of this earth without believing that we continue to exist after physical death. Just what, then, does a belief in survival add to the meaning of life for those who hold it? The added meaning, I think, lies in the spheres of moral conduct and personal relationships.

To explain what I have in mind I need to digress slightly and consider the different incentives for change in our behavior in childhood and adulthood. I believe that the last generation of western psychiatrists greatly exaggerated the influence of childhood events on the formation of character. It is incontestable, however, that a child is largely a prisoner of his parents and of the environment around them. The child's adaptations must perforce be to the parents and to that environment. The need to make such adaptations forces adjustments of character. Upon attaining adulthood, most persons assert their own authority and gain some control over their environment. As they achieve autonomy, however, the incentives to modify character by new adaptations rapidly diminish. Few persons change more than they need to change. And few indeed are the persons who change character fundamentally after reaching adulthood. The restrictions of childhood give rise to the fact that it is the main period of character formation and to the myth that it is the only one.

Certainly as a person grows older he may feel stimulated to make occasional additional adaptations. We all know of adults who study a foreign language in order to enjoy travel, or learn to dance in order to marry again, or take up skiing in order to get more exercise and excitement. These, however, are largely or entirely changes for our own immediate pleasure and gain, not changes to help other people. Our incentives for changing our moral conduct greatly diminish with age in the absence of any prospect for life after death. By the time of middle adulthood we have made our main friendships and intimacies; we have found ways of getting along with other people and if life ends at death, there seems little point in making further efforts to improve our conduct. On the other hand, a belief in life after death offers the incentive that efforts to change character and conduct (independent of present requirements for adaptation) will lead to later rewards in the "next world." This brings me to my next topic, that of "later rewards."

Superficial critics of the belief in life after death (who do not themselves share the belief) sometimes say that it is simply a means of coping with the fear of death. They forget that many more people believe in life after death than wish for it. And for the vast millions of Asia who believe in reincarnation, belief in survival after death provides no escape from a fear of death, for they fear rebirth more than death. The aim of their religious practices is to gain release from the "wheel of rebirth." They do accept, however, or believe they should try to accept, the burdens of today with the expectation of coming closer to the goal of sainthood and no rebirth later. They believe they must "pay now, or later." The saint is just as selfish as the rest of us in that he also wants to feel good. He differs from us in that he knows and constantly remembers that the quickest way to durable good feelings lies in service to others. The saint knows we are all part of one unity and that he can only rise by lifting others with him.

If the saint is correct in his belief that we must "pay now, or later" in service to others, we should try to imagine how such a system might work to help us change. The "pay now, or later" lesson might impinge in at least two ways: First, through our memories we can judge our own conduct. Many living persons have the experience of regretting some past action which at the time it happened they considered quite justified and "right." This self-judgment seems to be heightened under the influence of such drugs as LSD and in delirious states such as those of dying persons. It is therefore reasonable to speculate that after death we would be further exposed to guilty memories. Thus we would be punished *by* our sins rather than *for* them. Patanjali said that men are afraid of death because they vaguely remember what happened the last time they died; after dying they painfully reviewed the events and misdeeds of the life which they had just left. The fear of death, according to Patanjali (1953), is then really a fear of another unpleasant review of one's misconduct. It follows that as a man cultivates goodness, he loses his fear of death until, as Socrates taught, a truly good man has no fear of it at all (Plato, 1936, p. 115).

Then we may also be corrected by the company in which we find ourselves after death. Just as agent-percipient relationships among the living[2] derive mostly from loving relationships, so we might expect that after death we shall find ourselves among those persons with whom we deserve to be. Good mannered people shun boors; honest men avoid thieves. The worst deprivation to be imagined is a permanent separation from good people; the loss forever of their company and assistance. Yet, if I am correct, we only lose this companionship and support as a result of our own selfish conduct. And we may feel such separation and loss much more keenly after death than now.

There are two other respects in which materialism or physical monism differ in implications for our conduct from dualism with a belief in life after death. The dualist has little confidence in material progress as a remedy for our troubles. Western observers of the Asian belief in reincarnation often consider it responsible for the alleged sloth and for the lack of material progress in Asia compared to that developed by Europeans. In one sense this is true, but it is wrong to think that the belief in survival, and specifically in reincarnation, necessarily leads to passivity and inertia. These vices may be rationalized with reincarnation as may almost any other wickedness. In the main, however, the belief in survival and reincarnation leads to a realization that the only improvement worth achieving is one of moral self-betterment. And so more time would be allotted to meditation and other efforts at self-improvement, and less time to material objects. More and more people in the West are coming to realize that our material progress does not bring social progress or assure happiness for anyone. The "developed nations," we now begin to understand, have no philosophy to export to the less developed ones. "Development" is at last being seen a little more deeply.

The belief in survival also throws responsibility for moral improvement squarely on the individual. It does not oppose social changes which legislative and administrative action may help to bring about, but it does not look for improvement in anyone's emotional state from such changes. In the sphere of conduct and emotions, we can only change ourselves. The last generation in the West blamed parents for the troubles of their children; the present generation has exhausted that theory and turned to blaming social conditions. After the futility of this has been realized, there will finally come a return to the recognition of individual responsibility. I think we can see signs of this already in the increased interest western people now have in Asian religions, for these religions especially emphasize the individual as his own and only savior. No intermediary of priest or prophet stands between the individual and his advancement in Hinduism and Buddhism.

The insights of parapsychology, so far as we can claim to have developed any, do not offer easy solutions to the troubles of today. The way they point to is harder, indeed, than other ways, at least initially. Those of us who believe in the idea of "pay now, or later" feel obliged to put up with present sufferings and responsibilities that would gladly be rejected under the influence of another philosophy. One feels impelled to increase efforts at self-betterment and the provision of greater service to one's fellow-men with the hope that deferred pleasure will be followed by a deeper happiness later. I am myself convinced that the moral imperatives of parapsychological research into survival after death are heavier instead of lighter to carry in this world than those of beliefs which suppose man's life to end at death. It is indeed difficult to look at the evidence for survival after death without feeling both fear and hope.

I think the fear generated by the prospect of survival after death is an important factor accounting for some, perhaps much, of the opposition to parapsychology today, although this fear is probably not often consciously identified and even less often admitted. It is perhaps not our data as such that our opponents shun, but the implications of these data for their own conduct. We, of course, are not responsible for this, but we may be thought to be, and accordingly mistreated like those messengers of ancient days who brought news of defeats and were executed for doing so! In any case, for those who look deeper there seem to be more grounds for hope than for despair in the evidence for survival after death. That our message is not one of immediate joy helps to defend us from the charge already mentioned that we are engaged in wish-fulfilling fantasies; and that it is nevertheless a message of hope and eventual happiness makes it superior to most contemporary beliefs, especially to those derived from other branches of present-day psychology. Modern psychology seems to me to have become a very salty lake into which the stream of parapsychology may gradually introduce some sweetening.

There remain two other points to make before I close. To some readers these may not seem directly relevant to the question of survival after death, but I think they are sufficiently related to deserve brief mention at this time.

PARAPSYCHOLOGY AND THE UNITY OF ALL THINGS

I have already alluded to the emotional bonds which are usually a necessary (although not sufficient) condition for extrasensory perception among the living. And I have suggested that such bonds may importantly influence the company in which we will find ourselves after death. But these bonds, and the increasing evidence that extrasensory processes occur more commonly than most people have imagined, suggest that we are all somehow united with each other even now just as surely as all the islands and continents are united beneath the seas. But for most of us the evidence of this unity becomes apparent through extrasensory perception in relationships with some persons more readily than with others. The true saint, however, has risen above personal relationships and feels himself equally united with all people and all things. This idea of unity with everything in the universe is what we find in the perennial philosophy of the saints of all times and places. Thus an important implication of parapsychological research comes from its strong suggestion that there is indeed a ground of union between all people and things. This enables us to take more seriously the idea that by good wishes (call them prayers if you like) we can and do help each other, and that by failing in these good wishes we may help less than we can and should.

PARAPSYCHOLOGY AND DIRECT KNOWLEDGE

Finally, I wish to point out that in demonstrating the existence of extrasensory perception, parapsychology offers possibilities for acquiring knowledge directly without use of the scientific method (Thouless & Wiesner, 1948; Wheatley, 1961). Thus parapsychology is a science whose progress may lead to its own abolition, at least as regards the empirical methods of attaining knowledge it now employs. It is therefore not surprising that some parapsychologists, deeply affected by the material they study, have shown inclinations toward mysticism; that is, toward the idea of the direct attainment of knowledge as distinct from the empirical method of attaining it. Indeed, in the traditions of both western and eastern mysticism, paranormal phenomena are said to occur during progress toward the direct realization of truth. They are considered a sign of progress, but at the same time the aspirant is warned against being distracted by them.

This brings me in closing back to Chester Carlson, whom we are honoring tonight. No one was a more generous supporter of empirical investigations in parapsychology. And yet he also devoted much of his time to efforts aimed at the attainment of the direct realization of truth toward which our scientific investigations point, but to which they alone cannot take us.

NOTES

1. Excerpts from "Some Implications of Parapsychological Research on Survival After Death" (a symposium honoring Chester Carlson), *Proceedings of the American Society for Psychical Research, 28*, 18–35, 1969. Some other excerpts from this paper were reprinted in Part 4 in Chapter 14.—Ed.

2. Ian was here referring to a point he had made earlier in this paper, as well as elsewhere in his writings, that in both spontaneous cases and experimental studies the two people involved are often emotionally close.

REFERENCES

Patanjali (1953). *How to Know God: The Yoga Aphorisms* (Swami Prabhavananda, trans.). New York: Harper's.

Plato (1936). *Phaedo* (H. Cary, trans.). London: J. M. Dent.

Thouless, R. H., & Wiesner, B. P. (1948). The psi processes in normal and "paranormal" psychology. *Proceedings of the Society for Psychical Research, 48*, 177–196.

Wheatley, J. M. O. (1961). Knowledge, empiricism and ESP. *International Journal of Parapsychology, 3*, 7–19.

THIRTY-FOUR

Assumptions of Religion and Psychiatry

1955[1]

The comparison of religion and psychiatry is an act of boldness for which an author may not easily be forgiven by the partisans of both sides. For does anyone have authority to say who represents religion and what psychiatrists believe? Both religion and psychiatry have divided into multiple sects, each with its own doctrines, its own saints and apostolic successions, and its own propagandists. If, by this remark, I set psychiatry and religion on the same plane, I do not mean to devalue either. But since no one group of either psychiatry or religion has persuaded the whole world to acknowledge the truth of its doctrine alone, both psychiatry and religion should hold all their assumptions critically until further advances have been made. In this spirit we can say that to label scepticism of some assumptions "resistance" brings no advance on the use of the word "unregenerate" for persons who cannot accept other assumptions.

Despite the mentioned dissensions in both religion and psychiatry, certain themes in each may be compared as representative. No doubt many members of both groups will deny that they personally subscribe to some of the assumptions presented. I must take the responsibility for stating that the views presented are generally representative, although I do not claim that they are endorsed by all members of these two groups.

During the past 50 years psychiatry has developed, among many other things, a vigorous program for changing people by talking to them. The techniques used are called psychotherapy. If we look around us in space and time, we can readily see that the history of man's efforts to change himself did not begin 50 years ago. Nor does psychiatry have a monopoly of such efforts. On the contrary, countless men all over the world at all times have endeavored to change themselves and to help others change. Most of these men have related their efforts to some system of thought or belief and some associated ceremonial practices, which together are called a religion. Religion has thus become almost inextricably associated in our minds with a system of thought, especially a system explaining the larger or cosmic phenomena of our universe. Yet, as William James (1902) pointed out, all such systems of thought undoubtedly follow certain experiences, for the explanation of which they are secondarily devised. It is to these experiences and to the efforts religious people have made to change themselves, that I wish to direct attention.

Religious experiences have many varieties just as do musical or sexual experiences. Perhaps too arbitrarily, I should like to suggest that in the basic religious experience a person achieves a heightened sense of unity with everyone else, with everything else, and hence with God. Religious efforts at changing derive from this primary awareness of unity and at the same time strive to promote it. Which explains why genuine religious experiences resemble a self-fueling fire. From the sense of unity with other things and people arises different behavior toward them, the behavior of tender love.

In thus isolating what I consider to be the essence of religion from the many other activities, including excesses and crimes of all sorts which have occurred under that name, we commit no act of partisanship unfair to psychiatry. For psychiatry also has had, and still has, its follies and its fanaticisms, from the embarrassment of which all scientists wish to be delivered. And we can strip psychiatry also of its secondary doctrinal elaborations, and expose for consideration the simple principles whereby psychiatrists help people to change themselves.

For the details of religious efforts at personal changing we do not go to the theologians and philosophers. Nor do we even find help in the various official religious histories and revelations such as the Bible or the Koran. Rather we must turn to the records left by those men who have tried to change themselves, and to help others do so. Such works as *The Cloud of Unknowing* (Underhill, 1922), the *Bhagavad-Gita* (Prabhavananda & Isherwood, 1944), *The Imitation of Christ* (Thomas à Kempis, 1910), and *The Gospel of Sri Ramakrishna* ((Ramakrishna, 1947) repeat with a striking uniformity the same ideas and recommend the same techniques for changing oneself.[2]

The present comparison of religion can be seen already to differ from many of those to which we have become used. Numerous attempts have been made to reconcile psychiatry and religion. One of these maps out separate areas for each. According to this arrangement, religion is the subject of man's relations with God or with life, or some other concept of a super-individual nature, while psychiatry is the study of mental illness. The two subjects thus become politely separated into unimpinging spheres of influence. Such a division of interest might have had some plausibility so long as psychiatry confined itself to the grosser forms of mental illness such as psychoses. But the invasion by psychiatry of the field of character (and since religious people were already there it was an invasion) has made such a division no longer tenable. We must frankly admit that religion and psychiatry (in its psychotherapeutic activity) have the same task, that of helping man to be happy. They differ not in the goal but in their approaches.

But before we compare these differing approaches, I must answer one serious objection to religion, that which finds religion itself a pathological experience. According to this view, religion becomes a subject fit for psychiatric survey itself rather than one entitled to equal respect.

Psychiatrists critical of religion have usually taken up one of two positions. Some critics see religion as an escape from reality. They consider it a vestige of the fanciful formulations of natural events by which primitive men comforted themselves during their early ignorance of these events. According to them, the progress of science in bringing understanding of the universe around us, has removed the need for religion, which should now disappear. Certainly gross intellectual errors have been made under the name of religion, and their authors have had to endure a succession of ignominious retreats before the advance of science. But I have already mentioned that in religion, cosmological systems have always been secondary to particular experiences. The fanatical defense of such systems against other evidence forms no part of religious experiences, and indeed may be a sign of their absence. The basic religious experience brings a sense of unity with everything else—with other people, with other things, and with the whole universe. This experience does not come to one as an escape from the hazards of life. Rather, to those experiencing it, the sense of unity appears as a great enrichment of life, and brings an increasingly constructive attitude toward it. Undoubtedly many persons have escaped from the cruelties of life in the wagon of religion. Religion may indeed be used as an escape, but so may almost anything. Too many of our own adherents "intellectualize" their problems and we should hardly wish our efforts to be identified with their outpourings.

The second critical view of religion makes of it a mere repetition of infantile experiences. The infant, according to this opinion, feels a sense of unity with his mother because he cannot tell her from himself. The sense of unity in religious experiences is a recapitulation of the sense of unity with the parent. This reductionist interpretation of religion achieves an apparent plausibility by overlooking certain facts. We know nothing about the experiences of infancy which permits us to attribute definitely to it the assumed sense of unity. This speculation has been repeated cliche-like until its factual basis has become a quite unjustified belief.

Infants may have some sense of unity, but if so, we can be certain of a qualitative difference between this sense of unity and that of the adult. The infant may think of everything else as being a part of himself, but the religious sense of unity brings a conviction that the self is a part of everything else. The difference may seem subtle, but the significance for behavior tells us immediately that we must be dealing with two quite different sorts of experience. The infant is preoccupied with what is coming toward his observing self from the other parts of the totality which he senses. A genuine religious experience can be sharply distinguished from this (and from fictitious religious experiences) by the concern for the welfare of others which characterizes the subject.

SENSE OF UNITY

In early childhood, after infancy, we do indeed see a sense of unity rarely attained afterward. Children at this age approach other humans, animals and even inanimate objects on a basis of intimacy and equality. This ingenuousness fascinates us because it differs so strikingly from the isolation of the ordinary adult. Children do all this, it must be added, long after they have acquired a sense of personal identity, so that their sense of unity with other creatures and objects does not spring from a lack of differentiation of self from not-self.

The sense of unity exhibited by children (and by savages) may indeed be a primitive attitude which in ontogenetic maturation and in phylogenetic civilization has been lost to us. The religious sense of unity may therefore merely return us to a state with which we are already familiar (Custance, 1952, p. 254). It would not follow that this state is an undesirable or unfruitful one. Regression evokes connotations of morbidity, and we may have difficulty in thinking of regression as a recovery. Yet we psychiatrists assume that our patients have, through painful experiences, forgotten constructive attitudes and learned harmful ones. In our therapy we try to induce a regression, a revocation of earlier, constructive attitudes toward certain areas of life. Thus in our sexually inhibited patients we try to revive a natural expression of sexuality which has been driven under by thwarting experiences. Should we try to restore a childlike freedom for sexual expression and belittle the childlike sense of unity? Do we not make inconsistent value judgments if we encourage the one and deride the other? And in the last analysis does not the greatest satisfaction of the sexual impulse lie in a sense of unity with the partner? Whatever psychiatry may say of this problem, religion has always stated that the child's sense of unity expresses a more constructive attitude than the isolation so often shown by adults. "Except ye become as a little child again, ye shall in no wise enter into the Kingdom of Heaven." And in the language of Zen Buddhism: "When he is born, the person is like a new sword, shiny. But in the course of time the sword becomes tarnished and rusty, and similarly with a person in growing up. It is the purpose of the Zen training to remove the rust, so that the person can see himself as he really is" (Stunkard, 1951).

Freud (1930, 1949) was a principal exponent of the two mentioned criticisms of religion, but Freud did not create or even sustain the animus against religion. He merely articulated it. A strong antireligious trend in western civilization has existed for the past two hundred years. For this religion must blame itself and not its critics. The decline of religion has been largely occasioned by the substitution of ritualistic and ceremonial exercises for those inner experiences promoting the sense of unity which lead to personal change. However, this regrettable substitution of one thing for another (both labeled religion), should not lead to condemnation of one with the other, nor to withholding the courtesies of scientific method from the study of religious experiences.

People who have had meaningful religious experiences realize the impossibility of communicating the experience or its value to someone who has not had such experiences. They state simply that their experiences can be repeated by anyone who chooses to do so, provided he will repeat the steps which they have themselves taken. Critics of religion sometimes claim that they are asked to accept the statements of religious people on trust, whereas those of science can be verified (Freud, 1949). This betrays an ignorance of religion. The method of religion is no less scientific than that of physics. Only the subject matter differs. Those who care to repeat the steps prescribed can experience for themselves the states and changes described by religious persons. Those who do not do so should not say that the results are unverifiable.

Having thus, I hope, established religion as a respectable means of attaining the same ends as those for which psychiatry works, we may turn now to compare their differing approaches to these ends. Psychiatry and religion have many differing assumptions, but I shall mention only a few areas in which these assumptions may be usefully contrasted.

The first difference arises over the problem of what I call the superphysical needs of man. Psychiatric observations have clearly established the motivations of much of human behavior in the physical needs of the organism. Much of what formerly seemed purely gratuitous, or in the service of some other motive, has been found based on the needs of hunger, thirst, self-preservation and sex. Most psychiatrists today believe that these physical needs directly or indirectly motivate all human behavior. The behavior in question may be distantly removed from these needs but nevertheless reaches out from them, if only remotely or symbolically. According to this assumption, a man's affection for another man arises from his need to preserve friendly relations with other people so that he can hold his job, can buy food in the market place, and live in peace. Love has been defined from this point of view as "the feeling one has when some physiological need is about to be satisfied." Similarly, peace can be attributed to fear of being attacked and injured oneself.

Religion, on the other hand, assumes the independent existence of superphysical needs of humans. Love is considered existential, and a tendency to its expression a basic quality of humans. Whoever does not achieve the expression of genuinely altruistic love is accordingly an unfulfilled and incomplete person. Considerable evidence supports this view. First, tender love does in fact appear to be existential and to spring up in children even when they have not been taught it. And if they are taught it, how did the mother learn? This only removes the problem of its origin one generation back (Weigert, 1949). Secondly, tender love constantly exceeds the bounds of necessity which would be required if love were based on self-interest. Thirdly, tender love has a self-reinforcing quality not found in other emotions or in behavior designed to satisfy physical needs. No one feels pleasure in hostility, and it seems likely that the element of displeasure in hostility, more than any awareness of its social harmfulness or a fear of retaliation, drives persons to change themselves. In contrast, tender love carries with it a wish that this state might always remain and, in varying degrees, brings efforts to make it endure or to recapture it when it escapes.

Psychiatry and religion thus differ in their appraisal of the psychological needs of humans. Some psychiatrists naively believe that psychotherapy can somehow be divorced from the problem of values. Neglect of this problem has brought merited criticism on psychiatry (Fromm, 1950; Ginsburg, 1950; de Grazia, 1952).

The ambiguity about values in psychiatry arises, I believe, from the view that man's needs are circumscribed by his physical needs. So long as physical survival and comfort are the goals of therapeutic endeavor, opinions will differ in different cultures about the way in which this comfort can be achieved. These uncertainties do not plague religion. From the belief that each man has a center or Godhead of tender love within him, religion applies techniques which promote that love whether these make the patient more or less adaptive to the culture in which he lives.

TECHNIQUES OF CHANGING

Turning to those techniques whereby man does change himself, we find further differing assumptions in religion and psychiatry. Psychiatrists generally believe that man changes through interaction with some other person, notably the psychotherapist. Psychiatrists differ as to how this relationship changes the person who exposes himself to it, but they generally do agree that a man cannot change himself alone. This assumption may be related to the general preoccupation among psychiatrists with the influence of early experiences with parents on the development of personality. A reasonable accompaniment of this assumption would be the belief that what man does to man can only be undone by another man. Be that as it may, psychiatrists hardly ever consider the possibility that a man can change himself. Instances in which this has been attempted (notably Freud's self-analysis) are considered brilliant tour de forces hardly within the reach of ordinary beings.

Religious persons express astonishment on the opposite score—that men spend so much time talking to each other about themselves and so little time thinking about themselves alone. As Pascal wrote: "All of man's troubles come from his inability to sit in a room by himself." The principal religious techniques of changing are not, I need hardly say, attendance at church or participation in ceremonials. They are prayer and meditation. And prayer and meditation are, from the purely human point of view, solitary experiences. In their ultimate effect, however, not solitariness but an increased sense of unity with others appears.

Prayer and meditation often bring to the minds of their critics ideas of demands for some sort of material benefit or relief from suffering. Since the results of these petitions rarely match expectations, the whole concept of prayer is often written off as a residual of infantile magical thinking. But from the religious point of view, which I am trying to present, prayer and meditation are primarily instruments of self-change. They are simply a practical application of the thought that "as a man thinketh in his heart, so is he." Prayer and meditation are deliberate efforts to think something different in the heart and by so thinking change oneself.

For this, religion prescribes exercises of concentrating the attention upon those ideals which the subject has selected for development in himself. The ideal may be symbolized and visualized mentally. However, most religious exercises of this sort eventually strive for a transcendence of visual symbolization and move toward a sense of unity between the self and everything else in which visualization drops out. Our comparison of the assumptions of religion and psychiatry does not require details of these techniques. We are concerned here with principles only. The difference lies in the belief by religious people that one can change oneself by a conscious alteration of conscious thoughts. William James (1902) described this principle well:

> Let us, in speaking of the hot place in man's consciousness, the group of ideas to which he devoted himself, and from which he works, call it the habitual center of his personal energy. It makes a great difference to a man whether one set of ideas, or another, be the center of his energy; and it makes a great difference, as regards any set of ideas he may possess, whether they become central or remain peripheral in him. To say that a man is "converted" means, in these terms, that religious

> ideas previously peripheral in his consciousness, now take a central place, and that religious aims form the habitual center of his energy.

By "religious ideas" James means that which is referred to in this essay as the sense of unity and the expression of tender love. The essential techniques of religion bring these ideas from the periphery to the center of consciousness, from which position they naturally influence action much more effectively.

One may ask why these techniques of solitary self-changing are not more widely practiced than they are. We psychiatrists may be unaware of how extensively they are practiced. It may seem to us that religion has surrendered itself to obsessive rituals and perfunctory observances, whose neurotic aspects are all too apparent to our discernment. Yet, beside all this, there persists a great deal of participation in the sort of constructive religious experience that I have tried to describe. Moreover, we find today a growing interest in the inner experiences of religion in contrast to the outer ritualistic, symbolic and social aspects of religion. Nevertheless, religious practices still have a relatively small hold on the educated people of our time. The counterparts of these educated people occupied themselves quite differently in Europe in the Middle Ages, and for that matter do so in India today. No doubt this has something to do with what is acceptable to the culture as a whole. It is much easier to engage in some activity endorsed by one's fellowmen, than to run the risk of being thought eccentric or heretical to the prevailing intellectual doctrines. The separation of religion and psychology in the modern West has not always been found in other times. In the eighteenth century, John Wesley prescribed medicines equally for madness and irreligion (Wesley, 1790). Nor does this separation exist today in all other parts of the world. In Hinduism, for example, psychology and religion are the same subject and always have been (Akhilananda, 1951).

DIFFICULTIES OF SELF-CHANGING

A more significant reason for the relative neglect of personal efforts at self-changing lies in its greater difficulty. Casually one thinks that thinking must be easier than talking. This is true, if by thinking we mean allowing our thoughts to drift along association paths while we attend haphazardly now to perceptions of outer events and now to inner images. But concentrated thought and especially constructive examination of ourselves mean something else. All who have tried these agree that talking is a great deal easier. So we should not laugh at the little girl who said when reproved for talking without thinking: "How can I tell what I think until I hear what I say?" Most of us adults cannot tell what we think until we hear what we say. But knowing what we think before we speak is not impossible, it is only a great deal harder.

Psychoanalysis has an exercise known as self-analysis which is recommended to its students. Indeed personal analysis is sometimes said to be a mere preparation for continual self-analysis. But almost nothing has been written about this subject, and from my conversations with colleagues I question whether many psychiatrists engage in it. If they did, I think one would hear more about what they had been doing and whether it had helped. When something is generally recommended but never discussed in detail, one suspects that it remains an ideal rather than a fulfillment.

The lack of another person to keep our mind on the subject at hand makes self-analysis difficult. Concentration of thought and the techniques whereby a mind can be trained to this have been studied too little. But we know that the ability to concentrate comes only by training. When people first attempt to study themselves or to concentrate on some quality which they wish to imitate, their minds freely and obstinately wander off to other things. This happens so easily that, unless this wandering is itself made an object of study and accepted patiently, the beginner may soon give up the attempt in despair (Benoit, 1941).

A second, more significant obstacle to self-analysis lies in the well-known deceptiveness of our own observations of ourselves. Psychiatrists were late-comers in pointing out how distorted may be the picture which a man holds of himself. Modern psychiatrists could say nothing on this subject which would surprise La Rochefoucauld or Pascal. In efforts to change himself a man may easily begin with trivia and overlook glaring defects apparent to others. Religion has always recognized these hazards and guarded against them. The confessor and spiritual director of Catholicism, the guru of Hinduism (Akhilananda, 1951) and the master of Zen Buddhism (Kondo, 1952; Stunkard, 1951) testify to this.

In addition to these differences, an even greater one exists between self-analysis, as I understand it, and self-changing as practiced by religious people. The practitioner of self-analysis tries to explain the origin of his immature behavior. He assumes that, if he analyzes the origin of his behavior, he can change it. The religious self-changer tries to change his thoughts directly and through them his actions.

Which brings us to our last distinction between the assumptions of religion and psychiatry. Psychiatry believes that men ordinarily begin life healthy, but acquire inappropriate attitudes and behavior during their maturation. The removal of this unconstructive behavior frees the underlying healthy part of the personality for constructive action. This point of view may be stated in Freud's words: "The neurotic human being brings us his mind racked and rent by resistances; whilst we are working at analysis of it and removing the resistances, this mind of his begins to grow together; the great unity which we call his ego fuses into one all the instinctual trends which before had been split off and barred away from it. The psychosynthesis is thus achieved during analytic treatment without our intervention and inevitably" (Freud, 1950). This passage may be compared with one from an Indian saint and student of self-changing processes: "If you merely say, 'I will conquer lust, I will conquer anger and greed,' you can never conquer them; but if you fix your mind on God, the passions will leave you of themselves. Sri Ramakrishna used to say: 'The more you move eastward, the further you are from the west.' Call on God and pray to him. Then the objects of sense will no longer attract you" (Prabhavananda, 1948). I wish to direct attention not to the differing goals of these two psychologists but to their differing methods. In the simplest analogy, the one believes you can have no lawn unless you attack the weeds; the other recommends sowing a grass which will destroy the weeds.

CONCLUSION

I have made a comparison between some assumptions generally held in modern psychiatry and the corresponding beliefs held by religious persons. I do not believe that these views exclude each other, but rather that they can be supplementary. "What in the end," said William James (1902)

> are all of our verifications but experiences that agree with more or less isolated systems of ideas (conceptual systems) that our minds have framed? But why in the name of common sense must we assume that only one such system of ideas can be true? The obvious outcome of our total experience is that the world can be handled according to many systems of ideas and is handled by different men, and will each time give some characteristic kind of profit, for which he cares, to the handler, while at the same time some other kind of profit has to be omitted or postponed.

These remarks pertain even more today than 50 years ago. Psychiatry has gained much from adopting the methods and attitudes of science. But it should remember the limitations of science which derive from the fact that science itself is a creation of man and not something which stands outside him. As such, science, no less than religion, can have its fashions and its prejudices. In modern scientific psychology and psychiatry one such prejudice may be the tendency to reject introspective techniques of self-study and self-changing. The well-known (and previously mentioned) distortions in a man's perception of himself may explain this rejection of introspective techniques. But explanation is not justification. We know that a man may readily perceive deficiencies in other people, while overlooking the existence of the same defects in himself. And certainly we usually appraise others more accurately than ourselves. But this does not mean we must always do so. The immediate objects of scientific study are always our own perceptions. We never actually experience anything but ourselves, even when we think we are studying something outside ourselves. And whether we try to look inward or outward, the observer remains the same. Hence *a priori* we have no reason to believe that a man cannot come to know himself as well as he can know other men, or as well as other men know him.

Religious persons have always believed that a man can study and ultimately come to know himself and his true nature. In contrast, most psychiatrists have lost respect for what one can discover about himself. The study of those religious persons who have observed and changed themselves may teach us to cast off traditional restrictions and return to self-study and efforts at self-changing which can arise therefrom.

NOTES

1. Reprinted from the *Bulletin of the Menninger Clinic, 19,* 199–209, 1955.—Ed.
2. The essence of all these writings has been concentrated in an excellent anthology by Aldous Huxley (1945).

REFERENCES

Akhilananda, Swami (1951). *Mental Health and Hindu Psychology.* New York: Harper.

Benoit, H. (1941). Notes in regard to a technique of timeless realization. In C. Isherwood (ed.), *Vedanta for Modern Man* (pp. 387–394). New York: Harper.

Custance, J. (1952). *Wisdom, Madness and Folly.* New York: Pellegrini and Cudahy.

Freud, S. (1930). *Civilization and Its Discontents.* London: Hogarth.

Freud, S. (1949). *The Future of an Illusion.* New York Liveright.

Freud, S. (1950). Turnings in the ways of psychoanalytic therapy. In *Collected Papers* (vol. II, p. 392–402.) London: Hogarth.

Fromm, E. (1950). *Psychoanalysis and Religion.* New Haven: Yale University Press.

Ginsburg, S. W. (1950). Values and the psychiatrist. *American Journal of Orthopsychiatry, 20,* 466–478.

Grazia, S. De (1952). *Errors in Psychotherapy.* New York: Doubleday.

Huxley, A. (1945). *The Perennial Philosophy.* New York: Harper.

James, W. (1902). *The Varieties of Religious Experience.* New York: Longmans, Green.

Kempis, Thomas A. (1910). *The Imitation of Christ.* New York: E. P. Dutton.

Kondo, A. (1952). Intuition in Zen Buddhism. *American Journal of Psychoanalysis, 12,* 10–14.

Prabhavananda, Swami (1948). *The Eternal Companion.* Hollywood: Vedanta.

Prabhavananda, Swami, & Isherwood, C. (trans.) (1944). *Bhagavad-Gita: The Song of God.* Hollywood: Marcel Rodd.

Ramakrishna (1947). *The Gospel of Ramakrishna.* New York: Vedanta.

Stunkard, A. (1951). Some interpersonal aspects of an Oriental religion. *Psychiatry, 14,* 419–431.

Underhill, Evelyn (ed.). (1922). *The Cloud of Unknowing.* London: John M. Watkins.

Weigert, E. (1949). Existentialism and its relation to psychotherapy. *Psychiatry, 12,* 399–412.

Wesley, J. (1790). *Primitive Physic, or an Easy and Natural Method of Curing Most Diseases.* (Quoted in D. H. Tuke, *History of the Insane in the British Isles.* London: Kegan, Paul, Trench)

Conclusion: Toward a Tertium Quid[1]

EWK

Now that readers have become acquainted—or reacquainted—with the tenor and scope of Ian's work, they may well ask, What has been the effect of all this work? The easiest, and perhaps best, answer is that we cannot tell. Effects can only be felt over time, and particularly with regard to efforts as ambitious and potentially far-reaching as Ian's, that time may be of long duration. So we might ask instead, What has been the reception of Ian's work thus far?

Before trying to answer this question, however, I want to remind readers of the broad context in which Ian carried out his work. As I described in the General Introduction and in the introduction to part 5, Ian's work exemplified the important principle of "*tertium quid*." One of the founders of psychical research, Edmund Gurney, introduced a collection of his essays that he titled *Tertium Quid* as follows:

> Most of the papers deal with matters of contemporary controversy, as to which two antagonistic opinions have been strongly entertained and enforced. . . . In most of these questions I am conscious of "a great deal to be said on both sides", . . . [and] the truer view seems to me . . . not one that would extenuate differences . . . [but one whose] immediate tendency, on the contrary, is rather to make each of the duels triangular. In short, it is a *tertium quid*. (1887, pp. v–vii)

Similarly, the Oxford philosopher F. C. S. Schiller, himself active in early psychical research, noted that

> the shock of diametrically opposed views is generating in many thoughtful minds the conviction that their common ground and reconciliation must be sought deeper down than has been the fashion. (1891/1894, p. xi)

Central to this *tertium quid* approach is the belief that conflicts are resolved not by acrimonious debate but by moving beyond polarized positions to seek a broader perspective in which aspects of both (or all) sides may have a place.

Clearly, one of the most fundamental—and contentious—controversies has arisen and intensified over the three centuries since the birth of the scientific revolution: namely, that between science and religion. Especially during the past 150 years, as science has advanced in its description of the physical universe, religions have been forced to give up more and more territory in their own descriptions of the nature of the universe in which we live, and the two sides have responded by carving out their separate domains and ignoring what might be worthwhile on the other side. As a result, the rift has rapidly deepened, so that we in the 21st century find ourselves confronting an alarming bifurcation in modern society, one that began in the West but has spread with science and technology into much of the rest of the world. On the one hand, the world view that now prevails among many intellectual leaders, and that permeates all levels of our society, is that of a mechanistic and materialistic universe in which mind, consciousness, human personality, and the spiritual values by which many people try to live are, in the final analysis, mere byproducts of physical and biological processes. On the other hand, many people strongly feel that this materialistic world view cannot account for a wide variety of important human experiences, and that it fails to satisfy their hunger for a sense of meaning and dignity in human life.

This deepening conflict has fueled the rapid growth of fundamentalisms of varied kinds. Many people are keenly aware of the spread of *religious* fundamentalism and recognize it as rooted in a deep dissatisfaction with the currently dominant materialist world view. Not as many, however, recognize that a comparable fundamentalism has arisen on the other side, among people for whom currently prevailing scientific assumptions have hardened into an orthodoxy of unshakeable beliefs, a secular religion often labeled "scientism." These scientific fundamentalists have become just as vocal and strident as their religious counterparts—if not yet as violent—in promoting their beliefs and assumptions about the nature of reality. Scientific fundamentalism may in fact be even more pernicious than religious fundamentalism because of the revered, even exalted, position that science holds in much of contemporary society.

It seems increasingly clear that our most urgent need is for systematic efforts to bridge the gap between scientific and religious views of the nature of the universe, and to fill the gaps that remain in both sets of views. No one in the 20th century did more than Ian Stevenson to lead the effort to find a scientifically defensible yet humanly meaningful middle path between the religious and scientific fundamentalisms that threaten to engulf us, by applying the methods of science to the great questions about the origins, nature, and destiny of human personality that lie at the root of all religions. Unfortunately, those who try to take a broader and more comprehensive—or tertium quid—approach to such questions are too often lost in the clash and clamor of the warring fundamentalisms they seek to reconcile, and thus far Ian's work has been no exception. Among those who know his work, many have appropriated it, not to advance a tertium quid approach, but to advance their own entrenched positions. New Age aficionados may hail it as justification for believing wholly unfounded claims about hypnotic regression to past lives, while self-styled "skeptics" lambast it with all the similarly ill-founded or uninformed arguments they can muster. Even in the small arena of psychical research and parapsychology, where Ian is well known and respected, reactions generally fall into two camps, depending on whether one is primarily in the "psychical research" camp, where spontaneous experiences and survival research are taken seriously, or in the "parapsychology" camp, where experimental studies are considered the final—sometimes even the only—word.

In the larger intellectual community, however, Ian's work has been largely ignored, both by scientists and by religious leaders alike. Nevertheless, his books have been reviewed in mainstream (primarily medical) journals, and the reactions of the reviewers show the range of how thoughtful people confronted with work of this sort react. They also indicate what obstacles remain to be overcome before a true tertium quid approach can take root.

First of all, nearly all the reviewers agreed that Ian was a scientist not to be dismissed lightly, using such words to describe him as "serious," "scholarly," "cautious," "rigorous," and "well-credentialed." Nonetheless, there were, predictably, some reviews dismissing, even ridiculing, the work.[2] One reviewer, although acknowledging that "the material is fully documented and carefully presented," simply called the work "a rum enterprise" (Anon., 1981). Another said that "he has provided a set of interesting data" but does "not even give rationality its due"; and he concludes with the suggestive remark that the book "reads like fiction" (Frawley, 1985). Another ended his review by quoting Darwin as having said, in connection with Spiritualism, "the Lord have mercy on us all if we have to believe in such rubbish" (Prince, 1986, p. 434). A similar reaction is evident in a letter from an editor to whose journal Ian had submitted a research paper: "It is an interesting account of people's superstitions . . . [but] it cannot be taken seriously as a scientific contribution. . . . [A]s written, the reader is left with the impression that he is supposed to give credence to these accounts. . . . I have a hatred of superstition and see the whole scientific enterprise since Roger Bacon as being motivated to liberate people from this mediaeval curse." Needless to say, the paper was rejected.

Some of the negative reviewers, like their counterparts in popular skeptical magazines, seem to have dismissed the phenomena because they either are unfamiliar with the bulk of the research or have chosen to ignore much of it. A reviewer who found it to be "rubbish" also admitted that "the only fault I can find in the author's methodology was his approach to detecting fraud. Because of the controversial nature of such cases, they must be considered as deceptions (conscious or unconscious) until proven otherwise," and, for that, "one employs a detective and not a psychiatrist" (Prince, 1986, p. 434). Clearly, he failed to notice that Ian's methods were precisely those of a detective, showing that in the vast majority of instances conscious fraud was highly unlikely[3] and in an appreciable number of others even unconscious "fraud" is not an adequate explanation.[4] Another reviewer decided that the cases are the result of "a Freudian wobble: the reincarnated child turns out to be a newly embodied version of a relative who popped their clogs, and the new child comes back into their shoes. An obvious explanation is that a mourning family might either imagine this or teach the new child to fit the dead person's shoes" (Cohen, 1988, p. 68). Such an explanation is only "obvious" if one is unaware that many of the cases are *not* "same-family" cases and that Ian always deemphasized them in favor of "stranger" cases, in which the child gave veridical information about someone unknown to his family, or cases in which a physical birthmark or birth defect calls for some more adequate response than that "those who would dream up [that] they had been here before choose to have had interesting previous existences" (Cohen, 1988, p. 69).

I have perhaps given too much space to these negative reviews, but they do illustrate one of the major obstacles in the way of a more productive, tertium quid, analysis, and that is ignorance. One is simply not qualified to discuss, let alone derisively dismiss, a phenomenon without adequate knowledge of that phenomenon.

A more common, and more encouraging, reaction came from reviewers who found themselves caught on the fence and were at least honest enough to remain there. A well-known medical writer and editor at the *Journal of the American Medical Association* summarized succinctly the message in many of these reviews: "He may not convince skeptics but he has placed on record a large amount of data that cannot be ignored" (King, 1975). Another reviewer admitted that "one's first instinct is to dismiss these accounts as nonsense," but he then acknowledged that he honestly cannot (Meara, 1985).

A much more lengthy, and thoughtful, review starkly laid out the dilemma. The review was by Eugene Brody, long-time editor of the *Journal of Nervous and Mental Disease* and someone who knew Ian and respected him so much that, despite his own skepticism, he opened up the pages of his journal many times for papers and reviews on various aspects of psychical research, not only by Ian but by others. He stated that "we seem to be confronted with a real phenomenon" (Brody, 1979, p. 771), and he summarized his own position as "impressed" by the data but not convinced of the "paranormal hypotheses advanced to explain the data" (p. 770). For Brody, as for so many other people, "as someone reared in the dominant rational scientific culture of our time . . . paranormal phenomena in general and the theory of reincarnation are intrinsically unacceptable—there is no way to make them compatible with the total accumulated body of scientific knowledge" (pp. 769–770).

This unrelenting conviction that we are faced with a stark choice between two wholly incompatible sets of data, and that accepting one requires giving up the other, is clearly the major obstacle that blocks any true progress toward understanding the phenomena in question. The "fundamental question [is]: What are we to do with data that do not fit with 'mainstream' notions of how the world works?," and the overwhelming response so far has been that "*the evidence must be disposed of,*" usually by "relabeling, pathologizing, or simply ignoring it" (Bock, 1989, p. 445; italics in original). Fortunately, there are hopeful signs among the reviews of Ian's work that a seed may have been sown and that some people, feeling the discomfort, may be ready to move beyond the current polarization in which people "fall into two camps, the eager believers, who find his evidence convincing, and the scientifically minded who will not" (Carstairs, 1978). One fellow psychiatrist welcomed Ian's work as "a step on the road to discovery" by describing the difference between "controversy" and "innovation": "Controversy has a negative connotation implying polemics, disputation, and fanaticism. Innovation has a positive connotation implying rational introduction of new ideas, renovation of old ideas, expanding horizons, and breaking new ground. Dr. Stevenson . . . clearly belongs in the latter category" (Dean, 1978). Another reviewer concluded that "like a ghostly x-ray the painstakingly gathered descriptions Stevenson offers . . . [may] dissolve the fever of authority, belief and disbelief," and open up "a perspective from which one can glimpse some bone-deep truths about the human dilemma" (Briggs, 1976, p. 23).

There are also signs that, if the work of Ian and others facilitates a move toward a tertium quid in the search for those "bone-deep truths," then that move may ultimately take us beyond the current roster of explanations—beyond questions such as "are Dr. Stevenson's cases indeed recalling events of their past lives, or are they describing fantasies inspired by the prevailing beliefs of their surrounding culture?" (Carstairs, 1978). Some clearly recognize "the challenge [the cases] present to our current tacit assumptions about the nature of personality and individuality" (McHarg, 1969, p. 86). But many of them resisted Ian's interpretation of his data, however tentative, as evidence of survival in general or of reincarnation in particular; and a few did so not just because such a notion conflicts with current orthodoxy. Some instead seemed to have a sense that even the concept of reincarnation itself might be turn out to be inadequate for "the richness and diversity of the powerful data that Stevenson has so meticulously brought together" (Roth, 1998, p. 68). Like Gardner Murphy (1945), we might consider that even our questions about survival have not yet been "rightly stated," and that "it [is] probable that five hundred years hence the arguments both pro and con will sound childish and superficial, if indeed they sound relevant to the problem at all" (p. 93). Perhaps for now the best reaction to Ian's work is to admit that "no one knows for sure what causes the phenomena that Stevenson describes" (Roth, 1998, p. 67), and that "the time may have come to think of other approaches" (Brody, 1979, p. 774). If we do so, the "eventual interpretation may, in fact, shock us even more than the theory of reincarnation which, on the face of it, [the cases] seem to support" (McHarg, 1969, p. 86).

One reviewer seems to me to have best summed up where Ian's work currently stands, even though his words were written 45 years ago:

> If the first thing to be said about [his work] was that it is a work of major importance perhaps the final thing to be said about it is that it may be a long time before the world at large will recognize it as such. The fact is that not even a Dr. Stevenson can overnight break down the barriers. . . . However, Dr. Stevenson need not despair. No assumptions are sacrosanct. (Beloff, 1967, p. 93)

There are signs that even "the world at large," and not just reviewers in professional journals, may be slowly recognizing the potential importance of Ian's work; and it is particularly encouraging that two of those signs come from what would seem to be unlikely quarters. The astronomer Carl Sagan, a founder of a so-called skeptics' organization (once known as CSICOP, now as CSI) that has succeeded only in deepening the polarization of New Age superstition and fundamentalist scientism, suggested that "there are three claims in the ESP field which, in my opinion, deserve serious study"—one of these being Ian's cases of the reincarnation type (Sagan, 1996, p. 302). And Sam Harris, whose virulent attack on theistic religions seems directed more at those who believe something without evidence than at the deeper questions lying behind the religious impulse, insists that "anyone who wants to know how the world is, whether in physical or spiritual terms, will be open to new evidence" (Harris, 2004, p. 225). He is honest enough to say that there "seems to be a body of data attesting to the reality of psychic phenomena, much of which has been ignored by mainstream science" (p. 41); and among that body of data he, like Sagan, includes Ian's work (p. 242).

It remains to be seen whether other intellectual leaders follow the suggestion of Sagan and Harris to look seriously at the work of Ian and others like him and, if they do, whether that leads to any real progress in breaking down the current stark impasse in views about human nature. In the meantime, there is little doubt, in my view, that the neglect of Ian's work, as well as that of his predecessors in psychical research, has impoverished *both* science *and* religion. On the one hand, science has been narrowed and diminished by those who insist that its methods can be applied only to the physical universe, thus leaving out vast realms of human experience—and who then, in a peculiarly circular way, conclude that there *is* nothing but the physical universe. On the other hand, the basic religious sense that there are fundamental aspects of nature transcending finite existence has been unnecessarily discredited by religious persons who cling to specific ideological beliefs that are not, and probably *cannot*, be grounded in any evidential basis, while ignoring scientific evidence that might support the larger religious sense of our place in the universe.

Unfortunately, even among those who ostensibly are seeking common ground between science and religion, there is ignorance about the enormous amount of scientific evidence, accumulated over the past 130 years and indispensable to that task. Recently, the Templeton Foundation announced that it was giving a $5 million grant to study "immortality" because "anecdotal reports of glimpses of an afterlife abound, but there has been no comprehensive and rigorous, scientific study of global reports about near-death and other experiences" From an organization that is purportedly interested in the "big questions" about science and religion, including the question of survival, such ignorance about what has already been done is particularly disturbing. Clearly, one of the biggest challenges for the current generation of people interested in the survival question is to make that body of work more widely known.

Can science and religion be reconciled? Can we join modern society's respect for empirical science with the widely felt sense that our lives somehow transcend the boundaries of our current spatiotemporal existence? Unfortunately, the proposal that science and religion join forces in the search for a deeper understanding of ourselves and our universe too often provokes fear—and thus rejection—on both sides. Religious-minded persons fear that science will only continue to desecrate cherished beliefs, to "botanise upon his mother's grave," as Wordsworth lamented in "A Poet's Epitaph." Scientific-minded persons, on the other hand, fear that giving any ground to religion invites a return to irrational superstitions about "magic" or the "occult." But such consequences need not follow. As William James put it in *The Varieties of Religious Experience*: "Let empiricism once become associated with religion, as hitherto, through some strange misunderstanding, it has become associated with irreligion, and I believe that a new era of religion as well as philosophy will be ready to begin" (1902/1958, p. 270). Or, as James's colleague and friend F. W. H. Myers urged: "Religion, in its most permanent sense, is the adjustment of our emotions to the structure of the universe; and what we now most need is to discover what that structure is" (Myers, 1893/1961, p. 46).

If our society ever seriously attempts to push beyond the current polarization of science and religion, and reconcile them in a larger understanding of the world, then Ian Stevenson will surely be recognized as one of the great scientific pioneers of our age. He aimed for a true tertium quid—a science big enough to accommodate religious realities, and a religion grounded in scientific realities. But it is important to emphasize that such a tertium quid goes beyond any *particular* religion to address their common concerns. Ian, in short, provided a prime example of science working effectively in service of the truly fundamental interests of religion—and strengthening both in the process.

However Ian's *particular* body of work is ultimately judged, there can be no doubt that he pointed toward major issues that must be addressed and how they can best be attacked. He disliked the word "revolutionary" and would not want it applied to himself or his work. He continually walked that difficult fine line between broad vision and cautious claims. But the question now arises, as it does after every great pioneer is gone, who will come after? Few of us have his combination of far-reaching vision and meticulous attention to detail, of knowledge of history and belief in the power of science, indeed—I have to say it—of revolutionary thinking and conservative methods. Nonetheless, such people have had a way of appearing throughout history. With issues as challenging and crucial as those Ian tackled still remaining wide open, worthy successors will surely appear to take up where he left off.

NOTES

1. My comments in this conclusion are based in part on Kelly and Kelly (2008), in which we described our efforts to obtain recognition for Ian's work by nominating him repeatedly for the Templeton Prize for Progress Toward Research or Discoveries about Spiritual Realities—efforts that were, regrettably, unsuccessful.

2. Such reviews were perhaps surprisingly few, but that is almost certainly because journals whose editors and reviewers would not be open to entertaining such lines of research would also not be likely to solicit a review.

3. For reports of cases that Ian concluded *were* fraudulent, see Stevenson, Pasricha, and Samararatne (1988) and Stevenson and Beloff (1980).

4. These cases would include especially those 33 in which a written record of the child's statements was made before either the family or an outside investigator had verified them as accurate for one particular person (Keil & Tucker, 2005; Stevenson & Samararatne, 1988 [excerpts reprinted in Ch. 23]).

REFERENCES

Anonymous. (1981). Review of *Cases of the Reincarnation Type. Vol. III. Twelve Cases in Lebanon and Turkey*. *Psychological Medicine, 11*, 434.

Beloff, J. (1967). Review of *Twenty Cases Suggestive of Reincarnation*. *Journal of the Society for Psychical Research, 44*, 88–94.

Bock, P. K. (1989). Review of *Children Who Remember Previous Lives*. *Journal of Anthropological Research, 45*, 445–447.

Briggs, J. (1976). Review of *Cases of the Reincarnation Type. Vol. I: Ten Cases in India*. *The Academy, 20*, 22–23.

Brody, E. B. (1979). Review of *Cases of the Reincarnation Type. Vol. II: Ten Cases in Sri Lanka*. *Journal of Nervous and Mental Disease, 167*, 769–774.

Carstairs, G. M. (1978). Review of *Cases of the Reincarnation Type. Vol. II: Ten Cases in Sri Lanka*. *British Journal of Psychiatry, 33*, 475.

Cohen, D. (1988). Born-again children: Review of *Children Who Remember Previous Lives*. *New Scientist, 117*, 67–69.

Dean, S. R. (1978). Review of *Cases of the Reincarnation Type. Vol. II: Ten Cases in Sri Lanka*. *American Journal of Psychiatry, 135*, 1447.

Frawley, W. (1985). Review of *Unlearned Language: New Studies in Xenoglossy*. *Language, 61*, 739.

Gurney, E. (1887). *Tertium Quid: Chapters on Various Disputed Questions* (2 vols.). London: Kegan Paul, Trench.

Harris, S. (2004). *The End of Faith: Religion, Terror, and the Future of Reason*. New York: Norton.

James, W. (1958). *Varieties of Religious Experience*. New York: Mentor. (Original work published 1902)

Keil, H. H. J., & Tucker, J. B. (2005). Children who claim to remember previous lives: Cases with written records made before the previous personality was identified. *Journal of Scientific Exploration, 19*, 91–101.

Kelly, E. F., & Kelly, E. W. (2008). Where science and religion intersect: The work of Ian Stevenson. *Journal of Scientific Exploration, 22*, 73–80.

King, L. S. (1975). Reincarnation: Review of *Cases of the Reincarnation Type. Vol. 1: Ten Cases in India*. *Journal of the American Medical Association, 234*, 978.

McHarg, J. F. (1969). Review of *Twenty Cases Suggestive of Reincarnation*. *British Journal of Medical Psychology, 42*, 84–86.

Meara, P. (1985). Review of *Unlearned Language: New Studies in Xenoglossy*. *The Modern Language Review, 80*, 890–891.

Murphy, G. (1945). Difficulties confronting the survival hypothesis. *Journal of the American Society for Psychical Research, 39*, 67–94.

Myers, F. W. H. (1961). *Fragments of Inner Life*. London: Society for Psychical Research. (Original work published privately 1893)

Prince, R. (1986). Review of *Unlearned Language: New Studies in Xenoglossy*. *Journal of Nervous and Mental Disease, 174*, 433–434.

Roth, C. F. (1998). Review of *Where Reincarnation and Biology Intersect*. *Anthropology of Consciousness, 9*, 65–68.

Sagan, C. (1996). *The Demon-Haunted World: Science as a Candle in the Dark*. New York: Ballantine.

Schiller, F. C. S. (1894). *Riddles of the Sphinx: A Study in the Philosophy of Evolution* (2nd ed.). London: Swan Sonnenschein; New York: Macmillan. (Original work published 1891)

Stevenson, I., & Beloff, J. (1980). An analysis of some suspect drop-in communications. *Journal of the Society for Psychical Research, 50*, 427–447.

Stevenson, I., Pasricha, S., & Samararatne, G. (1988). Deception and self-deception in cases of the reincarnation type: Seven illustrative cases in Asia. *Journal of the American Society for Psychical Research, 82*, 1–31.

Stevenson, I., & Samararatne, G. (1988). Three new cases of the reincarnation type in Sri Lanka with written records made before verification. *Journal of Nervous & Mental Disease, 176*, 741.

Appendix: Publications of Ian Stevenson

BOOKS

(1969). *The Psychiatric Examination*. Boston: Little, Brown.

(1971). *The Diagnostic Interview* (2nd ed.). New York: Harper & Row. (Original work published in 1960 as *Medical History-Taking*. New York: Paul B. Hoeber)

(1970). *Telepathic Impressions: A Review and Report of Thirty-five New Cases*. Charlottesville: University Press of Virginia.

(1974). *Twenty Cases Suggestive of Reincarnation* (2nd rev. ed.) Charlottesville: University Press of Virginia, 1974. (Original work published in 1966)

(1974). *Xenoglossy*. Charlottesville: University Press of Virginia.

(1975). *Cases of the Reincarnation Type. Vol. I. Ten Cases in India*. Charlottesville: University Press of Virginia.

(1977). *Cases of the Reincarnation Type. Vol. II. Ten Cases in Sri Lanka*. Charlottesville: University Press of Virginia.

(1980). *Cases of the Reincarnation Type. Vol. III. Twelve Cases in Lebanon and Turkey*. Charlottesville: University Press of Virginia.

(1983). *Cases of the Reincarnation Type. Vol. IV. Twelve Cases in Thailand and Burma*. Charlottesville: University Press of Virginia.

(1984). *Unlearned Language: New Studies in Xenoglossy*. Charlottesville: University Press of Virginia.

(1997). *Reincarnation and Biology: A Contribution to the Etiology of Birthmarks and Birth Defects* (2 vols.). Westport, CT: Praeger Scientific Publishers.

(1997). *Where Reincarnation and Biology Intersect*. Westport, CT: Praeger Scientific Publishers.

(2001). *Children Who Remember Previous Lives: A Question of Reincarnation (rev. ed.)*. Jefferson, NC: McFarland. (Original work published in 1987, Charlottesville: University Press of Virginia)

(2003). *European Cases of the Reincarnation Type*. Jefferson, NC: McFarland.

(2005). *A World in a Grain of Sand: The Clairvoyance of Stefan Ossowiecki* (with M. R. Barrington & Z. Weaver). Jefferson, NC: McFarland.

PAPERS

Autobiographical

(1990). Some of my journeys in medicine. The Flora Levy Lecture in the Humanities 1989. University of Southwestern Louisiana Printing Services.

(1993–1994). Ian Stevenson: An Omega Interview (with R. Kastenbaum). *Omega, 28*, 165–182.

(1994). A few memories and a look into a blurred future. *Psi Today*, no. 3, 10–13.

(2006). Essay: Half a career with the paranormal. *Journal of Scientific Exploration, 20*, 13–31.

Drug Studies

(1957). From mescaline to eternity. *The New Republic, 136,* 22.
(1957). Serenity without somnolence. *G.P., 15,* 95–101.
(1957). Tranquilizers and the mind. *Harper's Magazine, 215,* 21–27.
(1957). Comments on the psychological effects of mescaline and allied drugs. *Journal of Nervous & Mental Disease, 125,* 438–442.
(1957). The antidotal action of sodium succinate in the mescaline psychosis (with A. J. Sanchez Jr.). *American Journal of Psychiatry, 114,* 328–332.
(1958). A further note on the mechanism of the antidotal action of sodium succinate in the mescaline psychosis (with L.C. Mokrasch). *American Journal of Psychiatry, 114,* 1038–1039.
(1958). Interviewing with narcosis. *G.P., 18,* 133–137.
(1959). The metabolism of mescaline with a note on correlations between metabolism and psychological effects (with L .C. Mokrasch). *Journal of Nervous & Mental Disease, 129,* 177–183.
(1960). Prolonged reactions to mescaline (with T. W. Richards). *Psychopharmacologia, 1,* 241–250.
(1961). Consistency in the psychologic reaction to mescaline (with T. W. Richards). *Southern Medical Journal, 54,* 1319–1320.
(1966). Effectiveness and processes of interviewing with drugs (with J. D. Hain & B. M. Smith). *Journal of Psychiatric Research, 4,* 95–106.
(1969). Emotional expression, memory and feelings during and after interviews with drugs (with B. M. Smith & J. D. Hain). *Behavorial Neuropsychiatry, 1,* 10–14.
(1970). Controlled interviews using drugs (with B. M. Smith & J. D. Hain). *Archives of General Psychiatry, 22,* 2–10.
(1973). Controlled interviews using drugs. II. Comparisons between restricted and freer conditions (with J. Buckman, J. D. Hain, & B. M. Smith). *Archives of General Psychiatry, 29,* 623–627.
(1974). The use of drugs in psychiatric interviews: Some interpretations based on controlled experiments (with J. Buckman, B. M. Smith, & J. D. Hain). *American Journal of Psychiatry, 131,* 707–710.

Medicine, Psychiatry, and Science

(1942). The third circulation: Cerebrospinal fluid (with E.M. Webb). *McGill Medical Journal, 11,* 23–55.
(1943). Paroxysmal hemoglobinuria with report of a case. *McGill Medical Journal, 12,* 192–210.
(1943). Some aspects of itching. *McGill Medical Journal, 12,* 292–300.
(1946). Sickle cell anemia. *Arizona Medicine, 3,* 161–163.
(1947). Modern management of oedema. *Arizona Medicine, 4,*105–113.
(1947). The therapeutic effect of the climate of Arizona. *Archives of Physical Medicine, 28,* 644–652.
(1947). Bronchial lavage for bronchiectasis. *American Review of Tuberculosis, 56,* 279–286.
(1948). The influence of oxygen tension upon the respiration of rat kidney slices (with L. Smith). *Archives of Biochemistry, 17,* 61–73.
(1948). Studies on cardiac function: Occurrence of extrasystoles with variation in the emotional state in man (with C. H. Duncan & S. Wolf). *Bulletin of the New York Academy of Medicine, 24,* 393.
(1948). Changes in form and function of mucous membranes occurring as part of protective reaction patterns in man during periods of life stress and emotional conflict (with H. G. Wolff, S. Wolf, W. J. Grace, T. E. Holmes, L. Straub, H. Goodell, & P. Seton). *Transactions of the Association of American Physicians, 61,* 313–334.

(1948). The constitutional approach to medicine. *New York State Journal of Medicine, 48,* 2156–2159.
(1949). Rest and exercise in the management of rheumatic fever. *Arizona Medicine, 6,* 13–18.
(1949). Why medicine is not a science. *Harper's Magazine, 198,* 36–39.
(1949). Life situations, emotions, and bronchial mucus (with H.G. Wolff). *Psychosomatic Medicine, 11,* 223–227.
(1949). Life situations, emotions, and extrasystoles (with C. H. Duncan, S. Wolf, H. S. Ripley, & H. G. Wolff). *Psychosomatic Medicine, 11,* 257–272.
(1949). Circulatory dynamics before and after exercise in subjects with and without structural heart disease during anxiety and relaxation (with C. H. Duncan & H. G. Wolff). *Journal of Clinical Investigation, 28,* 1534–1543.
(1949). Variations in the secretion of bronchial mucus during periods of life stress. *Proceedings Association for Research in Nervous and Mental Disease, 29,* 596–601.
(1949). Alterations in cardiac function and circulatory efficiency during periods of life stress as shown by changes in the rate, rhythm, electrocardiographic pattern and output of the heart in those with cardiovascular disease (with C. H. Duncan). *Proceedings Association for Research in Nervous and Mental Disease, 29,* 799–817.
(1950). Life situations, emotions, and paroxysmal auricular arrhythmias (with C. H. Duncan & H. S. Ripley). *Psychosomatic Medicine, 12,* 23–37.
(1950). Physical symptoms during pleasurable emotional states. *Psychosomatic Medicine, 12,* 98–102.
(1950). The relation of life stress to cardiovascular symptoms and disease (with C. H. Duncan, S. Wolf, & H. G. Wolff). *Medical Clinics of North America, 34,* 817–831.
(1950). Paroxysmal arrhythmias: A psychosomatic study (with C. H. Duncan). *Geriatrics, 5,* 259–267.
(1950). The art of interviewing (with R. A. Matthews). *G.P., 2*(4), 59–69.
(1951). Life situations, emotions, and exercise tolerance (with C. H. Duncan & H.G. Wolff). *Psychosomatic Medicine, 13,* 36–50.
(1951). Variations in the electrocardiogram changes in emotional state (with C. H. Duncan & H. S. Ripley). *Geriatrics, 6,* 164–178.
(1951). A new day for the general practitioner. *G.P., 4*(4), 29–31.
(1951). Evaluating psychosomatic disorders. *G.P., 4*(5), 1–5.
(1951). Analyzing psychosomatic relationships. *G.P., 4*(5), 6–16.
(1952). Detection of the dangerous paranoid patient (with R. A. Matthews). *Postgraduate Medicine, 11,* 12–16.
(1952). Illness from the inside. *Harper's Magazine, 204,* 61–67.
(1952). Observations on illness from the inside (bronchiectasis). In M. Pinner & B. F. Miller (eds.), *When Doctors Are Patients* (pp. 223–235). New York: W. W. Norton.
(1952). "Spells": The causes and diagnosis of a common complaint. *New Orleans Medical and Surgical Journal, 104,* 352–359.
(1952). The medical review team in the evaluation of welfare applicants (with C. A. Potter Jr.). *Louisiana Welfare, 12,* 5.
(1952). Hypertension as a reaction pattern to stress (with C. H. Duncan, J. T. Flynn, & S. Wolf). *American Journal of the Medical Sciences, 224,* 286–299.
(1952). Variations in respiration and in respiratory symptoms during changes in emotion (with H. S. Ripley). *Psychosomatic Medicine, 14,* 476–490.
(1952). Psychotherapy—How to begin. *G.P., 6*(6), 57–63.
(1952). The diagnosis of the complaint of "spells." *Medical Horizons, 3*(2),1–5.
(1953). Psychotherapy—How to guide interviews. *G.P., 7*(1), 69–79.
(1953). Evaluation of disability in applicants for welfare assistance (with C. A. Potter Jr.). *Journal of the Louisiana State Medical Society, 105,* 116–123.
(1953). Why people change. *Harper's Magazine, 207,* 55–60.
(1953). Psychiatry and social work in the vocational rehabilitation of psychiatric patients (with T. Morris). *Social Welfare Forum, 80,*148–157.

(1953). Fact and theory in psychosomatic medicine (with R. A. Matthews). *Journal of Nervous & Mental Disease, 118*, 289–306.
(1954). Management of common psychiatric problems. *G.P., 9*(1), 69–75.
(1954). Psychosomatic medicine. Part I: What we know about illness and the emotions. *Harper's Magazine, 209*, 34–37.
(1954). As a man thinketh . . . Psychosomatic medicine, Part II. *Harper's Magazine, 209*, 83–87.
(1954). The diagnosis of cardiac disturbances of emotional origin. *Medical Clinics of North America, 38*, 1535–1545.
(1954). Techniques in the vocational rehabilitation of chronically unemployed psychiatric patients (with T. M. Fisher). *American Journal of Psychiatry, 111*, 289–300.
(1954). The nurse and her patient in long-term cases. *American Journal of Nursing, 54*, 1462–1464.
(1955). Psychiatry. *Annual Review of Medicine, 6*, 201–210.
(1955). The use of home visits in teaching psychological attitudes to medical students (with T. M. Fisher). *Journal of Medical Education, 30*, 203–214.
(1955). Recovery from dementing psychoses of old age (with R. A. Matthews). *Journal of the American Geriatrics Society, 3*, 720–724.
(1955). Assumptions of religion and psychiatry. *Bulletin of the Menninger Clinic, 19*, 199–209.
(1956). Psychotherapy by the general practitioner. *Journal of the Louisiana State Medical Society, 108*, 129–134.
(1956). Southern attitudes on desegregation. *The New Republic, 134*(20), 22.
(1956). Theory and the great game of words. *The New Republic, 135*(12), 22.
(1957). Psychiatric aspects of school desegregation (with other members of Committee on Social Issues, Group for the Advancement of Psychiatry). GAP Publication No. 37. New York: Group for the Advancement of Psychiatry.
(1957). Schizophrenia: What we are finding out about our worst mental illness. *Harper's Magazine, 215*, 59–65.
(1957). Is the human personality more plastic in infancy and childhood? *American Journal of Psychiatry, 114*, 152–161.
(1957). What am I? *Vedanta and the West, 127*, 7.
(1958). How children learn behavior. *Mental Health in Virginia, 8*, 15–19.
(1958). Psychological aspects of prejudice with special reference to desegregation (with H. I. Lief). *American Journal of Psychiatry, 114*, 816–823.
(1958). Scientists with half-closed minds. *Harper's Magazine, 217*, 64–71.
(1959). Direct instigation of behavioral changes in psychotherapy. *A.M.A. Archives of General Psychiatry, 1*, 99–107.
(1959). The challenge of results in psychotherapy. *American Journal of Psychiatry, 116*, 120–123.
(1959). The psychiatric interview. In S. Arieti (ed.), *American Handbook of Psychiatry* (pp. 197–214). New York: Basic Books.
(1959). The psychiatric examination (with W. M. Sheppe Jr.). In S. Arieti (ed.), *American Handbook of Psychiatry* (pp. 215–234). New York: Basic Books.
(1959). A note on the shortage of first-rate research in psychiatry. *Clinical Research, 7*, 375–377.
(1960). People are not born prejudiced. *Parents Magazine, 35*, 39.
(1960). Recovery from sexual deviations through overcoming non-sexual neurotic responses (with J. Wolpe). *American Journal of Psychiatry, 116*, 737–742.
(1961). The role of wishes in the origin of dreams and the psychoses. *Psychiatric Quarterly, 35*, 49–59.
(1961). Processes of "spontaneous" recovery from the psychoneuroses. *American Journal of Psychiatry, 117*, 1057–1064.
(1961). A case of multiple personality illustrating the transition from role-playing (with M. H. Congdon & J. Hain). *Journal of Nervous and Mental Disease, 132*, 497–504.

(1962). The use of rewards and punishments in psychotherapy. *Comprehensive Psychiatry, 3,* 20–28.
(1962). Explaining the results of examinations to patients, Part 1. *Postgraduate Medicine, 31,* 517–521.
(1962). Explaining the results of examinations to patients, Part 2. *Postgraduate Medicine, 32,* 31–35.
(1962). Summary report: Measuring personality change. In H. H. Strupp & L. Luborsky (eds.), *Research in Psychotherapy* (pp. 269–270). Washington, DC: American Psychological Association.
(1963). Disease as response to life stress. I. The nature of the evidence (with D. T. Graham). In H. I. Lief, V. F. Lief, & N. R. Lief (eds.), *The Psychological Basis of Medical Practice* (pp. 115–136). New York: Harper & Row.
(1963). Disease as response to life stress. II. Obtaining the evidence clinically (with D. T. Graham). In H. I. Lief, V. F. Lief, & N. R. Lief (eds.), *The Psychological Basis of Medical Practice* (pp. 137–153). New York: Harper & Row.
(1963). Techniques of interviewing (with W. M. Sheppe Jr.). In H. I. Lief, V. F. Lief, & N. R. Lief (eds.), *The Psychological Basis of Medical Practice* (pp. 181–192). New York: Harper & Row.
(1963). The preservation of a vanishing species: The part-time chairman. *Journal of Nervous and Mental Disease, 137,* 21–524.
(1964). Criteria for the evaluation of the results of the psychotherapies. *American Journal of Psychotherapy, 18*(Supp.1),128–131.
(1965). On the irrational among the rational: Incredulity in scientists. *Virginia Quarterly Review, 41,* 40–57.
(1965). Sequential treatments in a case of Gilles de la Tourette's syndrome (with D. J. Polites & D. Kruger). *British Journal of Medical Psychology, 38,* 43–52.
(1966). Systematic desensitization therapy: An analysis of results in twenty-seven patients (with J. D. Hain & R. H. G. Butcher). *British Journal of Psychiatry, 112,* 295–307.
(1966). New channels for grants [correspondence]. *Science, 153,* 816–817.
(1967). The need for research on mental illness in Virginia. *Virginia Medical Monthly, 94,* 104–106.
(1967). On the different meanings of apparently similar symptoms, illustrated by varieties of barber shop phobia (with J. D. Hain). *American Journal of Psychiatry, 124,* 399–403.
(1969). Single physical symptoms as residues of an earlier response to stress. *Annals of Internal Medicine, 70,* 1231–1237.
(1969). Assumptions of religion and psychiatry. *Pastoral Psychology, 20,* 41–50.
(1970). Physical symptoms occurring with pleasurable emotional states. *American Journal of Psychiatry, 127,* 175–179.
(1974). The psychiatric interview. In S. Arieti (ed.), *American Handbook of Psychiatry,* 2nd ed. (vol. 1, pp. 1138–1156). New York: Basic Books.
(1974). The psychiatric examination (with W. Sheppe Jr.). In S. Arieti (ed.), *American Handbook of Psychiatry,* 2nd ed. (vol. 1, pp. 1157–1180). New York: Basic Books.
(1979). Comments on "Is outcome for schizophrenia better in non-industrial societies? The case of Sri Lanka." *Journal of Nervous & Mental Disease, 167,* 159–160.
(1983). Do we need a new word to supplement "hallucination"? *American Journal of Psychiatry, 140,* 1609–1611.
(1984). On preserving the healing power of hope. *Pharos, 47,* 20–22.
(1985). The end of patient abuse in medical care. *Virginia Quarterly Review, 61,* 565–583.
(1994). Response to Wirth *et al. Journal of Scientific Exploration, 8,* 379–380.

PSYCHICAL RESEARCH

General

(1965). Sensitives, scientists, and clergymen: Liaison the strategic role of the minister. *Gate Way: Journal of the Spiritual Frontiers Fellowship, 10,* 201–208.
(1966). Criticism in parapsychology: An informal statement of some guiding principles (with W. G. Roll). *Journal of the American Society for Psychical Research, 60,* 347–356.
(1969). Establishment of a Division of Parapsychology at the University of Virginia. *Journal of the American Society for Psychical Research, 63,* 210–211.
(1971). The substantiality of spontaneous cases (Presidential Address). In W. G. Roll, R. L. Morris, & J. D. Morris (eds.), *Proceedings of the Parapsychological Association 5, 1968* (pp. 91–128). Durham, NC: Parapsychological Association.
(1977). An authenticity rating scale for reports of spontaneous cases (with J. Palmer & R. Stanford). *Journal of the American Society for Psychical Research, 71,* 273–288.
(1978). Some comments on automatic writing. *Journal of the American Society for Psychical Research, 72,* 315–332.
(1981). Can we describe the mind? (Presidential Address) In W.G. Roll & J. Beloff (eds.), *Research in Parapsychology 1980* (pp. 130–142). Metuchen, NJ: Scarecrow Press.
(1983). Cryptomnesia and parapsychology. *Journal of the Society for Psychical Research, 52,* 1–30.
(1984). Are parapsychology journals good for parapsychology? (Guest editorial). *Journal of the American Society for Psychical Research, 78,* 97–104.
(1986). Investigating the paranormal (Correspondence). *Nature, 322,* 680.
(1987). Changing fashions in the study of spontaneous cases. (Guest editorial). *Journal of the American Society for Psychical Research, 81,* 1–10.
(1987). Why investigate spontaneous cases? (Guest editorial). *Journal of the American Society for Psychical Research, 81,* 101–109.
(1988). Was the attempt to identify parapsychology as a separate field of science misguided? (Guest editorial). *Journal of the American Society for Psychical Research, 82,* 309–317.
(1990). Thoughts on the decline of major paranormal phenomena (Presidential Address). *Proceedings of the Society for Psychical Research, 57,* 149–162.
(1996). Guest column: On the necessity of medical documents in claims of paranormal phenomena in diseases. *Journal of Scientific Exploration, 10,* 299–306.

Apparitions

(1964). The blue orchid of Table Mountain. *Journal of the Society for Psychical Research, 42,* 401–409.
(1965). The case of the "teddy bear" suit. *Journal of the Society for Psychical Research, 43,* 92–93.
(1982). The contribution of apparitions to the evidence for survival. *Journal of the American Society for Psychical Research, 76,* 341–358.
(1995). Six modern apparitional experiences. *Journal of Scientific Exploration, 9,* 351–366.

Extrasensory Perception

(1959). A proposal for studying rapport which increases extrasensory perception. *Journal of the American Society for Psychical Research, 53,* 66–68.
(1959). The uncomfortable facts about extrasensory perception. *Harper's Magazine, 219,* 19–25.
(1960). A review and analysis of paranormal experiences connected with the sinking of the *Titanic. Journal of the American Society for Psychical Research, 54,* 153–171.

(1961). An example illustrating the criteria and characteristics of precognitive dreams. *Journal of the American Society for Psychical Research, 55,* 98–103.

(1963). A postcognitive dream illustrating some aspects of the pictographic process. *Journal of the American Society for Psychical Research, 57,* 182–202.

(1965). Seven more paranormal experiences associated with the sinking of the *Titanic*. *Journal of the American Society for Psychical Research, 59,* 211–225.

(1966). The connections between previous experiences and an apparently precognitive dream (with Rosalind Heywood). *Journal of the American Society for Psychical Research, 60,* 32–45.

(1968). A survey of spontaneous psychical experiences in school children of Uttar Pradesh, India (with Jamuna Prasad). *International Journal of Parapsychology, 10,* 241–261.

(1968). Identification of concealed randomized objects through acquired response habits of stimulus and word association (with J. G. Pratt, W.G. Roll, J. G. Blom, G. L. Meinsma, H. H. J. Keil, & N. Jacobson). *Nature, 220,* 89–91.

(1969). Identification of concealed randomized objects (with J. G. Pratt). *Nature, 221,* 586.

(1970). Three-experimenter ESP tests of Pavel Stepanek during his 1968 visit to Charlottesville (with J. G. Pratt & H. H. J. Keil). *Journal of the American Society for Psychical Research, 64,* 18–39.

(1970). Precognition of disasters. *Journal of the American Society for Psychical Research, 64,* 187–210. (First published as Proceedings of a 1969 MEND symposium on the psychological aspects of stress. Washington, DC: Government Printing Office)

(1972). EEG correlates of free-response GESP in an individual subject (with R. G. Stanford). *Journal of the American Society for Psychical Research, 66,* 357–368.

(1972). An electroencephalographic study of free-response GESP in an individual subject (with R. G. Stanford) (abstract). In W. G. Roll, R. L. Morris, & J. D. Morris (eds.), *Proceedings of the Parapsychological Association 8, 1971* (pp. 82–84). Durham, NC: Parapsychological Association.

(1974). The Soal-Goldney experiments with Basil Shackleton: A discussion. VIII. The credibility of Mrs. Gretl Albert's testimony. *Proceedings of the Society for Psychical Research, 56,* 117–129.

(1992). Comment on the Hansen critique. *Journal of Parapsychology, 56,* 370.

(1992). A series of possibly paranormal recurrent dreams. *Journal of Scientific Exploration, 6,* 281–289.

Mediumship

(1965). New evidence on an important detail in the case of Abraham Florentine. *Journal of the American Society for Psychical Research, 59,* 47–55.

(1968). The analysis of a mediumistic session by a new method. *Journal of the American Society for Psychical Research, 62,* 334–355.

(1970). A communicator unknown to medium and sitters. *Journal of the American Society for Psychical Research, 64,* 53– 65.

(1973). A communicator of the "drop in" type in France: The case of Robert Marie. *Journal of the American Society for Psychical Research, 67,* 47–76.

(1974). An experiment with the Icelandic medium Hafsteinn Björnsson (with E. Haraldsson). *Journal of the American Society for Psychical Research, 68,* 192–202.

(1975). A communicator of the "drop in" type in Iceland: The case of Runolfur Runolfsson (with E. Haraldsson). *Journal of the American Society for Psychical Research, 69,* 33–59.

(1975). The case of Robert Marie: An additional note. *Journal of the American Society for Psychical Research, 69,* 167–168.

(1975). A communicator of the "drop in" type in Iceland: The case of Gudni Magnusson (with E. Haraldsson). *Journal of the American Society for Psychical Research, 69,* 245–261.

(1980). An analysis of some suspect drop-in communications (with J. Beloff). *Journal of the Society for Psychical Research, 50*, 427–447.

(1990). The case of Giuseppe Riccardi: An unusual drop-in communicator in Italy (with S. Ravaldini & M. Biondi). *Journal of the Society for Psychical Research, 56*, 257–265.

Near-Death and Out-of-Body Experiences

(1979). Near-death experiences: Relevance to the question of survival after death (with B. Greyson). *Journal of the American Medical Association, 242*, 265–267.

(1980). Comments on "the reality of death experiences: A personal perspective." *Journal of Nervous & Mental Disease, 168*, 271–272.

(1980). The phenomenology of near-death experiences (with B. Greyson). *American Journal of Psychiatry, 137*, 1193–1196.

(1986). Near-death experiences in India: A preliminary report (with S. Pasricha). *Journal of Nervous & Mental Disease, 174*, 165–170.

(1989–1990). Are persons reporting "near-death experiences" really near death? A study of medical records (with E. W. Cook & N. McClean-Rice). *Omega, 20*, 45–54.

(1990). Features of "near-death experience" in relation to whether or not patients were near death (with J. E. Owens & E. W. Cook). *The Lancet, 336*, 1175–1177.

(1991). Near-death experience (with J. E. Owens & E. W. Cook) [correspondence]. *The Lancet, 337*, 1167–1168.

(1994). Absence of tunnel sensation in near-death experiences from India (with A. Kellehear, S. Pasricha, & E. W. Cook). *Journal of Near-Death Studies, 13*, 109–113.

(1995). Involuntary memories during severe physical illness or injury (with E. W. Cook). *Journal of Nervous and Mental Disease, 183*, 452–458.

(1998). Do any near-death experiences provide evidence for the survival of human personality after death? Relevant features and illustrative case reports (with E. W. Cook & B. Greyson). *Journal of Scientific Exploration, 12*, 377–406.

(1999–2000). Can experiences near death furnish evidence of life after death? (with E. W. Kelly & B. Greyson). *Omega, 40*, 513–519.

Psychokinesis, Poltergeists, and Psychic Surgery

(1968). Exploratory investigations of the psychic photography of Ted Serios (with J. G. Pratt). *Journal of the American Society for Psychical Research, 62*, 103–129.

(1969). Further investigations of the psychic photography of Ted Serios (with J. G. Pratt). *Journal of the American Society for Psychical Research, 63*, 352–364.

(1972). Are poltergeists living or are they dead? *Journal of the American Society for Psychical Research, 66*, 233–252.

(1972). Inferences about processes derived from unusual occurrences during "psychic photography" (with L. F. Barcus & J. G. Pratt) (abstract). In W. G. Roll, R. L. Morris, & J. D. Morris (eds.), *Proceedings of the Parapsychological Association 8, 1971* (pp. 17–18). Durham, NC: Parapsychological Association.

(1976). An instance of possible metal-bending indirectly related to Uri Geller (with J. G. Pratt). *Journal of the American Society for Psychical Research, 70*, 79–93.

(1981). Distortions in the photographs of Ted Serios (with J. Eisenbud & J. G. Pratt). *Journal of the American Society for Psychical Research, 75*, 143–153.

(1982). Some investigations of claims of PK effects on metal and film by Masuaki Kiyota. III. The Charlottesville experiments (with J. Keil, E. W. Cook, M. Dennis, & C. Werner). *Journal of the American Society for Psychical Research, 76*, 236–250.

(1985). The Kern City poltergeist: Comments on the critique by Hövelmann and Zorab. *Journal of the Society for Psychical Research, 53*, 96–99.

(1987). Difficulties confronting investigators of "psychic surgery" in the Philippines (with N. Azuma). *Parapsychology Review, 18*(2), 6–8.

(1988). "Psychic surgery" in the Philippines as a form of group hypnosis (with N. Azuma). *American Journal of Clinical Hypnosis, 31,* 61–67.

Survival

(1965). Some psychological principles relevant to research in survival. *Journal of the American Society for Psychical Research, 59,* 318–337.
(1969). Some implications of parapsychological research on survival after death. *Proceedings of the American Society for Psychical Research, 28,* 18–35.
(1972). Is there a case for disembodied survival? Discussion of Professor Flew's paper. II. Survival and embodiment. *Journal of the American Society for Psychical Research, 66,* 154–161.
(1977). Research into the evidence of man's survival after death. *Journal of Nervous & Mental Disease, 165,* 152–170.
(1977). Reply to the comments of Dr. Lief and Dr. Ullman. *Journal of Nervous & Mental Disease, 165,* 181–183.
(1980). The possible nature of post-mortem states: A discussion (with C. Tart & M. Grosso). *Journal of the American Society for Psychical Research, 74,* 413–424.
(1982). Survival after death: Evidence and issues. In Ivor Grattan-Guinness (ed.), *Psychical Research: A Guide to Its History, Principles and Practices* (pp. 109–122). Wellingborough, Northamptonshire, England: Aquarian Press.

Survival: Combination Lock Test

(1968). The combination lock test for survival. *Journal of the American Society for Psychical Research, 62,* 246–254.
(1976). Further observations on the combination lock test for survival. *Journal of the American Society for Psychical Research, 70,* 219–229.
(1989). Two tests of survival after death: Report on negative results (with A. T. Oram & B. Markwick). *Journal of the Society for Psychical Research, 55,* 329–336.
(1992). Survival or super-psi: A reply. *Journal of Scientific Exploration, 6,* 145–150.

Xenoglossy and Possession

(1976). A preliminary report of a new case of responsive xenoglossy: The case of Gretchen. *Journal of the American Society for Psychical Research, 70,* 65–77.
(1979). A case of secondary personality with xenoglossy (with S. Pasricha). *American Journal of Psychiatry, 136,* 1591–1592.
(1980). A preliminary report on an unusual case of the reincarnation type with xenoglossy (with S. Pasricha). *Journal of the American Society for Psychical Research, 74,* 331–348.
(1989). A case of the possession type in India with evidence of paranormal knowledge (with S. Pasricha & N. McClean-Rice). *Journal of Scientific Exploration, 3,* 81–101.

Reincarnation

(1960). The evidence for survival from claimed memories of former incarnations. Part I. Review of the data. *Journal of the American Society for Psychical Research, 54,* 51–71.
(1960). The evidence for survival from claimed memories of former incarnations. Part II. Analysis of the data and suggestions for further investigations. *Journal of the American Society for Psychical Research, 54,* 95–117.
(1960). Criteria for the ideal case bearing on reincarnation. *Indian Journal of Parapsychology, 2,* 149–155.
(1961). A Western view of karma. *Vedanta and the West, 147,* 11–22.

(1961). Reincarnation—East-West views. *Tomorrow, 9*(1), 26–34.
(1962). Introduction to "A Case Suggestive of Reincarnation in West Bengal" by Professor P. Pal. *Indian Journal of Parapsychology, 3,* 1–4.
(1962). Comments on parapsychology and "reincarnation" by Professor C. T. K. Chari. *Indian Journal of Parapsychology, 3,* 22–26.
(1966). Cultural patterns in cases suggestive of reincarnation among the Tlingit Indians of Southeastern Alaska. *Journal of the American Society for Psychical Research, 60,* 229–243.
(1967). A case of the reincarnation type in Ceylon (with F. Story). *Journal of the American Society for Psychical Research, 61,* 130–145.
(1970). Characteristics of cases of the reincarnation type in Turkey and their comparison with cases in two other cultures. *International Journal of Comparative Sociology, 11,* 1–17.
(1970). A case of the reincarnation type in Ceylon: The case of Disna Samarasinghe (with F. Story). *Journal of Asian and African Studies, 5,* 241–255.
(1971). Some personal aspects of case studies in India. *Parapsychology Review, 2*(6), 7–8.
(1971). Preliminary investigations of the correspondences in Samskars (personality traits) of the present and previous personalities in cases of the reincarnation type in India (with J. Prasad) (abstract). In W. G. Roll, R. L. Morris, & J. D. Morris (eds.), *Proceedings of the Parapsychological Association 6, 1969* (pp. 4–6). Durham, NC: Parapsychological Association.
(1971). The belief in reincarnation and related cases among the Eskimos of Alaska (abstract). In W. G. Roll, R. L. Morris, & J. D. Morris (eds.), *Proceedings of the Parapsychological Association 6, 1969* (pp. 53–55). Durham, NC: Parapsychological Association.
(1972). Some new cases suggestive of reincarnation. I. The case of Rajul Shah. *Journal of the American Society for Psychical Research, 66,* 288–309.
(1972). Some new cases suggestive of reincarnation. II. The case of Bishen Chand. *Journal of the American Society for Psychical Research, 66,* 375–400.
(1973). Carington's psychon theory as applied to cases of the reincarnation type: A reply to Gardner Murphy. *Journal of the American Society for Psychical Research, 67,* 130–146.
(1973). Some new cases suggestive of reincarnation. III. The case of Suleyman Andary. *Journal of the American Society for Psychical Research, 67,* 244–266.
(1973). Some new cases suggestive of reincarnation. IV. The case of Ampan Petcherat. *Journal of the American Society for Psychical Research, 67,* 361–380.
(1973). Characteristics of cases of the reincarnation type in Ceylon. *Contributions to Asian Studies, 3,* 26–39.
(1973). The "perfect" reincarnation case (abstract). In W. G. Roll, R. L. Morris, & J. D. Morris (eds.), *Research in Parapsychology 1972* (pp. 185–187). Metuchen, NJ: Scarecrow Press.
(1974). Some new cases suggestive of reincarnation. V. The case of Indika Guneratne. *Journal of the American Society for Psychical Research, 68,* 58–90.
(1974). The investigation of cases of the reincarnation type in India (with J. Prasad, L. Mehrotra, & K. Rawat). *Contributions to Asian Studies, 5,* 36–49.
(1974). Some questions related to cases of the reincarnation type. *Journal of the American Society for Psychical Research, 68,* 395–416.
(1975). Dr. R. L. Soni as an investigator of rebirth cases (a personal tribute). *The Maha Bodhi, 83,* 167–169.
(1975). Introduction and verifications in Ryall, E. *Second Time Round*. London: Neville Spearman. (American edition, *Born Twice*. New York: Harper & Row, 1975)
(1977). The belief and cases related to reincarnation among the Haida. *Journal of Anthropological Research, 31,* 364–375. (Reprinted with revisions in *Journal of the American Society for Psychical Research, 71,* 177–189, 1977)
(1977). The explanatory value of the idea of reincarnation. *Journal of Nervous & Mental Disease, 164,* 305–326.

(1977). Reincarnation: Field studies and theoretical issues. In B. B. Wolman (ed.), *Handbook of Parapsychology* (pp. 631–663). New York: Van Nostrand Reinhold.
(1977). The Southeast Asian interpretation of gender dysphoria: An illustrative case report. *Journal of Nervous & Mental Disease, 165,* 201–208.
(1977). Three cases of the reincarnation type in India (with S. Pasricha). *Indian Journal of Psychiatry, 19,* 36–42.
(1979). The search for the less than perfect case of the reincarnation type. *Journal of Indian Psychology, 2,* 30–34.
(1979). A partly independent replication of investigations of cases suggestive of reincarnation (with S. Pasricha). *European Journal of Parapsychology, 3,* 51–65.
(1983). A review and analysis of "unsolved" cases of the reincarnation type: I. Introduction and illustrative case reports (with E. W. Cook, S. Pasricha, G. Samararatne, & U Win Maung). *Journal of the American Society for Psychical Research, 77,* 45–62. (Abstract in W. G. Roll, J. Beloff, & J. McAllister [eds.], *Research In Parapsychology 1980* [pp. 111–113]. Metuchen, NJ: Scarecrow Press, 1981)
(1983). A review and analysis of "unsolved" cases of the reincarnation type: II. Comparison of features of solved and unsolved cases (with E. W. Cook, S. Pasricha, G. Samararatne, & U Win Maung). *Journal of the American Society for Psychical Research, 77,*115–135. (Abstract in W. G. Roll, J. Beloff, & J. McAllister [eds.], *Research In Parapsychology 1980* (pp. 214–217). Metuchen, NJ: Scarecrow Press, 1983)
(1983). Sickle cell anaemia and reincarnation beliefs in Nigeria (with S. J. Edelstein) (letter to the Editor). *Lancet, 322,* 1140.
(1983). American children who claim to remember previous lives. *Journal of Nervous & Mental Disease, 171,* 742–748.
(1985). Birth defects from cursing? A case report. *British Medical Journal, 290,* 1813.
(1985). The belief in reincarnation among the Igbo of Nigeria. *Journal of Asian & African Studies, 20,*13–30.
(1986). Characteristics of cases of the reincarnation type among the Igbo of Nigeria. *Journal of Asian & African Studies, 21,* 204–216.
(1987). Indian cases of the reincarnation type two generations apart (with S. Pasricha). *Journal of the Society for Psychical Research, 54,* 239–246.
(1988). Deception and self-deception in cases of the reincarnation type: Seven illustrative cases in Asia (with S. Pasricha & G. Samararatne). *Journal of the American Society for Psychical Research, 82,* 1–31.
(1988). Two correlates of violent death in cases of the reincarnation type (with N. K. Chadha). *Journal of the Society for Psychical Research, 55,* 71–79.
(1988). Three new cases of the reincarnation type in Sri Lanka with written records made before verification (with G. Samararatne). *Journal of Nervous & Mental Disease, 176,* 741.
(1988). Three new cases of the reincarnation type in Sri Lanka with written records made before verifications (with G. Samararatne). *Journal of Scientific Exploration, 2,* 217–238.
(1989). A case of severe birth defects possibly due to cursing. *Journal of Scientific Exploration, 3,* 201–212.
(1990). Can children be stopped from speaking about previous lives? Some further analyses of features in cases of the reincarnation type (with N. K. Chadha). *Journal of the Society for Psychical Research, 56,* 82–90.
(1990). Phobias in children who claim to remember previous lives. *Journal of Scientific Exploration, 4,* 243–254.
(1992). A new look at maternal impressions: An analysis of 50 published cases and reports of two recent examples. *Journal of Scientific Exploration, 6,* 353–373.
(1993). Birthmarks and birth defects corresponding to wounds on deceased persons. *Journal of Scientific Exploration, 7,* 403–416.
(1994). Afterthoughts. Addition for reprinting of "Cultural patterns in cases suggestive of reincarnation among the Tlingit Indians of Southeastern Alaska." In A. Mills & R.

Slobodin (eds.), *Amerindian Rebirth* (pp. 256–260). Toronto: University of Toronto Press.
(1994). A case of the psychotherapist's fallacy: Hypnotic regression to "previous lives." *American Journal of Clinical Hypnosis, 36,* 188–193.
(1994). Response to Chamberlain. *American Journal of Clinical Hypnosis, 37,* 78–79.
(1997). Reincarnation. In T. Barfield (ed.), *The Dictionary of Anthropology* (pp. 400–401). Oxford: Blackwell.
(1998). Does the socio-psychological hypothesis explain cases of the reincarnation type? (with S. A. Schouten). *Journal of Nervous & Mental Disease, 186,* 504–506.
(1999). Do cases of the reincarnation type show similar features over many years? A study of Turkish cases a generation apart (with J. Keil). *Journal of Scientific Exploration, 13,* 189–198.
(1999). Past lives of twins. *Lancet, 353,* 1359–1360.
(2000). The phenomenon of claimed memories of previous lives: Possible interpretations and importance. *Medical Hypotheses, 54,* 652–659.
(2000). The stability of assessments of paranormal connections in reincarnation-type cases (with J. Keil). *Journal of Scientific Exploration, 14,* 365–382.
(2000). Unusual play in young children who claim to remember previous lives. *Journal of Scientific Exploration, 14,* 557–570.
(2001). Ropelike birthmarks on children who claim to remember past lives. *Psychological Reports, 89,* 142–144.
(2001). Godwin Samararatne and the study of rebirth cases in Sri Lanka. In N. Senanayake (ed.), *Trends in Rebirth Research: Proceedings of an International Seminar.* Ratmalana, Sri Lanka: Sarvodaya Vishva Lekha.
(2003). The similarity of features of reincarnation type cases over many years: A third study (with E. Haraldsson). *Journal of Scientific Exploration, 17,* 283–289.
(2005). Reincarnation. In J. Henry (ed.), *Parapsychology: Research on Exceptional Experiences* (pp. 224–232). London: Routledge.
(2005). Children of Myanmar who behave like Japanese soldiers: A possible third element in personality (with J. Keil). *Journal of Scientific Exploration, 19,* 171–183.
(2005). Some bodily malformations attributed to previous lives (with S. K. Pasricha, J. Keil, & J. B. Tucker). *Journal of Scientific Exploration, 19,* 359–383.

TRIBUTES AND OBITUARIES

(1941). William Harvey. *McGill Medical Journal, 10,* 19–47.
(1941). The medical aspects of Oliver Wendell Holmes. *McGill Medical Journal, 11,* 97–107.
(1947). John Ray and his contributions to plant and animal classification. *Journal of the History of Medicine and Allied Sciences, 2,* 250–261.
(1953). Sir James Mackenzie, 1853–1953. *American Heart Journal, 46,* 479–484.
(1969). Chester F. Carlson: An appreciation. *Journal of the American Society for Psychical Research, 63,* 115–122.
(1970). A tribute to Curt John Ducasse, 1881–1969. *Journal of the American Society for Psychical Research, 64,* 148–153.
(1971). Eileen J. Garrett—an appreciation. *Journal of the American Society for Psychical Research, 65,* 336–343.
(1980). Gardner Murphy and the question of survival of human personality after death. *Journal of the American Society for Psychical Research, 74,* 78–88.
(1980). Gaither Pratt—an appreciation. *Journal of the American Society for Psychical Research 74,* 277–295.
(1981). Remembering Rosalind Heywood. *Journal of the American Society for Psychical Research, 75,* 267–271.
(1981). James S. McDonnell and the support of parapsychology. *Journal of the American Society for Psychical Research, 5,* 321–324.

(1983). In praise of Laura Dale. *Journal of the American Society for Psychical Research, 77,* 276–278, October 1983.
(1998). Paranormal cognition in the style of Dorris Carlson. *Journal of the American Society for Psychical Research, 92,* 172–173.

Index

About the Author

Emily Williams Kelly (PhD, University of Edinburgh) is research assistant professor in the Division of Perceptual Studies, Department of Psychiatry and Neurobehavioral Sciences, at the University of Virginia.

www.ingramcontent.com/pod-product-compliance
Lightning Source LLC
LaVergne TN
LVHW101444200926
848483LV00001B/44